D1446599

# MULTIPLE SCLEROSIS

## CURRENT STATUS AND STRATEGIES FOR THE FUTURE

Janet E. Joy and Richard B. Johnston, Jr., *Editors*

Committee on Multiple Sclerosis:
Current Status and Strategies for the Future

Board on Neuroscience and Behavioral Health

INSTITUTE OF MEDICINE

NATIONAL ACADEMY PRESS
Washington, D.C.

**NATIONAL ACADEMY PRESS • 2101 Constitution Avenue, N.W. • Washington, DC 20418**

NOTICE: The project that is the subject of this report was approved by the Governing Board of the National Research Council, whose members are drawn from the councils of the National Academy of Sciences, the National Academy of Engineering, and the Institute of Medicine. The members of the committee responsible for the report were chosen for their special competencies and with regard for appropriate balance.

Support for this project was provided by the National Multiple Sclerosis Society. The views presented in this report are those of the Institute of Medicine Committee on Multiple Sclerosis: Current Status and Strategies for the Future and are not necessarily those of the funding agencies.

Additional copies of this report are available for sale from the National Academy Press, 2101 Constitution Avenue, N.W., Box 285, Washington, D.C. 20055. Call (800) 624-6242 or (202) 334-3313 (in the Washington metropolitan area), or visit the NAP's home page at **www.nap.edu.** The full text of this report is available at **www.nap.edu.**

For more information about the Institute of Medicine, visit the IOM home page at: **www.iom.edu.**

**Library of Congress Cataloging-in-Publication Data**

Multiple sclerosis : current status and strategies for the future /
Janet E. Joy and Richard B. Johnston, Jr., editors.
    p. ; cm.
Includes bibliographical references and index.
  ISBN 0-309-07285-9 (hardcover)
  1. Multiple sclerosis.
  [DNLM: 1. Multiple Sclerosis—therapy. 2. Multiple
Sclerosis—physiopathology. 3. Research. WL 360 M956378 2001] I. Joy,
Janet E. (Janet Elizabeth), 1953- II. Johnston, Richard B., 1935-
  RC377 .M8455 2001
  616.8'34—dc21

                                2001002431

Copyright 2001 by the National Academy of Sciences. All rights reserved.

Printed in the United States of America.

The serpent has been a symbol of long life, healing, and knowledge among almost all cultures and religions since the beginning of recorded history. The serpent adopted as a logotype by the Institute of Medicine is a relief carving from ancient Greece, now held by the Staatliche Museen in Berlin.

*"Knowing is not enough; we must apply.
Willing is not enough; we must do."*

—Goethe

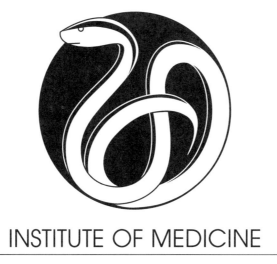

## INSTITUTE OF MEDICINE

Shaping the Future for Health

# THE NATIONAL ACADEMIES

National Academy of Sciences
National Academy of Engineering
Institute of Medicine
National Research Council

The **National Academy of Sciences** is a private, nonprofit, self-perpetuating society of distinguished scholars engaged in scientific and engineering research, dedicated to the furtherance of science and technology and to their use for the general welfare. Upon the authority of the charter granted to it by the Congress in 1863, the Academy has a mandate that requires it to advise the federal government on scientific and technical matters. Dr. Bruce M. Alberts is president of the National Academy of Sciences.

The **National Academy of Engineering** was established in 1964, under the charter of the National Academy of Sciences, as a parallel organization of outstanding engineers. It is autonomous in its administration and in the selection of its members, sharing with the National Academy of Sciences the responsibility for advising the federal government. The National Academy of Engineering also sponsors engineering programs aimed at meeting national needs, encourages education and research, and recognizes the superior achievements of engineers. Dr. William A. Wulf is president of the National Academy of Engineering.

The **Institute of Medicine** was established in 1970 by the National Academy of Sciences to secure the services of eminent members of appropriate professions in the examination of policy matters pertaining to the health of the public. The Institute acts under the responsibility given to the National Academy of Sciences by its congressional charter to be an adviser to the federal government and, upon its own initiative, to identify issues of medical care, research, and education. Dr. Kenneth I. Shine is president of the Institute of Medicine.

The **National Research Council** was organized by the National Academy of Sciences in 1916 to associate the broad community of science and technology with the Academy's purposes of furthering knowledge and advising the federal government. Functioning in accordance with general policies determined by the Academy, the Council has become the principal operating agency of both the National Academy of Sciences and the National Academy of Engineering in providing services to the government, the public, and the scientific and engineering communities. The Council is administered jointly by both Academies and the Institute of Medicine. Dr. Bruce M. Alberts and Dr. William A. Wulf are chairman and vice chairman, respectively, of the National Research Council.

# COMMITTEE ON MULTIPLE SCLEROSIS: CURRENT STATUS AND STRATEGIES FOR THE FUTURE

RICHARD B. JOHNSTON, JR. (*Chair*), Professor of Pediatrics, National Jewish Medical and Research Center, University of Colorado School of Medicine

JACK P. ANTEL, Professor of Neurology and Neurosurgery, Montreal Neurological Hospital and Institute, McGill University, Quebec, Canada

SAMUEL BRODER, Executive Vice President for Medical Affairs, Celera Genomics, Rockville, Maryland

JESSE M. CEDARBAUM, Vice President of Clinical Affairs, Regeneron Pharmaceuticals, Tarrytown, New York

PATRICIA K. COYLE, Professor of Neurology, State University of New York, Stony Brook

STEPHEN L. HAUSER, Professor of Neurology, University of California, San Francisco School of Medicine

LISA I. IEZZONI, Professor of Medicine, Harvard Medical School, Beth Israel Deaconess Medical Center, Boston, Massachusetts

SUZANNE T. ILDSTAD, Director of Institute for Cellular Therapeutics, University of Louisville, Kentucky

SHARON L. JULIANO, Professor of Anatomy and Cell Biology and Neurosciences Program, Uniformed Services University of the Health Sciences, Bethesda, Maryland

DONALD L. PRICE, Professor of Pathology, Neurology and Neuroscience, Johns Hopkins University School of Medicine, Baltimore, Maryland

RAYMOND P. ROOS, Professor of Neurology, University of Chicago, Illinois

ALAN J. THOMPSON, Professor of Neurology, University College, London, England

STEPHEN G. WAXMAN, Professor of Neurology, Yale Medical School, New Haven, Connecticut

HARTMUT WEKERLE, Director, Max-Planck-Institut fur Neurobiologie, Planegg-Martinsreid, Germany

## Study Staff

JANET E. JOY, Study Director
JOHN A. ROCKWELL, Research Assistant
AMELIA B. MATHIS, Project Assistant
LINDA LEONARD, Administrative Assistant (until 9/2000)
LORA K. TAYLOR, Administrative Assistant (from 9/2000)
TERRY C. PELLMAR, Board Director
CARLOS GABRIEL, Financial Associate

## BOARD ON NEUROSCIENCE AND BEHAVIORAL HEALTH

ANN M. GRAYBIEL *(Chair)*, Massachusetts Institute of Technology, Cambridge
KENNETH B. WELLS *(Vice-Chair)*, Neuropsychiatric Institute, University of
     California, Los Angeles
NANCY E. ADLER, University of California, San Francisco
RICHARD J. BONNIE, University of Virginia School of Law, Charlottesville
WILLIAM E. BUNNEY, University of California, Irvine
RICHARD G. FRANK, Harvard Medical School, Boston, Massachusetts
JEROME KAGAN, Harvard University, Cambridge, Massachusetts
HERBERT D. KLEBER, Columbia University and New York State Psychiatric
     Institute, New York, New York
BEVERLY B. LONG, World Federation for Mental Health, Atlanta, Georgia
KATHLEEN R. MERIKANGAS, Yale University, New Haven, Connecticut
STEVEN M. MIRIN, American Psychiatric Association, Washington, D.C.
STEVEN M. PAUL, Lilly Research Laboratories, Indianapolis, Indiana
DAVID REISS, George Washington University Medical Center, Washington, D.C.
RHONDA J. ROBINSON-BEALE, Blue Cross/Blue Shield of Michigan, Southfield
STANLEY J. WATSON, University of Michigan, Ann Arbor
STEPHEN G. WAXMAN, Yale Medical School, New Haven, Connecticut
NANCY S. WEXLER, Columbia University, New York, New York
ANNE B. YOUNG, Massachusetts General Hospital, Boston

# Preface

Multiple sclerosis (MS) is not a new disease. Its effects on the brain were described in the 1830s, and it was identified as a distinct clinical entity in the 1860s. In fact, writings from the Middle Ages appear to describe individuals with this condition. MS is the most common neurological disorder of young adults; there are approximately 350,000 people with MS in the United States and an estimated 2 million patients worldwide.

Research on the disorder has been energetic over recent decades. In 1996, the U.S. National Institutes of Health (NIH) spent almost $83 million on MS research. This sum exceeded the NIH expenditure that year on asthma, tuberculosis, or cervical cancer. MS has not been neglected by researchers in this country or worldwide.

As a result, important progress has been made in defining the pathologic changes of MS, in using new imaging techniques for evaluation, and in developing treatments that can modify its course. Yet, despite concerted effort on the part of many good researchers, the fundamental elements of MS are still not understood, and the path toward consistently preventing its progression or curing it remains obscure. For example, we do not know what causes MS to appear in one person and not another. We do not know what role genes play. We have known for decades that MS has a widely variable clinical expression and unpredictable course, but do the variations reflect different causative agents or different responses to the same basic cause? Most investigators consider MS to be an autoimmune disease, but what incites the autoimmune response—a change in the cells of the nervous system so that they appear foreign or a microbial agent that mimics a cell component? Why is it approximately twice as common in women as in men? How can we most effectively relieve the various troubling symptoms of MS such as pain and fatigue? How can we help people with MS adapt to the disease and live their lives to the fullest level possible?

The National Multiple Sclerosis Society was founded in 1946 to address these and other questions about MS. Its mission is simple and forthright: "To end the devastating effects of multiple sclerosis." Through the efforts of its 650,000 members and staff, it has made extraordinary contributions to understanding MS by a series of highly imaginative programs in research and patient services, including almost $300 million in research grants. The report that you see here is the result of a request from the Society to the Institute of Medicine (IOM) for guidance in developing a strategic plan to direct future investments in MS research.

The multidisciplinary committee convened by the IOM in response to this request was charged to review current knowledge of all aspects of MS from cells to symptoms; to identify techniques, resources, and innovations used outside the field that might be applied to the MS challenge; and to recommend strategies that might push MS research forward most effectively.

To address its charge, the committee, with the support of IOM staff, reviewed the scientific literature related to all aspects of MS and received input from 45 outside consultants: 9 of these wrote state-of-the-art commentaries on symptom management, some told us what they needed most as MS patients, and 17 described the newest science during three workshops. Most of the workshop participants were not primarily involved in MS research or with MS patients but agreed to brainstorm with us about how the best of their disciplines might be applied to MS. We clearly could not have accomplished our work without the help of these consultants, and their listing in the Acknowledgments badly understates our gratitude. Finally, the committee recognizes with the deepest appreciation the support given by the extraordinary staff assigned to us by the IOM—Janet Joy, John Rockwell, Amelia Mathis, and Terry Pellmar. In particular, Janet Joy, study director and neuroscientist by training, with intelligence, humor, and an exceptional intensity of commitment, inspired and guided us to the completion of our task.

Richard B. Johnston, Jr., M.D.
*Chair*

# Acknowledgments

People live with multiple sclerosis (MS) for decades, making it a disease of selves as well as cells. The committee's assessment of the current status of progress against MS thus entailed a review from biomedical perspectives, as well as from psychological and social perspectives. This massive undertaking could not have been accomplished without the help of an array of experts as multifaceted as the disease itself. The committee is deeply indebted to these many people for their valuable contributions.

The following people wrote invaluable background papers for the committee: Dedra Buchwald (fatigue), Howard Fields (pain), Robert W. Hamill (bladder and bowel control), David E. Krebs (assistive technology), T. Jock Murray (cognitive impairment), Peggy Neufeld (assistive technology), Trevor Owens (genetic animal models), Robert G. Robinson (depression and brain injury), William Z. Rymer (spasticity and weakness), and Marca Sipski (sexual function).

Another group presented a series of excellent talks on new approaches to MS research at workshops for the committee. This group includes Mindy Aisen, Michael Conneally, Scott E. Fraser, Chien Ho, Ole Isacson, Elliott D. Kieff, Jeffery Kocsis, Henry McFarland, Deborah Miller, Rhona Mirsky, Marc Peschanski, John C. Roder, Jay Siegel, Joy Snider, Lawrence Steinman, Barbara Vickrey, and Michael Weinrich. (Topics are listed individually in Appendix C.)

The following people provided technical comments on draft sections of the report: Robert Burke, Mary Horwitz, Peggy Neufeld, John Roder, and Richard Rudick. Still others served as technical consultants either in meetings with the committee, sharing unpublished reports, or in consultations with Institute of Medicine (IOM) staff. This group includes Elaine Collier, Gary Karp, Lorna Layward, Ian McDonald, Sarah Minden, Audrey Penn, and Albert van der Pol.

All of these people gave generously of their time and made a tremendous and much appreciated contribution to the breadth and depth of this report.

Stephen Reingold, Vice President of Scientific Programs, and Nicholas LaRocca, Director of Health Care Delivery and Policy Research, at the National Multiple Sclerosis Society were indispensable to the committee's efforts. They provided the committee with volumes of background material and fielded an endless stream of inquiries from IOM staff. They were unfailingly quick to reply to queries and provided stores of information.

Miriam Davis and Jane Durch provided substantive editing for sections of the report, Amy Fluet wrote material for several of the explanatory boxes in the report, and Florence Poillon edited the uncorrected proofs. Each of them greatly enhanced the readability of the report and we are grateful for their excellent work.

This report has been reviewed in draft form by individuals chosen for their diverse perspectives and technical expertise, in accordance with procedures approved by the National Research Council's Report Review Committee. The purpose of this independent review is to provide candid and critical comments that will assist the institution in making the published report as sound as possible and to ensure that the report meets institutional standards for objectivity, evidence, and responsiveness to the study charge. The review comments and draft manuscript remain confidential to protect the integrity of the deliberative process. We wish to thank the following individuals for their participation in the review of this report:

**Fred Barkhof**, Diagnostic Radiology, Vrije Universiteit Hospital, Amsterdam, Netherlands

**George Ebers**, Professor, Department of Clinical Neurology, Oxford University

**Jill S. Fischer**, Director, Psychology Program (1985-2000), Mellen Center for MS Treatment and Research Cleveland Clinic

**Zach W. Hall**, Vice Chancellor, Office of Research, University of California, San Francisco

**Charles A. Janeway, Jr.**, Department of Immunobiology, Yale School of Medicine

**Alan M. Jette**, Dean, Sargent College of Health and Rehabilitation Services, Boston University

**Jurg Kesselring**, Professor and Head, Department of Rehabilitation Centre, Valens, Switzerland

**Samuel K. Ludwin**, Professor, Pathology Department, Queens University, Ontario, Canada

**Robert H. Miller**, Associate Professor, Case Western Reserve University School of Medicine

**Mary Beth Moncrief**, Manager, Associate National Scientific Program
　　Juvenile Diabetes Foundation International
**John Newsom-Davis**, Professor, Clinical Neurology, University of Oxford
**Michael B.A. Oldstone**, Professor, Department of Neuropharmacology,
　　Division of Virology, The Scripps Research Institute
**Jerry Wolinsky**, Professor, Department of Neurology, University of Texas,
　　Houston Medical Center Health Science Center

　　Although the individuals listed above have provided constructive comments and suggestions, they were not asked to endorse the conclusions or recommendations nor did they see the final draft of the report before its release. The review of this report was overseen by Joseph B. Martin, Dean, Harvard Medical School and Floyd R. Bloom, Chair, Department of Neuropharmacology, the Scripps Research Institute, who were responsible for making certain that an independent examination of this report was carried out in accordance with institutional procedures and that all review comments were carefully considered. Responsibility for the final content of this report rests entirely with the Committee on Multiple Sclerosis: Current Status and Strategies for the Future and the Institute of Medicine.

# Contents

# List of Tables and Figures

## TABLES

## FIGURES

# Executive Summary

Multiple sclerosis (MS) is a complex disease that has been much more difficult to cure than was expected when the National Multiple Sclerosis Society (the MS Society) was founded in 1946 by Sylvia Lawry "to end the devastating effects of multiple sclerosis." Yet optimism is possibly greater than it has ever been since those early years, in large part due to the development of the first treatments that can slow the progress of MS. Services for people with MS have also improved. "Diagnose and adios," Labe Scheinberg's famously disparaging quote about the options available to MS neurologists in the 1970s, no longer rings true. Nor does the advice to young researchers that "if you want to ruin your career, go into MS." Much has changed since 1946. Still, no cause or cure for MS has been found. It remains a mysterious disease with no known pathogen or even known determinants of its severity and course.

MS is not alone in this regard. Neurological diseases are among the most difficult to study, and although beneficial therapies have been developed in the last decades for Parkinson's disease, Alzheimer's disease, and epilepsy, there is still no cure for any of the degenerative neurological diseases. Advances on key fronts, such as improved ability to create images of the living brain and spinal cord, new understanding of the brain's capacity for repair, and an overall accelerated pace of new discoveries about the cellular machinery of the brain, have renewed the optimism of many investigators about the possibility of developing effective therapeutic strategies for MS patients. New therapeutic strategies, such as gene therapy, stem cell transplantation, and neuroprotection strategies, rising on the horizon have emerged from recent advances in these areas.

Over the years, the specific targets of MS research have been refocused and revised. The MS Society has reconsidered and remained committed to its focus on research. At the same time, the scope of research topics has expanded, as have perspectives of the Society's role. Although MS research has traditionally been conducted on behalf of patients who remained in the background, now—to a small, but increasing degree—patient perspectives have stimulated new areas of research. New disciplines have emerged. Health care policy, functional status measurement, and quality-of-life assessment are all relatively new areas of research and are critically important for improving the lives of people with MS. The spectrum of current MS research ranges from strategies to develop treatments that impede the disease process, to treatments for specific symptoms, to research aimed at promoting successful adaptations to the illness, including optimizing the abilities of people with MS to function in their daily lives.

In December 1998, the National Multiple Sclerosis Society asked the Institute of Medicine to undertake a strategic review of MS research on its behalf. This report presents the research strategies and programs that the committee believes are likely to be the most productive and most important in the near future. Throughout the study, the committee sought to identify windows of opportunity for research, such as those created by new discoveries about the self-repair mechanisms of the brain or new disease-specific changes in gene activation. The committee also sought to identify research needs where the windows of opportunity are less transparent, such as the development of evidence-based approaches to address varied information needs of people with MS and to treat the fatigue and pain that so often accompany MS. Ideas for the future are built on the review of current knowledge and gaps in the biomedical and social science of MS. The intended audience of this report includes the architects and developers of MS research programs, as well as people with MS and their families who want to learn what is currently known about MS and what might lie ahead.

The report covers three broad areas: (1) biomedical aspects of the disease, causes, course, and treatments (Chapters 2, 5, and 6); (2) adaptation and management (combination of medical, technological, and psychosocial aspects) (Chapters 3 and 4); and finally, (3) proposals for research managers to facilitate research progress (Chapter 7).

## DISEASE CAUSES, COURSE AND TREATMENTS

The ultimate goal of research in MS is the development of interventions that can improve the lives of those living with MS and can prevent or cure MS. However, understanding of the MS disease process is not yet sufficient to predict which therapeutic strategies will be most effective. Although the new disease-modifying drugs are a major leap forward, it is important to remember that they are not a cure, nor are they effective for all patients. The recommendations described below summarize the committee's conclusions about which directions appear most likely to provide the fundamental knowledge that can lead to the development of effective therapies (see Box 1 for summary).

> RECOMMENDATION 1: **Research on the pathological changes underlying the natural course of MS should be emphasized, because it provides the key to predicting disease course in individual patients, understanding the physiological basis of MS, and a basis for developing improved therapeutic approaches.**

Unpredictability imposes a particularly acute burden on people with MS. They have no way of knowing when a relapse will occur, how impaired they will be, or whether they will recover from the relapse. Yet it is now clear that disease activity precedes relapses. Understanding these pathological changes is the first step toward predicting—at least in the short term—disease progression in individual patients.

Research on the natural course of MS would include defining the relationship between cellular and molecular changes and the progression of disability, as well as determining the physiological basis for different clinical manifestations of MS. Changes in gene expression should be analyzed in individual cell types, particularly those in and at the borders of lesions. Such information will also improve the ability to develop more refined diagnostic tools, provide benchmarks against which to measure the effect of therapeutic interventions, and provide the scientific basis to identify new therapeutic approaches.

Research on pathological changes occurring early in the disease should be particularly emphasized. This should also include the development of improved diagnostic criteria (most likely, criteria based on neuroimaging) that allow early and more accurate diagnoses of MS. If aggressive treatment is to be instituted at the onset of disease, early and accurate diagnosis is especially important.

> RECOMMENDATION 2: **Research should be pursued to identify how neurons are damaged in MS, how this damage can be prevented, and how oligodendrocytes and astrocytes are involved in damage and repair processes.**

Oligodendrocytes, astrocytes, and neurons can, in a sense, all be regarded as the cellular "victims" in multiple sclerosis. It is clear that oligodendrocytes and the myelin sheaths they form are damaged, astrocytes respond by forming a glial scar, and in some cases, axons (outgrowths of neurons) degenerate in MS. However, a better understanding of the neuronal response to injury and capacity for repair, the capacity of myelin-forming cells to remyelinate neurons and restore function, and the contribution of astrocytes is essential to deciphering the neuropathology of MS. Although much is known, many questions remain, and their answers have important implications for therapy.

**BOX 1**
**Recommendations for Research on Causes,**
**Course, and Treatments**

Recommendation 1: Research on the pathological changes underlying the natural course of MS should be emphasized, because it provides the key to predicting disease course in individual patients, understanding the physiological basis of MS, and a basis for developing improved therapeutic approaches.

Recommendation 2: Research should be pursued to identify how neurons are damaged in MS, how this damage can be prevented, and how oligodendrocytes and astrocytes are involved in damage and repair processes.

Recommendation 3: The genes that underlie genetic susceptibility to MS should be identified, because genetic information offers such a powerful tool to elucidate fundamental disease processes and prognosis, and to develop new therapeutic approaches.

Recommendation 4: Because the discovery of an MS pathogen would likely provide the single most important clue for identifying effective treatments, this search must remain a high priority, but it should be conducted using powerful new and efficient methods.

Recommendation 5: Research to identify the cascade of immune system events that culminates in the destruction of myelin should remain a priority.

Recommendation 6: The power of neuroimaging as a tool for basic research and for clinical assessment should be taken advantage of more extensively.

Recommendation 7: Animal models should be developed that more faithfully mirror the features of MS and permit the analysis of how specific molecules and cells contribute to the disease process.

Recommendation 8: Strategies for protection and repair of neural cells, including the use of neuroprotective factors as well as stem cells, hold great promise for the treatment of MS and should be a major research priority.

Recommendation 9: New, more effective therapeutic approaches to symptom management should be pursued, including those directed at neuropathic pain and sensory disturbances.

Recommendation 10: In the absence of any fully effective therapies, integrated approaches for the delivery of currently available therapeutic agents should be investigated.

Recommendation 11: Better strategies should be developed to extract the maximum possible scientific value from MS clinical trials.

RECOMMENDATION **3: The genes that underlie genetic susceptibility to MS should be identified, because genetic information offers such a powerful tool to elucidate fundamental disease processes and prognosis, and to develop new therapeutic approaches.**

Compelling data indicate that MS is a complex genetic disorder. The identification of susceptibility genes for MS represents a significant challenge but also a major opportunity to elucidate the fundamental disease process. Genetic discoveries are likely to contribute to a better understanding of heterogeneity, clinical course, prognosis, and response to therapy. Even the discovery of a new gene with a very small genetic effect on MS could have major implications for the development of entirely new therapies based on the genetic mechanism. The committee believes that an aggressive effort in human genetics is essential.

The critical importance of identifying rare families with monogenic variants of MS cannot be overstated; this approach has been extraordinarily fruitful in neurodegenerative diseases such as Alzheimer's disease and Parkinson's disease.

RECOMMENDATION **4: Because the discovery of an MS pathogen would likely provide the single most important clue for identifying effective treatments, this search must remain a high priority, but should be conducted using powerful new and efficient methods.**

Conventional tissue culture approaches to isolate pathogens in MS have consistently failed to find any convincing result, possibly because some pathogens do not grow in tissue culture. Newer approaches should be used, such as those that involve the identification of genomic information relevant to the pathogen and those that have the potential to reveal a broader range of pathogens than are detectable in tissue culture. The methods include polymerase chain reaction (PCR), representational difference analysis, and sequence screening using the host immune response. These powerful new methods have not yet been applied to investigations of MS tissues in any concerted and organized way, and their use should be a high priority.

Discovery of a trigger for the first MS event would likely provide the single most important clue for identifying a cure and means of prevention. This event might precede clinically observable symptoms and might be different from the events that drive subsequent autoimmune attacks. Thus, despite the long and thus far unsuccessful search, research to identify the trigger event(s) of MS must remain a high priority.

RECOMMENDATION **5: Research to identify the cascade of immune system events that culminates in the destruction of myelin should remain a priority.**

The most striking pathology in MS is the immune system's attack and destruction of the body's own myelin sheath. What causes the immune system to attack myelin is unknown. Although myelin basic protein (MBP) might trigger a particularly vigorous autoimmune response, it is not the only autoantigen, nor does it account for the full autoimmune response. Any brain protein is a potential autoantigen, although not all are equal in their consequences. Two critical foci for research in the immunopathology of MS include:

- identification of the most important autoantigen triggers for autoimmune responses in MS and
- increased understanding of pathogenic immune cells.

One of the first pathological processes leading up to MS attacks is thought to be activation of autoreactive T lymphocytes, or T cells, and their migration into the central nervous system. However, T cells and the inflammatory molecules they secrete are not the only players. Many cells and molecules of the immune system—likely unleashed by T-cell activation—participate in demyelination. The entire cascade of immune system events eventually culminates in myelin destruction. The key features of this cascade are not fully understood, including the precise ordering of events, the precise antigens targeted by T cells, and the precise contributions of B lymphocytes and other cells of the immune system.

RECOMMENDATION 6: **The power of neuroimaging as a tool for basic research and for clinical assessment should be taken advantage of more extensively.**

Neuroimaging is an invaluable adjunct to clinical exam and patient reports for evaluating the effects of therapeutic intervention. Research should emphasize the application of various accepted and evolving neuroimaging techniques to understand the evolution of MS lesions from pre- or asymptomatic stages through the progression to permanent tissue alteration or recovery from disability. Understanding of the MS disease process will be enhanced by expanded use of imaging techniques such as magnetic transfer imaging (MTI), magnetic resonance spectroscopy (MRS), diffusion tensor imaging (DTI), functional magnetic resonance imaging (fMRI), and positron emission tomography (PET) scanning.

RECOMMENDATION 7: **Animal models should be developed that more faithfully mirror the features of MS and permit the analysis of how specific molecules and cells contribute to the disease process.**

An animal model for a particular disease or condition can provide the understanding to design therapies based on biological knowledge, rather than shotgun testing. For example, mouse models with targeted mutations in the cystic fibrosis gene are providing a means for testing gene therapy delivered by aerosol into the lungs. Characterization of mouse models of various dwarfing syndromes, cloning of mutated genes, and parallel comparative genetic mapping and cloning of genes for similar human syndromes have led to an understanding of various human dwarfing conditions.

Generation of a reliable animal model of MS has been a long-standing goal in MS research. Current animal models of MS fall into a group of diseases like experimental autoimmune encephalomyelitis (EAE) and animal models of virus-induced demyelination. Although the models that are presently available have yielded a tremendous amount of information relevant to MS, better animal models can be developed. Key advantages of current animals models include the fact that the initiating trigger is known, the exact time of the initiating event is known, a great deal is known about the genetics and the immune system in the case of rodents, and finally, the availability of animal mutants with "knockouts" of genes for particular arms of the immune system or those that carry a transgene perturbing a protein that is relevant to MS.

A key disadvantage of available models is that they do not replicate the cellular or molecular pathology of MS. Some types of EAE, for example, produce brisk demyelination, whereas others produce little demyelination. In addition, these models are not very tractable for studies of the electrophysiology and biophysics of neuronal function, a serious limitation in a disease such as MS in which symptoms and signs arise from impaired nerve function.

RECOMMENDATION 8: **Strategies for protection and repair of neural cells, including the use of neuroprotective factors as well as stem cells, hold great promise for the treatment of MS and should be a major research priority.**

Specific neuroprotective strategies to be investigated include:

- elucidation of the pathways leading to cell death in the central nervous system;
- identification of neuroprotective and repair strategies that will reduce or repair axonal injury;
- development of therapeutic approaches that will induce restoration of conduction in demyelinated axons, for example, by inducing expression of appropriate densities of the appropriate subtype(s) of sodium channels among them;
- development of approaches to stimulate re-growth of damaged axons; and
- development of systems for the delivery of neuroprotective and repair factors to the central nervous system.

An effective delivery system is an essential link in the development of neuroprotective or restorative therapies. Thus, the development of such delivery tools, for example, cells that have been genetically engineered to produce specific neuroprotective factors, or molecular packaging systems, is a high priority.

Specific goals to identify the cellular and molecular pathways that control the death of myelin-forming oligodendrocytes include the identification of the following:

- therapeutic strategies that can protect oligodendrocytes from immune attack;
- strategies to activate endogenous oligodendrocyte precursor cells to promote remyelination (endogenous stem cells); and
- strategies for the transplantation of myelin-forming cells into the demyelinated CNS. This includes using precursor cells or genetically engineered cells (exogenous stem cells).

The last two strategies must be considered in the context of the specific features of MS. For example, newly formed myelin might be destroyed through the same immune response that destroyed the original myelin.

RECOMMENDATION 9: **New, more effective therapeutic approaches to symptom management should be pursued, including those directed at neuropathic pain and sensory disturbances.**

- The pathophysiology of pain and paraesthesia in MS is not understood. Although neuronal hyperexcitability appears to underlie these symptoms, it is not known why it occurs in MS. The cellular and molecular basis for neuronal hyperexcitability in MS should be investigated.
- Molecular targets should be identified; for example, inappropriately expressed ion channels that cause abnormal impulse trafficking in MS. After identification of such targets, pharmacological methods can be developed for regulating the activity of these critical molecules.
- The impact of electrical activity within neurons and of exercise and physical therapy should be investigated in regard to disease progression and functional capacities. This will require the development of better tools to measure function.

RECOMMENDATION 10: **In the absence of any fully effective therapies, integrated approaches for the delivery of currently available therapeutic agents should be investigated.**

Since there are, as yet, no treatments that cure MS or halt disease progression entirely, it is important to develop integrated approaches to testing those agents that can at least modify the course of the disease. Such trials are expensive and lengthy, and they require large numbers of patients. Agents of different classes will have to be tested in sequence and in combination. Such trials are also best done when the dose range and safety profile of each individual agent to be employed in the trial are known, and the potential for adverse drug interactions should be carefully monitored. Separate end points might be required for each agent as appropriate to its individual pharmacological profile. Most importantly, standardized protocols and assessments will have to be devised and agreed upon, including Phase II studies that will allow abandonment of ineffective combinations before incurring the time, expense, and exposure to risk that are inherent in large, multicenter efficacy trials.

RECOMMENDATION **11: Better strategies should be developed to extract the maximum possible scientific value from MS clinical trials.**

The committee noted that many of the pivotal MS clinical trials on disease-modifying therapies were terminated early, usually because of predetermined stopping rules, and, thereby, lost unique opportunities to obtain critical data. Although it is not generally feasible for voluntary health organizations such as the National MS Society to lead their own clinical trials, they can and should continue to play an advisory in the design of large-scale clinical trials.

## DISEASE ADAPTATION AND MANAGEMENT

At the moment of being diagnosed, the patient is forever transformed into a "person living with MS." Even in the absence of signs or symptoms, this person will forever after live with the knowledge that he or she can be unpredictably impaired. Sometimes a person will recover, sometimes not. For most people, living with MS will become one of the major challenges of their life. Given the millions of people currently living with MS, and those expected to do so in the future, it is important that the focus on curing MS not come at the expense of efforts to address the disruptions that pervade routine daily activities, personal relationships, family life, work responsibilities, and social involvement.

Improving the lives of people with MS rests on better understanding of both their needs and their successes, specifically research into the conditions of life with MS, which requires objective, reliable research tools. The most essential tools are the various survey instruments that measure abilities to function and quality of life, which are discussed in the latter part of this chapter. These tools not only provide for objective assessment of the needs of people with MS, but also are an essential element of measuring the effectiveness of any sort of therapeutic intervention—be it a rehabilitation process, a self-help program, or a disease-modifying therapy. Quality-of-life measures can also reveal aspects of the disease process that are not readily captured in standard clinical measures and can often provide more sensitive outcome measures of the clinical efficacy of new therapies. Perhaps most importantly, they measure the outcomes that concern patients the most (see Box 2 for summary).

RECOMMENDATION **12: Health status assessment methods for people with MS should be further developed and validated to increase the reliability and power of clinical trials and to improve individual patient care.**

**BOX 2**
**Recommendations on Disease Adaptation and Management**

Recommendation 12: Health status assessment methods for people with MS
should be further developed and validated to increase the reliability and power of clinical trials and to improve individual patient care.

Recommendation 13: Research strategies aimed at improving the ability of people
with MS to adapt and function should be developed in partnership with research practitioners, managers, and patients; toward this end, a series of
forums to identify the most pressing needs experienced by people with MS
should be convened.

Quantifying health status, including functional status and quality of life, for
persons with MS is essential for several reasons. Given the chroicity and uncertain course of MS, tracking its impact over time can assist with care of individual
patients, suggesting near-term prognoses and the need for various interventions.
Tabulating these findings across individuals offers insight into the burden of MS-
related disability within populations, information increasingly used to set research, health, and social policy priorities. Longitudinal studies of the trajectory
of functioning and quality of life should help to define the natural history of the
disease and expand understanding of its clinical epidemiology and patterns of
progression. Finally, functional status and quality of life are critical end points in
measuring the effectiveness of therapy, both for clinical trials and for routine
patient care.

Clinical neurology should move toward adopting as a standard of care a
concise measurement of health status that includes quality-of-life measures, as
well as impairment and disability measures. This could serve as the basis for
communication between physicians and other caregivers and for increasing the
efficiency and thoroughness of consultations between patients and physicians,
particularly if filled out by patients before meeting with the physician. If long-
term records of such data were maintained in a data registry, they would also
provide much-needed insights into the natural course of the illness. Individual
records would provide information about patient health that would not normally
be collected in routine clinical exam.

The development and validation of new impairment and disability measures
should continue to be supported. Validation of the MS Functional Composite
Scale should continue, particularly to measure its sensitivity to changes in patient
condition over time.

RECOMMENDATION 13: **Research strategies aimed at improving the
ability of people with MS to adapt and function should be developed**

**in partnership with research practitioners, managers, and patients; toward this end, a series of forums to identify the most pressing needs experienced by people with MS should be convened.**

The goal of such forums would be to define research needed to identify ways to help people with MS adapt to the illness and enhance their ability to function. The committee did not include the expertise to develop a research agenda to meet needs as experienced by patients. Indeed, there is such a small body of empirical research on this topic that the committee felt it was perhaps premature to specify the most appropriate research strategies. Rather, the committee recommends that the MS Society work in partnership with people with MS to guide the development of specific research strategies that will identify the most effective approaches toward improving their everyday lives. A series of forums could provide the needed perspective to defining those research strategies and should include the following constituencies:

- patients and their families;
- health care providers;
- allied health professionals, such as physical therapists, occupational therapists, and social workers;
- health services researchers, including survey scientists and clinical epidemiologists;
- social scientists, including sociologists, anthropologists, and psychologists; and
- representatives of organizations of patients with other disorders that present some of the same challenges faced by people with MS.

The MS Society should identify specific individuals, including those whose work focuses on related issues outside the field of MS. Since the research community that deals with these issues is so small and has so many fewer funding resources than biomedicine, it is essential to look more broadly for resources. The needs of people with other chronic, debilitating diseases have much in common with those of people with MS. The MS Society should work with other relevant societies and government funding agencies to identify the most important research questions to address the goal of improving the lives of people with chronic and debilitating diseases, such as MS.

New strategies are needed to improve dissemination of the latest research information and the best methods of informing patients so they can take the fullest advantage of treatment options and available assistance. This includes developing a better understanding of the most effective timing, settings, and modes of delivering information. Some information is important to deliver at the time of diagnosis (for example, what to expect in the next few years, how to ensure health care); other information is only of interest to patients much later in the disease course (for example, how to obtain and choose a wheelchair). Modes and settings are also important determinants of effective communication. Certain information is best imparted by a health care provider during a private, scheduled visit; other information is best gained in a group setting. Some information has to be processed and molded to fit individual needs, and this is often accomplished more effectively in the back-and-forth exchange of a group setting. Uses of computers, including the Internet and chat groups, should be researched.

## RESEARCH MANAGEMENT

The foundations of scientific progress are laid in the building and maintenance of the research enterprise. In simplest terms, this means getting the "right" people in the "right" places, and this is the essential role of research managers (see Box 3 for summary).

RECOMMENDATION **14: New researchers should be actively recruited to work in MS, and training programs should be designed to foster**

---

**BOX 3**
**Recommendations to Build and Support**
**the MS Research Enterprise**

Recommendation 14: New researchers should be actively recruited to work in MS, and training programs should be designed to foster productive interactions with established investigators both within and outside the MS research community.

Recommendation 15: Concerted efforts should be made to stimulate enduring interdisciplinary collaborations among researchers in the biological and non-biological sciences relevant to MS and to recruit researchers from other fields into MS research.

Recommendation 16: Programs to increase research efficiency should be developed, including collaborations to enable expensive large-scale projects (e.g., clinical trials, genome screens) and to organize collection of scarce resources (e.g., human tissue).

Recommendation 17: New strategies should be developed to encourage more integration among the different disciplines that support and conduct research relevant to improving the quality of life for people with MS.

Recommendation 18: To protect against investing research resources on false leads, there should be an organizational structure to promote efficient testing of new claims for MS pathogens and disease markers.

**productive interactions with established investigators both within and outside the MS research community.**

In the last few decades there has been a tremendous influx of talented researchers into the field of neuroscience. Yet committee members observed that this burgeoning pool of researchers has not been drawn to MS research in the same numbers as they have to other neurological diseases. To bring new researchers into MS, it is not enough to rely on those who have already shown an interest in it. Active outreach is necessary. Funding new researchers is of little value without the ability to sustain the investment. Attracting new researchers should be balanced with reasonable expectations that successful researchers can continue. In the 1990s, more Ph.D.s were awarded than could be employed in research. During such periods, recruitment efforts by private research foundations might be more productive if they were to shift the balance of their efforts towards reducing support for training Ph.D. students and increasing their efforts to recruit and support postdoctoral fellows.

RECOMMENDATION **15: Concerted efforts should be made to stimulate enduring interdisciplinary collaborations among researchers in the biological and non-biological sciences relevant to MS and to recruit researchers from other fields into MS research.**

Concerted efforts should be made to stimulate enduring cross-pollination among the different research areas relevant to MS. It is not enough to bring in researchers from other fields to participate in isolated workshops. Rather, sustained interactions that promote productive collaborations or the development of new ideas must be fostered.

The committee felt that giving a small amount of funding (for example, $100,000) to an established laboratory, which has been done in the past, is not enough to encourage researchers to pursue MS research. Programs to encourage cross-pollination should target individual researchers. This has been tried successfully by other private health foundations (for example, the Hereditary Disease Foundation, CaP CURE, and the ALS Association).

More cross-talk between clinical and basic scientists is needed. One means of stimulating more exchange between basic researchers and clinicians would be to provide special funding for sabbaticals in which basic scientists could work with clinicians. There was a sense among the committee that MS has attracted less interest from basic neuroscientists than other neurological diseases. This should be actively encouraged by organizing symposia at scientific meetings, such as those of the Society for Neuroscience where MS research has received relatively little attention.

RECOMMENDATION **16: Programs to increase research efficiency should be developed, including collaborations to enable expensive large-scale projects (for example, clinical trials, genome screens)**

**and to organize collection of scarce resources (for example, human tissue).**

The committee recommends that the MS Society consider exploring less conventional approaches such as those tried by other health care foundations. The MS societies should consider leading an effort to identify and develop successful models of collaboration. Although these societies cannot fund many clinical trials, it might be able to work as a catalyst to facilitate more effective, far-reaching clinical trials, for example, by bringing together the right people.

This would also include the development of data registries that would apply to natural history studies and long-term therapeutic evaluations.

RECOMMENDATION **17: New strategies should be developed to encourage more integration among the different disciplines that support and conduct research relevant to improving the quality of life for people with MS.**

This would include research on the instruments used to assess quality of life, employment issues, personal independence, and the identification of optimal models of caring for people with MS. Research in these areas has too often proceeded in parallel paths with little apparent recognition of the work of others. For example, many articles about the psychosocial aspects of MS are published in nursing, psychology, physiotherapy, and neuroscience journals, and yet they often fail to cite articles on the same topic published outside their professional disciplines.

Because the health policy research field is relatively small and research funds are limited, partnerships should be developed among MS societies and with other health research organizations that target diseases that confront patients with similar challenges. Although each of these diseases has some unique features, for the most part, the research techniques, patients' needs, and even the investigators themselves overlap across different diseases, particularly chronic, debilitating diseases. Examples of such diseases include rheumatoid arthritis, diabetes, Parkinson's disease, Alzheimer's disease, and amyotrophic lateral sclerosis (ALS). Much of the research on quality-of-life issues for any of these diseases is likely to be relevant to people with MS. Indeed the development of partnerships among the related health care organizations should benefit a far greater number of patients than each could serve alone. Partnerships could take a variety of forms from collaborative development and funding of requests for proposals (RFPs) to collaborations in convening symposia and workshops.

RECOMMENDATION **18: To protect against investing research resources on false leads, there should be an organizational structure to promote efficient testing of new claims for MS pathogens and disease markers.**

Over the years, various viruses, bacteria, and toxins have been proposed as possible causes of MS. None of them have withstood the scrutiny of careful research, although, in a few cases, they have not been ruled out as causes. Although erroneous claims in MS research are relatively rare—there have been fewer than five in the last five years—their effects can be far-reaching. In some cases, erroneous claims have misdirected research, resulting in a substantial but unproductive investment in time and money. These erroneous claims have also led to the treatment of patients with inappropriate, expensive, and potentially harmful therapies. For example, the claim that metal toxicity causes MS induced some patients to have teeth extracted and amalgam fillings removed. New claims of MS pathogens, when appropriate, should be resolved as quickly as possible.

The MS societies are the most likely organizations to undertake such tests of newly proposed pathogens on an ad hoc basis. One possible approach is that following a potentially credible claim implicating a particular pathogen in MS, a society could oversee a project whereby the investigator making the claim, as well as an expert in the particular pathogen, could review clinical samples. A similar approach could be taken in terms of other claims related to diagnosis or treatment of MS in situations in which a quick confirmation of the results would be important to MS patients or to the neurological and scientific community. This approach should reduce costs to patients, researchers, and even the MS societies. The key elements of such a program would be:

- evaluation of credible claims that are judged to have the potential for influencing research strategies or treatments,
- rapid response, and
- generation of replicate data sets, necessary for establishing the reliability of claims.

If the validation experiments were conducted in established laboratories equipped with the necessary expertise and research tools, the costs should be relatively low. It might also be possible to offer the possibility of confirming such path-breaking claims prior to their initial publication in order to increase the immediate impact of the discoveries or spare investigators embarrassment should their data be incorrect.

# 1

# Introduction

Nancy Mairs was barely aware she had developed a limp.* It had come on so gradually and she had been so busy over the past months that she had given it little heed. She had just moved with her husband and two young children from Boston to Tucson to start a new life as a graduate student in English literature. During the past year, she had had countless bouts of exhaustion, but what working mother of young children doesn't? Indeed, she was startled and somewhat offended when a fellow graduate student asked her why she was limping. Had she hurt herself? It was that question that finally jarred her enough to consult her family doctor who then referred her to a neurologist.

Readers of this report will immediately suspect that this woman has multiple sclerosis (MS). She does, but like so many other people with MS, it was the last thing she suspected. Multiple sclerosis sneaks up on people. The earliest symptoms are usually mild enough to be blamed on temporary causes such as fatigue or stress. It is often only after someone is diagnosed that they recall their history of episodic clumsiness, deep fatigue, or blurred vision.

Although multiple sclerosis sneaks up on individuals, it is fairly predictable in populations. Approximately 1 in 1,000 people develop MS, usually in their late twenties, and about two-thirds of them are women. It is more common among people of Northern European heritage and more common among people who live in the high latitudes during childhood (Figure 1.1). Genetic factors can increase

---

*Taken with Nancy Mairs' permission from her autobiographical book on life with multiple sclerosis, *Waist High in the World*.[3]

*17*

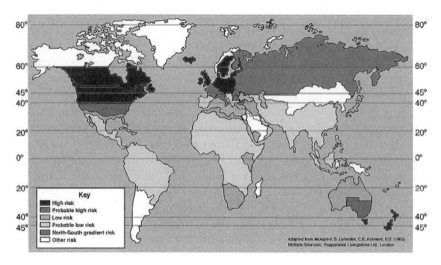

**FIGURE 1.1** MS distribution map. SOURCE: Adapted from McAlpine D, Lumadan CE, Acheson ED. 1967. Multiple Sclerosis a Reappraisal. Livingstone Ltd., London. Courtesy of John Rose and the Knowledge Weavers, University of Utah.

the risk of developing MS, but the precipitating event that somehow results in the immune system's attack on the nervous system remains unknown. The attacks may be few and far between with little or no impact on a person's ability to function, or they may cause a rapid progression toward severe disability. Most people with MS fall between these extremes and, on average, live only a few years less than the general population.

MS is probably an autoimmune disease, meaning that the body's natural defenses are turned against itself. Instead of destroying foreign cells, the immune system destroys the body's native cells. For example, in the autoimmune disease, Type 1 diabetes, the insulin-producing cells of the pancreas are destroyed. In MS, the myelin sheath that insulates nerve cells is destroyed (see Figure 1.2). Without the myelin sheath, nerve cells lose their ability to conduct nerve impulses. As the number of damaged nerve cells increases, the body loses its ability to perform the functions controlled by these cells.

This attack on the myelin sheath is believed to be orchestrated by blood-borne immune cells that invade the brain through the blood-brain barrier, the physical-chemical barrier that surrounds the brain and normally protects it from foreign and toxic substances circulating in the blood. The brain is thus normally resistant to infections that afflict the rest of the body. MS is one of the few diseases in which the blood-brain barrier is breached.

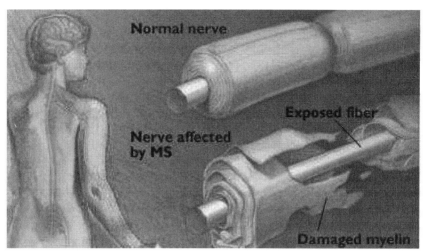

FIGURE 1.2  The nerve fiber in multiple sclerosis. SOURCE: Mayo Clinic Health Letter. Multiple Sclerosis: New leads into its cause and treatment. November 1995. Reprinted with permission of Mayo Foundation for Medical Education and Research.

## THE U.S. NATIONAL MULTIPLE SCLEROSIS SOCIETY

The National MS Society (the MS Society) was founded in 1946 by Sylvia Lawry "to end the devastating effects of multiple sclerosis." Her brother had been diagnosed with MS and doctors told her there was nothing they could do for him. In response, she established a foundation that would be devoted to research on MS. It was an optimistic era. Fatal diseases were being conquered in rapid succession. In the late 1920s, it was discovered that vitamin $B_{12}$ could both prevent and cure pernicious anemia. By 1940, insulin was being used to control diabetes. Also, with the discovery of the curative powers of penicillin and streptomycin in the 1930s and 1940s, a major revolution in public health and medicine had been launched—the "age of antibiotics." Each of these triumphs, marked by Nobel prizes, inspired the search for clear-cut cures.

However, much has changed since 1946. Many diseases, including MS, have disappointed those hoping to discover simple answers. Nevertheless, the study of MS has led to many improvements, in both quality and longevity, in the lives of people with MS. For the first time ever, treatments that can slow the progress of the disease are available, but still no cause or cure for MS has been found. MS remains a mysterious disease.

**BOX 1.1**
## Recent Research Advances with Far-Reaching Implications for People with MS

**THERAPEUTIC DEVELOPMENTS**

*   Development of the first therapies that can modify the course of MS. These therapies include the beta-interferons (Betseron, Rebif, and Avonex), anti-inflammatory agents that suppress cell migration into the central nervous system (CNS); and glatiramer acetate (Copaxone), a mixture of peptide fragments thought to act as a decoy for the immune system to spare myelin from further attack.

*   Development of neuroimaging techniques that allow much more sensitive detection of pathological changes associated with the MS disease process than was possible in the past
    *   Allows noninvasive exploration of pathological changes in MS patients
    *   Provides a tool to measure the effect of therapeutic interventions at an earlier stage than was previously possible

*   Discovery that neurologic function can fully recover after acute inflammation, despite persistent demyelination

*   Discovery of endogenous pluripotent neural stem cells and their potential to be used to repair damaged neural cells in the brain

*   Discovery of the therapeutic potential for neural, glial, and stem cell transplantation in the brain and spinal cord

*   Development of standardized methods for conducting clinical trials

*   Increased awareness of the need for objective evaluation of patient perspectives in health care assessment and clinical trials, and the incorporation of quality-of-life measures into research on MS

*   Introduction of rigorous evaluation of therapy and rehabilitation in MS patients

**BASIC RESEARCH DISCOVERIES THAT ARE IMPORTANT FOR NEW THERAPEUTIC STRATEGIES IN MS**

*   Recognition of involvement of axonal pathology in MS and its association with the development of disability

*   Characterization of the formation and function of the myelin sheath, including:
    *   Discovery of the myelin cell lineage
    *   Understanding of how demyelination interferes with nerve conduction
    *   Discovery that a number of different cell types can remyelinate neurons

*   Molecular dissection of myelinated axons, leading to an understanding of mechanisms of electrical impulse conduction in normal myelinated axons and of the restoration of conduction in demyelinated axons

*continued*

- Increased understanding of the role of the immune system in MS
  - Demonstration of autoreactive T cells in MS
  - Understanding of the steps involved in T-cell trafficking in the CNS
  - Refinement of animal models, both immune and virally mediated
  - Application of tolerance strategies to animal models and to MS
  - Appreciation of a role for humoral mechanisms for MS
  - Identification of myelin gene products that can act as autoimmunogens
  - Discovery of the relevance of cytokines to MS pathogenesis, including their involvement in inflammation, immune responses, and cellular repair in brain
- Establishment of the infrastructure necessary to identify genes involved in susceptibility to MS

## Recent Advances in MS

In recent years, progress in MS research has accelerated (see Box 1.1). The 1990s saw the development of the first therapies that can modify the course of the disease. Admittedly, these therapies are not a cure, nor do they work equally well for all patients, but they are a major breakthrough. Twenty-five years ago, the possibility that human nerves damaged by disease could be repaired was almost unthinkable. Now, the many years of basic research on the development and function of nerve cells are beginning to bear fruit. A number of therapeutic strategies to repair nerve cells are under serious investigation to treat a variety of diseases and injuries. For the most part, these strategies are still experimental and remain to be proven safe and effective for human use, but they have the potential to revolutionize the treatment of neurological disorders.

## Origin of the Study

In December 1998, the National Multiple Sclerosis Society asked the Institute of Medicine (IOM) to undertake a strategic review of MS research on its behalf. The society selected the IOM because, in its words, the IOM offered a uniquely "broad, intellectual perspective." The selection goes both ways. IOM studies are undertaken only upon approval from the National Research Council (NRC) Governing Board that oversees all studies of the National Academies, which includes the Institute of Medicine. To be approved, a study must be timely and of national significance. While this study is clearly significant for MS patients and the research community, its value also lies in its potential as a model for the development of similarly broadly based strategic research plans for other health fields.

By the end of 2000, the MS Society will have spent more than $285 million to support research on MS. People with MS, their families, and friends are understandably discouraged that no cure has resulted from this 50-year effort. During this period, many diseases have succumbed in the face of concerted research efforts. Polio and smallpox are diseases of the past. Where cancer was once diagnosed with a prognosis of "years to live," many people now recover to live many years after their diagnosis. Neurological diseases, however, are among the most difficult to study, and although beneficial therapies have been developed in the last decades for Parkinson's disease, Alzheimer's disease, and epilepsy, there is still no cure for any of the degenerative neurological diseases. MS is not alone in this regard. This is, nonetheless, a period of tremendous optimism about future therapeutic strategies, due in large part to the accelerating pace of new discoveries about the cellular machinery of the brain and spinal cord, as well as the information explosion emanating from the human genome project.

## Previous Reviews of MS Research Programs

Since 1973, various groups have met to review the status of research in multiple sclerosis. Each group had a somewhat different goal and each resulted in different initiatives.

### 1973 National Advisory Commission on Multiple Sclerosis

This commission laid out a detailed set of recommendations, to the point of recommending how much the MS Society should spend on specific projects.[4] Among other proposals, it recommended that

- $150,000 be spent in 1975, $300,000 in 1976, and $300,000 in 1977 for research on the demyelination and remyelination process of nerve cells in culture;
- $10,000 be spent to disseminate information to physicians and nurses on the prevention and treatment of bedsores; and
- $225,000 be spent in 1975, $400,000 in 1976, and $500,000 in 1977 for support of the first comprehensive treatment center devoted to the prevention of complications and disabling effects of MS rather than research on the disease process (all dollars are 1975 dollars).

Other recommendations included the establishment of a dedicated staff member to oversee multiple sclerosis research at the National Institute of Neurological Disease and Stroke (which was implemented and continues to this day), and the integration of MS research across the National Institutes of Health (which was not implemented).

## 1986 IOM Workshop

In the mid-1980s, some members of the MS Society argued that more of the their funds should be spent directly on patient services and less on supporting basic research. At the invitation of the MS Society Board of Directors, the IOM convened a workshop to discuss the question, Should the hard-won dollars of single-disease-oriented voluntary agencies be spent on patient services or on lobbying to obtain a larger NIH budget, rather than on research?[1] The participants included leaders of various health care foundations, and they strongly endorsed a continued commitment to the MS Society's support for basic research. They also recommended that the society set funds aside for innovative research projects that might not have enough preliminary data to be considered "safe" enough to risk a large investment. This was the origin of the pilot research program of the MS Society, which awards about 20 small grants (less than $30,000) each year. (Grants to individual investigators are generally funded at about $200,000 to $400,000 for three years.)

## 1996 MS Society Strategic Planning Retreat

The 1996 report reviewed the portfolio of MS Society research programs, which it strongly supported.[5] The report recommended that the Society encourage research on gender-related issues and that programs be developed to encourage more physicians to do research. Both recommendations reflected current trends that transcended research in multiple sclerosis. Gender-based differences in immune responses had recently been recognized as more important than previously understood, and the combination of unprecedented levels of medical school debt, low grant funding rates, and changes in the U.S. health care system had all contributed to making a research career a discouraging prospect for potential physician-researchers. Although that report strongly supported the MS Society's research programs, there was some sentiment that it was inherently biased in having been written by a committee that was composed only of MS "insiders," that is, members of the MS research elite who were unlikely to be critical of a society in whose decisions they were deeply involved and that also supported their own research.

## 1998 Review of the MS Society of Great Britain and Northern Ireland

The 1998 review identified results from the British MS Society's funding of research in the previous decade, as an accounting of how effectively it had used its resources during that period and, also, as a basis for considering future strategies to support research.[2] The three primary recommendations on research funding were that (1) support of investigator-initiated projects should remain the backbone of the research program, (2) training mechanisms should be supported to recruit talented young investigators, and (3) a research advisory group should be established that would be composed of experienced scientists who are less dependent on MS Society funding than the current advisory council and that would include distinguished investigators in cognate fields. Overall, many of that committee's recommendations were that the British MS Society should operate more like its larger counterpart across the Atlantic Ocean, the National MS Society.

## THE IOM COMMITTEE AND ITS MANDATE

The IOM committee was asked to review current scientific knowledge and to recommend strategic plans for future research, including laboratory and clinical research. In developing research strategies for the future, the committee was asked to look beyond both national and disciplinary boundaries to identify new ideas and new techniques that can be enlisted in the fight against MS. The committee was also asked to consider the roles played by different types of organizations that sponsor MS research. Private health organizations such as the MS Society, private firms, and the federal government each occupy different niches both in the scientific research community and for health care consumers or caregivers. Identifying how these different organizations can use their resources most productively toward "ending the devastating effects" of MS is important for everyone concerned. Further details of what the committee was asked to do are listed under the "Statement of Task" (see Box 1.2).

The committee was *not* asked to evaluate the MS Society's research program or grant review process. As noted earlier in this chapter, that has been done before. Indeed, the MS Society's research program has helped to model programs of other voluntary health organizations including the Arthritis Foundation, Cystic Fibrosis Foundation, Hemophilia Foundation, and the British MS Society.

Forming the study committee involved recruiting an intricate balance of a broad range of professional expertise and individual perspectives. The foremost consideration was that all members be considered by their peers to be among the very best in their areas of expertise. A second consideration was to form a committee whose thinking was not limited to the well-established research strategies in MS, but nonetheless included the in-depth knowledge of past and present research in MS and related fields needed to provide a solid foundation upon which new ideas could be weighed. Anyone currently in a policy-setting position at the MS Society was excluded from consideration.

The committee included people whose primary field of expertise is research on multiple sclerosis and those who worked in other fields; it included clinicians and basic researchers; people from academe and industry; those with experience managing research in government and private foundations; and researchers from the United States, Canada, Britain, and Germany (see Appendix A for committee

---

**BOX 1.2**
**Statement of Task**

The Institute of Medicine will review current knowledge about the cause and treatment of MS and will develop a strategic plan to guide future investments. The goal of the study is to identify the potentially most productive research strategies for the field of MS as a whole; in particular, to identify the resources and strategies from disciplines not generally considered to be involved in MS research, but that might nonetheless expand the intellectual and technological resources from which researchers might draw in the fight against MS. The IOM will assemble a study committee of outstanding scientists and other experts from academia, industry, and other research and medical organizations that include health care practitioners, who are knowledgeable about the fields relevant to MS research, but whose careers are generally not focused on this disease. The committee will be charged with the following:

- Assess the current status of progress against MS. The review will describe what is known about the etiology, pathogenesis, and clinical management of MS, as well as identify the information most needed to understand the mechanisms underlying the cause and progression of MS. Studies funded from domestic and international sources (National MS Society, the National Institutes of Health, industry, and other research organizations) will be considered in the review.
- Identify research areas and disciplines that have the greatest potential for the future of MS scientific progress, which will include: (1) identifying advances in related fields that might prove to be beneficial for the cure and treatment of MS, (2) exploring opportunities for innovations that have prospects for creating significant scientific and clinical advances, and (3) identifying areas that have not previously been involved in MS and might contribute new insights.
- Consider strategies to facilitate application of new scientific findings to treatment protocols and to enhance communication of research advances to caregivers.
- Develop recommendations regarding the direction of future research investments to attract interest from researchers that have not previously focused on the disease and to draw some of the brightest young researchers to this field.
- Highlight the most effective role for the NMSS in contributing to the recommended strategies. Recommendations will consider the distinctive contributions that could be made by the NMSS in the context of total research supported by the NMSS, NIH, other domestic and international organizations, including private industry.

---

biographies). Different ways of knowing MS were also represented on the committee: those of someone living with MS, clinicians who treat MS patients, and scientists at the cutting edge of research, ranging from the study of fundamental brain mechanisms to clinical trials of treatments for neurological disease.

## How the Committee Carried Out Its Task

The committee supplemented its expertise through a series of background papers and three workshops. The background papers were written for the committee by experts on the different complications of MS such as pain, fatigue, and bladder problems (see Appendix B for the list of expert consultants). Each workshop was organized as a combined information-gathering and brainstorming session on one of the following themes: new technologies and research on the mechanism of disease in MS, new opportunities for the treatment of neurological disease, and research toward improving the quality of life for people with MS (see Appendix C for a list of workshop participants). To supplement the committee members' own experience treating MS patients, they also met with several people—some of whom have MS themselves—who work with MS patients in a variety of nonresearch settings, including nursing, outdoor adventures, and the Jimmie Heuga Center, an exercise and life-style management facility for people with MS.

Among the important audiences for this report are the architects and developers of multiple sclerosis research programs. The report covers a broad spectrum of MS research, ranging from strategies to develop treatments that impede the disease process, to treatments for specific symptoms, to research aimed at promoting successful adaptations to the illness including optimizing the abilities of people with MS to function in their daily lives. Throughout the study, the committee sought to identify windows of opportunity for research, such as those created by new discoveries about the self-repair mechanisms of the brain or new disease-specific changes in gene activation. The committee also sought to identify research needs where the windows of opportunity are less transparent, such as the development of evidence-based approaches for addressing the varied information needs of people with MS and for treating the fatigue and pain that so often accompany MS.

Ultimately, however, this report is for people with MS. It represents another chapter in the efforts of the National Multiple Sclerosis Society to conquer MS. Thus, the report also attempts to provide a readable, comprehensive review of what is currently known about MS, what needs to be learned, and the promises that research holds in the near future.

## Organization of the Report

Chapter 2 reviews what is known about the clinical and biological aspects of MS, including possible causes of the disease and the destructive mechanisms that leave the brain and spinal cord unable to perform their normal functions. It also reviews the research tools that hold the greatest promise to reveal those underlying disease mechanisms.

Chapter 3 reviews what is known about the prevalence, causes, impact, and treatment of specific symptoms of MS such as fatigue, spasticity, and visual disturbances.

Chapter 4 focuses on the lives of people with MS and strategies for adapting to the illness. It also reviews the tools that are most important for research aimed at improving the lives of people with MS, specifically the tools that measure quality of life and functional status.

Chapter 5 looks forward and discusses research strategies and techniques that have the greatest potential to reveal new insights into the biology of the disease, insights that are likely to be crucial in the development of effective treatments.

Chapter 6 also looks forward, in this case reviewing critical issues and research for developing specific therapeutic strategies, with an emphasis on disease-modifying therapies. This chapter includes a discussion of challenges inherent in designing appropriate clinical trials in MS research.

Chapter 7 discusses building and supporting the research enterprise necessary to facilitate the most effective research strategies for MS.

Finally, Chapter 8 collates the key recommendations that emerge from discussions in the preceding chapters.

## REFERENCES

1. Asbury AK, Goldsmith CH. 1987. The role of voluntary agencies in the funding of biomedical research. *N Engl J Med.;* 316:1665.
2. Ewart WR, Silberberg DH, Wekerle H. 1998. Review and development of a strategic plan of MS research. London, UK: MS Society of Great Britain and Northern Ireland.
3. Mairs N. 1996. Waist-high in the world. A life among the nondisabled. Boston, MA: Beacon Press.
4. National Advisory Commission on Multiple Sclerosis. 1974. *Report and Recommendations: An Overview.* Bethesda, Maryland: National Institutes of Health; Volume One.
5. National Multiple Sclerosis Society. 1996. Strategic Planning Retreat for Research and Training Programs. Washington, DC: National Multiple Sclerosis Society.

# 2

# Clinical and Biological Features

Multiple sclerosis (MS) literally means "many scars," which refers to the lesions that accumulate in the brain and spinal cord throughout the course of the disease. These scars, or lesions, consist mostly of dead nerve cells, whose axons have been denuded of the myelin sheaths that normally protect them and permit the conduction of nerve impulses. MS is a chronic, degenerative disease that usually begins in young adulthood and most visibly destroys muscular control, although many other brain functions are affected. Most people will live with MS for decades after their diagnosis. MS reduces life expectancy after onset (as measured by current diagnostic criteria) by only about 10-15 years, and about half of the patients survive 30 years or more from onset.[110]

## THE CLINICAL PICTURE: SYMPTOMS, DISEASE COURSE, VARIATION, AND DIAGNOSIS

### Disease Activity and Progression

MS, as defined by ongoing central nervous system (CNS) lesion formation and increasing cumulative damage, is now recognized as a disease that is active in most patients most of the time. Disease activity has reversible and irreversible sequelae; irreversible sequelae ultimately lead to progressive impairment and disability in most patients. MS takes a variety of forms, distinguished by the clinical pattern of disease activity (Table 2.1, Figure 2.1). Accumulated deficit can produce sustained worsening in both relapsing and progressive MS. In re-

**TABLE 2.1** Varieties of MS

| | |
|---|---|
| **Asymptomatic MS** | Autopsy studies indicate there are individuals without any known clinical history who have neuropathologic changes typical of MS. It is difficult to get an accurate estimate of subclinical disease, but one recent review suggested asymptomatic MS might account for up to 25% of all cases. |
| **Relapsing-remitting MS** | This is the major MS subtype. Approximately 85% of patients with a diagnosis of MS start out with relapsing MS. Overall, this subtype accounts for 55% of MS. Relapsing MS patients show a high rate of inflammatory lesion activity (gadolinium-enhancing lesions). |
| **Benign relapsing MS** | This category represents a subset of relapsing patients who have few attacks and make an excellent recovery. They show minimal impairment and disability, even after 20-30 years. The proportion of MS patients with benign disease is controversial. Reasonable studies suggest 10-20% of people with MS fit into this category. |
| **Primary progressive MS** | This subtype accounts for 10% of MS. Patients show gradual worsening from onset, without disease attacks. These patients tend to be older and often present with a spinal cord dysfunction without obvious brain involvement. This subtype is the least likely to show inflammatory lesion activity on MRI (gadolinium-enhancing). Unlike the other subtypes of MS, men are as likely as women to develop primary progressive MS. |
| **Progressive relapsing MS** | This subtype accounts for 5% of MS. Patients show slow worsening from onset, with superimposed attacks. Recent studies suggest these patients are similar to primary progressive patients. |
| **Secondary progressive MS** | This is the major progressive subtype and accounts for approximately 30% of MS. Relapsing MS patients usually transition to secondary progressive disease. They show gradual worsening, with or without superimposed relapses. Natural history studies of untreated relapsing MS indicate 50% of patients will be secondary progressive at 10 years and almost 90% by 25 years. This form of MS shows a lower rate of inflammatory lesion activity than relapsing MS, yet the total burden of disease continues to increase. This most likely reflects ongoing axonal loss. |
| **Acute MS** | Also referred to as Marburg variant MS, this is the most severe form of MS. Significant disability develops much more rapidly than usual, over weeks to months. Pathologic changes are widespread and destructive. These cases are rare and generally occur in young people. |
| **Clinically isolated syndromes** | This refers to patients who present with an isolated CNS syndrome (optic neuritis, incomplete transverse myelitis, brainstem or cerebellar lesion), which is often the first MS attack. Clinical, MRI, and CSF studies indicate that such patients with normal brain MRI and CSF have a low risk of developing MS. In contrast, those with abnormal MRI have a high risk of developing MS. |

NOTE: CSF = cerebrosinal fluid; MRI = magnetic resonance imaging

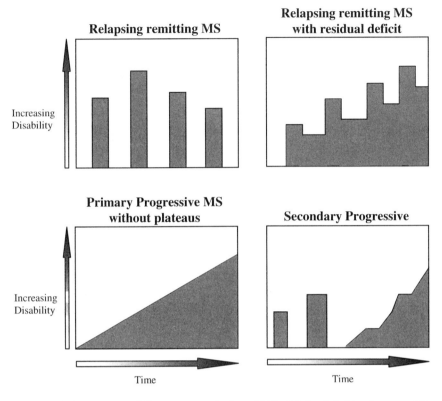

**FIGURE 2.1** Spectrum of disease course (refer to Table 2.1 for definitions). SOURCE: Adapted from Lublin and Reingold, 1996.[125]

lapsing MS, worsening occurs in most patients during acute attacks with incomplete recovery. In progressive MS, the dominant pattern is a gradual accumulation of neurologic deficits, with slow clinical worsening.

Disease activity and progression have both clinical and subclinical components. Clinical disease activity and progression are judged by observation and neurologic examination. Subclinical components refer to pathological changes that are not observable in a clinical examination but are observed using a variety of laboratory tests, predominantly neuroimaging parameters.

## Clinical Activity

**Relapses.** Relapses are variously referred to as acute attacks, exacerbations, or disease flare-ups. They involve the acute, or sudden onset, of focal neurological disturbances. Examples of typical MS relapses include blurring of vision in one eye (optic neuritis), persistent numbness or tingling of a body part (sensory system relapse), weakness of a body part (motor system relapse), or loss of coordination (cerebellar system relapse). Early in the MS disease process, relapses are likely to involve sensory, motor, cerebellar, or visual system abnormalities (Figure 2.2, Table 2.2). Later in the disease process, relapses are likely to involve bladder, bowel, cognitive, and sexual function abnormalities. Acute disease attacks are a characteristic feature of the relapsing-remitting MS subtype. Relapses also occur in patients with progressive relapsing disease and in a number of patients with secondary progressive disease. The only clinical disease subtype in which relapses never occur is primary progressive MS.

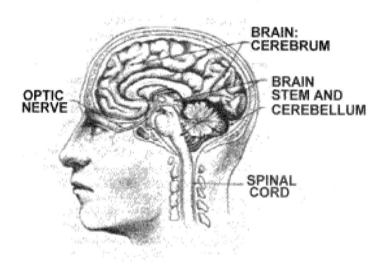

**FIGURE 2.2** Areas of the CNS often affected by MS. Reprinted with permission from University of Delaware.

**TABLE 2.2** Initial Signs and Symptoms of MS

| COMMON | UNCOMMON |
|---|---|
| • Sensory problems (numbness or tingling of a body part)<br>• Weakness<br>• Difficulty walking<br>• Monocular decreased vision<br>• Poor coordination | • Bladder problems<br>• Bowel problems<br>• Sexual dysfunction<br>• Cognitive difficulties<br>• Pain |

Relapses generally consist of three phases. There is a period of worsening, with onset of new deficits or increasing severity of old deficits. This is followed by a period of stability, with no change in deficits. The final phase is the period of recovery, with variable degrees of improvement in deficits. Most patients recover within six weeks, although for some, improvements can continue over months. Recovery can be complete return to baseline status, partial return, or no improvement. However, some degree of improvement is typical, particularly early in the disease. Relapsing patients then remain clinically stable until the next disease attack.

To be considered a relapse, deficits must persist for a minimum of 24 hours. This avoids confusion with deficits lasting only minutes to hours, which are believed to be a consequence of impaired nerve conduction through old lesion areas rather than the formation of a new lesion. Alternatively, new abnormalities that last seconds to minutes, such as Lhermitte's sign (a tingling sensation radiating down the arms, neck, or back on neck flexion), or paroxysmal attacks (stereotypic neurologic deficits occurring multiple times a day that last less than a minute) are also considered relapses if they occur repeatedly over several weeks. Sequential relapses are considered distinct only when they occur at least 30 days apart with a month of clinical stability in between. Although clinical relapses always produce changes in a patient's condition, they are always associated with changes on neurologic examination. Maximal deficit in an MS relapse typically develops over several days but in some cases can develop much faster, over hours or even minutes, or much more slowly, over a period as long as several weeks.

Physiologic factors such as temperature, pH, or electrolyte balance can temporarily disrupt nerve conduction and produce neurologic abnormality. A relapse must be distinguished from a *pseudoexacerbation*, which is a neurologic deterioration associated with a physiologic change such as infection or fever. This condition can last for days, mimicking a true relapse. Pseudoexacerbation deficits disappear once the precipitating factor has been corrected. They reflect a temporary disruption in nerve conduction, rather than the formation of a new lesion.

Approximately 85 percent of MS patients begin with relapsing-remitting disease.[222] MS relapses can involve a single neural system, as in optic neuritis, or several anatomically distinct systems at the same time, for example, combined motor and sensory problems. Attacks involving single neural systems are somewhat more common in the first MS relapse.

Most patients experience their second attack within two to three years of the first, but 5 percent of patients remain free of relapses for 15 years or more. In most cases, there is substantial recovery from the first relapse; only 4 percent of patients show no improvement. The average relapse rate is one to two attacks a year, but this rate normally declines over time. The longer a person has MS, the less likely it is that relapses will be followed by complete recovery and the more likely it is that relapses will be associated with residual deficits and increasing disability.

**TABLE 2.3** Prognostic Relapse Indicators

| Feature | Favorable Prognosis | Unfavorable Prognosis |
|---|---|---|
| Relapse rate in first 2 years | <5 relapses | ≥5 relapses |
| Relapse rate after 5 years | No increase | Increasing |
| Duration between relapses | Long | Short |
| Number of neural systems involved | One | Multiple |
| Relapse recovery | Complete | Incomplete |
| Type of systems involved | Visual, sensory, brainstem | Motor, cerebellar, bowel or bladder |

Relapse features have prognostic significance (Table 2.3). In the first few years after disease onset, the number and type of relapses, as well as the degree of recovery, help predict future disease course.[8] Relapses that involve visual, sensory, or brainstem systems have a better prognosis than those that involve cerebellar, motor, or sphincter systems. In the first two years of disease, a low relapse rate with excellent recovery indicates a better prognosis than a high relapse rate with poor recovery. Relapses restricted to single neural systems are prognostically better than those involving multiple systems. The relapse rate also has prognostic significance in the later stages of MS. With a disease duration of five or more years, an increasing relapse rate, polyregional relapses that involved multiple systems, and incomplete recovery from relapses indicate a worse prognosis.[8]

**Progression.** The relapsing form of MS is characterized by acute disease exacerbations. In contrast, progressive MS is characterized by slow deterioration and increasing neurological deficits. There are three forms of progressive MS. Approximately 15 percent of MS patients show slow deterioration from onset. In the second form, 10 percent have either primary progressive MS and never experience acute disease attacks or progressive relapsing MS (5 percent), and have occasional subsequent attacks. The third form, secondary progressive MS, is the major progressive subtype. These are relapsing patients who begin to slowly worsen 5 to 15 years after the first relapse. Once relapsing patients enter a progressive phase, they either stop having relapses or continue to experience exacerbations superimposed on slow worsening.

Documentation of a progressive course requires at least six months of observation. Observation over a year or two is often necessary to be confident of progression, since deficits can accumulate at a very gradual rate. The major defining feature of progressive MS is slow deterioration that occurs independently of acute disease relapses and does not reflect residual deficits from acute disease attacks. An analysis of the disease course among 1,844 patients indicated that the presence or absence of relapses during the progressive phase does not significantly affect the progression of irreversible disability[45] (4 percent of patients in this study had been treated for up to one year with beta-interferon, but this did not affect the study results). Progressive MS patients can be clinically stable for up to several years at a time and can even show slight improvement for a period of time. Ultimately, however, all progressive MS patients develop disability with limited ability to walk. Progressive MS is a more severe form than benign or relapsing-remitting MS and has a worse prognosis.

## Subclinical Disease Activity and Progression

Clinical parameters such as relapses and progression underestimate the actual damage to tissue that occurs in MS. When macroscopically normal-appearing brain tissue is looked at under the microscope, one can detect inflammation, gliosis (scarring), and myelin damage. Chemical studies of normal-appearing brain tissue often reveal changes in organelles such as lysosomes, in enzymes, and in myelin constituents. In addition, a number of the new research neuroimaging techniques can detect changes in brain and spinal cord areas that appear free of lesions on conventional magnetic resonance imaging (MRI). Some of these abnormalities are detectable several months to years before they can be seen with conventional MRI. Changes in normal-appearing brain tissue are generally pronounced in MS patients with severe impairment. As a group, secondary progressive MS patients show more abnormalities in normal white matter and brain tissue than relapsing patients. (White matter corresponds to brain regions where axons are ensheathed in myelin; gray matter corresponds to brain regions that are rich in cell bodies.) Primary progressive patients often show subtle but diffuse changes in normal-appearing brain areas.

Even conventional MRI indicates that most new lesion formation is clinically silent, meaning that clinical exam does not reveal any corresponding symptoms. Approximately 80 to 90 percent of new brain lesions do not produce identifiable relapses. They might, however, be associated with subtle cognitive changes or other neuropsychological changes that are not detected in clinical examination. The total lesion burden increases in MS patients, on average, 5 to 10 percent per year, reflecting in large part the development of clinically silent lesions. (This does not apply to patients on the disease-modifying therapies discussed later in this section.) Atrophy of both brain and spinal cord can be detected even in patients with minimal symptoms. Atrophy can progress without obvious lesion formation, most likely reflecting loss of axons. MS patients show an accelerated rate of age-related brain and spinal cord atrophy that is three- to tenfold higher than the rate in control populations.[76]

Spinal cord lesions are generally similar to those in the brain except for the absence of "black holes" (see discussion in Box 2.1 of T1-weighted lesions).[69] Spinal MS lesions rarely cover more than half of the cross-sectional area of the cord or exceed two vertebral segments in length. They are found more often in the cervical spinal cord (neck region) than thoracic region (midback) and are most

## BOX 2.1
### Basic Technical Principles of MRI

MRI involves application of a magnetic field to the body that causes nuclei with odd numbers of protons, such as hydrogen nuclei, to behave like tiny magnets. These protons align themselves either parallel or antiparallel to the applied external magnetic field. The net magnetization induces an electric current that forms the basic MR signal. An MR image is formed by determining the spatial distribution of the signal and reconstructing the data into detailed images. The signals are picked up by a very sensitive antenna and forwarded to a computer for processing.

Two time constants, T1 and T2 relaxation times, are important in determining the appearance of MR images. T1, or the longitudinal relaxation time, is the time constant when 63 percent of the original longitudinal magnetization is regained as the nuclei return to alignment with the external magnetic field. T2 or the transverse relaxation time, is the time constant when the transverse magnetization decreases to 37 percent of its original value as the nuclei lose alignment with each other following the initial application of an external magnetic field (a radio-frequency pulse).

By altering the imaging parameters and pulse sequences used, differences between tissues with intrinsically different proton densities and T1 and T2 relaxation times can be highlighted or obscured. Image contrast can be either T1 weighted or T2 weighted in order to emphasize the differences between normal and pathological tissues. For example, cerebrospinal fluid (CSF) is dark on T1-weighted images and bright on T2-weighted images. White matter is bright on T1-weighted images, whereas a matter is dark but not as dark as CSF.

common in the midcervical region. Disease activity is much less frequent in the spine than in the brain.

In summary, the clinical manifestations of MS possibly represent only the "tip of the iceberg," with most of the CNS damage occurring much earlier and being detectable only when the accumulated damage overwhelms the ability of the CNS to compensate. The mechanisms through which CNS tissue is damaged or destroyed are discussed in greater detail later in the chapter.

## Disease Markers

At the present time, neuroimaging provides the best assessment of disease activity in MS (Box 2.1, Figure 2.3).

### Neuroimaging Abnormalities

A number of neuroimaging techniques can measure distinct pathologic changes and thereby provide markers for different aspects of the MS disease

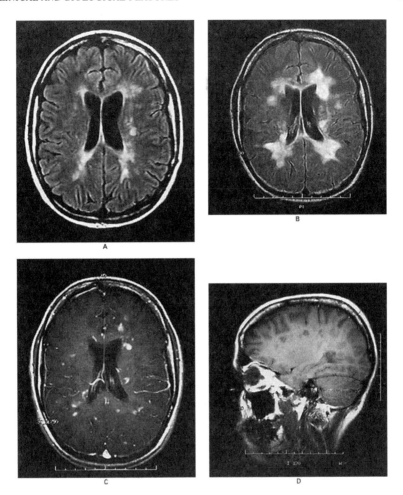

**FIGURE 2.3** MRI scans of the brain of a 25-year-old woman with relapsing-remitting multiple sclerosis.
(A) An MRI image shows multiple ovoid and confluent hyperintense lesions in the white matter surrounding the ventricles (the ventricles appear in the center of this image as a dark butterfly shape; they are the spaces through which cerebrospinal fluid [CSF] flows). (B) Nine months later, the number and size of the lesions have increased substantially. (C) After the administration of gadolinium, many of the lesions demonstrate ring or peripheral enhancement, indicating the breakdown of the blood-brain barrier. (D) A parasagittal T1-weighted MRI scan shows multiple regions in which the signal is diminished (referred to as "black holes") in the periventricular white matter and corpus callosum. These regions correspond to the chronic lesions of multiple sclerosis. SOURCE: Reprinted with permission from Noseworthy et al.[154] Copyright 2000 Massachusetts Medical Society. All rights reserved.

process (Table 2.4). Magnetic resonance imaging is a technique that creates cross-sectional images of the brain using a magnetic field and radio waves (Box 2.1). It is a versatile, powerful, and sensitive tool for measuring abnormalities in the brain. This is especially valuable with MS, because so much of the pathological activity of the disease is neurologically asymptomatic.

Indeed, until neuroimaging results proved otherwise, the disease appeared to be quiescent during remissions. Neuroimaging has revealed a previously unsuspected level of activity and pathology throughout the course of disease.

**Contrast-Enhanced Lesions.** Contrast agents are used in MRI in cases where contrast between two tissues is poor. The contrasting agent, gadolinium, is normally excluded from the brain by the blood-brain barrier. Its presence in the

**TABLE 2.4** Information Provided by Neuroimaging

| Observation or Method | What it Reveals |
| --- | --- |
| T1 gadolinium-enhancing lesions | Detects blood-brain barrier leakage, inflammatory disturbances, and recent ($\leq 6$ weeks) activity, with lesion formation. |
| T2 hyperintense lesions | Provides total burden of disease measure, including reversible and irreversible pathologies. Most predictive of disease course in early MS. |
| T1 hypointense lesions (black holes) | Reflects more severe tissue pathology, including axon loss, and correlates with disability. |
| Atrophy | Reflects axon loss, as well as other tissue component loss. Correlates with disability. Atrophy is detectable in both brain and spinal cord of MS patients. CNS atrophy is ongoing and accelerated compared to normal age-related changes. |
| MR spectroscopy measure of *N*-acetyl aspartate (NAA) levels | Decreased NAA levels reflect axon damage. Often shows abnormalities in normal brain tissue. Can be measured in whole brain or in region of interest. |
| Magnetization transfer imaging and magnetization transfer ratio | Indicates more severe lesions, with tissue destruction. Abnormalities noted within both lesions and normal-appearing CNS tissue. Marker for disability. Can be measured in whole brain or in region of interest. |
| Diffusion-weighted MRI | Detects abnormalities in both lesions and normal-appearing CNS tissue. Detects white matter changes. |
| High field MRI | Increased sensitivity for MS lesions. Can be used in conjunction with MS spectroscopy or magnetization transfer imaging. |
| Functional MRI | Measures critical circuitry involved in response to injury, activation, loss of function, and recovery of function. |

brain, therefore, indicates a breakdown of the blood-brain barrier. Gadolinium-enhancing activity on MRI correlates with clinical relapses and predicts increased risk or further disease activity. However, since most new brain MRI lesions are clinically silent, gadolinium-enhanced lesions are seen more often than clinical relapses.

**T2-Weighted Hyperintense Lesions.** In T2-weighted images, MS lesions appear as very bright white areas against a gray or more neutral background and are the most readily visualized MS lesions by MRI. They reflect lesions with different pathology and of various ages, and reversible as well as irreversible abnormalities. T2-weighted hyperintense lesions can be used to measure the total lesion volume (burden-of-disease). The variable pathology, which is not distinguished in T2 burden-of-disease measures, is probably a determinant of associated disability. Only a modest relationship has been observed between T2 burden of disease and clinical disability in relapsing and secondary progressive MS. However, in patients with clinically isolated syndromes who are in the early stages of MS, T2 burden-of-disease has been correlated with the development of MS, as well as the clinical subtype of MS and disability 10 years later. The magnitude of T2 burden-of-disease changes very early in the disease process and may be valuable for predicting subsequent course.

**Atrophy.** Atrophy of both brain and spinal cord can be detected in MS patients, including relapsing patients with minimal neurologic deficits.[200] Both axon and myelin loss contribute to tissue atrophy. Recent studies suggest that CNS atrophy may be the best neuroimaging correlate for clinical disability (reviewed in 1999 by Trapp et al.[213]). A number of different methodologies are used to measure atrophy. Current advances involve measurement of the whole brain and improved automation, but the optimal technique has not been decided.

**MR Spectroscopy.** Axonal injury can be measured on proton MR spectroscopy by estimating $N$-acetyl aspartate (NAA) levels in brain tissue. NAA is a molecule that is virtually confined to axons and neurons. Levels of NAA can fluctuate, suggesting that they can be used to measure reversible as well as irreversible damage. Persistent reduction of NAA on MR spectroscopy correlates with axon loss, damage, or dysfunction. Reduced NAA is found not only within MS lesions but also in the normal-appearing white matter of relapsing-remitting, secondary progressive, and primary progressive MS patients. The reduction in NAA is more severe in secondary progressive MS than in relapsing MS. In addition, NAA decrease in cerebellar white matter has been correlated with clinical ataxia.[51] NAA can be measured in a discrete region of interest within the brain. Recently, whole-brain NAA has been measured in MS. This appears to be a more meaningful neuroimaging marker to evaluate axon damage. MR spectroscopy can also be used to measure lipid changes within both lesions and normal-appearing brain tissue, but these studies are very preliminary and NAA measurements are the major focus of current MR spectroscopy studies in MS.

**T1-Weighted Hypointense Lesions.** Also referred to as black holes, T1-weighted hypointense lesions have lower signal intensity than the surrounding white matter. T1 hypointense lesions are most common in the supratentorial region (cerebral hemispheres). They are much less common in the infratentorial (brainstem and cerebellum) region and are not reported in the spinal cord. Compared to T2-weighted lesions, they represent more severe tissue pathology, with axon loss, demyelination, and extracellular edema.[24] In postmortem studies of progressive MS, T1-weighted hypointense lesions correlate strongly with axon density measurements. T1-weighted hypointense lesions show a stronger correlation with disability than T2-weighted hyperintense lesions.

**Magnetization Transfer Imaging.** Magnetization transfer imaging (MTI) can be used to study global brain function or to measure changes within a local region of interest.[71,198] Populations of bound and soluble protons produce different signals in response to the external magnetic field. The magnetization transfer ratio (MTR) is the ratio of the different signals produced by these two populations. It is reduced in MS and is believed to reflect both demyelination and axon loss, thereby producing an index of tissue destruction. MTR measurements are correlated with MS disability, as measured by the Expanded Disability Status Scale (EDSS; see Appendix D), as well as cognitive measures. MTI shows great promise as a disease marker. Lower MTR values occur with disease worsening in relapsing, secondary progressive, and primary progressive MS patients and even in patients with clinically isolated MS syndromes. In primary progressive patients who have a relatively small T2 burden of disease, MTR is significantly reduced, suggesting that axon damage is significantly greater in this clinical subtype.

Differences in MTRs are associated with different lesion pathology. Lesions that are more destructive (as indicated by T1 hypointensity) have reduced MTR values. Lesions that remain hypointense show a persistent reduction in MTR, whereas lesions that become isointense recover in MTR. New lesions in secondary progressive patients have a lower MTR than those in relapsing patients. The decline in MTR over three years is significantly greater in secondary progressive MS than in relapsing MS, supporting a relationship between MTR changes and disease progression. MTR measures allow more significant lesions to be detected and may provide a better potential correlate with clinical disability. Reduction in MTR can precede the development of new lesions on conventional MRI.

**Diffusion-Weighted MRI.** Diffusion-weighted MRI is sensitive to the diffusion, or random motion, of water molecules in tissue. It can detect subtle pathological changes that are not seen on conventional MRI. This technique might allow detection of pathological change in white matter tracts, including demyelination and loss of axons,[223] by quantifying anisotropy through a measure of diffusion tensor imaging (DTI). DTI can identify significantly altered diffusion properties in normal-appearing white matter. Lesions with the highest diffusion are the more destructive black holes, while the greatest change in anisotropy is seen in acute inflammatory lesions. Coincident with new lesion formation, diffusion-weighted imaging has shown changes in contralateral normal-appearing white matter.

**High-Field-Strength MRI.** High-field-strength magnets, which are 4 tesla (T) or higher, increase the signal-to-noise ratio (conventional imaging machines are 1.5 T). They allow enhanced detection of small (less than 5 mm) MS lesions, particularly those aligned along blood vessels. Both MR spectroscopy and MTI can be conducted on high-field machines with enhanced sensitivity.

**Functional MRI.** Functional magnetic resonance imaging, or fMRI, is a technique for determining which parts of the brain are activated by different types of sensation such as sight or sound, by different types of tasks such as moving one's fingers or legs, or by different mental tasks such as adding sums, reading, or memorizing. This "brain mapping" is achieved by using an MRI scanner to measure changes in blood flow to different areas of the brain. When a particular brain region is activated, blood flow into the region increases. The incoming arterial blood is rich in oxygenated hemoglobin, and there is a corresponding decrease in local deoxygenated hemoglobin. Changes in the MRI signal are derived from regional changes in the concentration of deoxygenated hemoglobin, which is a paramagnetic molecule (reviewed in Hirsch et al.[91]). The fMRI signal is, thus, determined by the balance between oxygenated and deoxygenated hemoglobin.

FMRI can provide second-by-second images of changes in response to different stimuli and during performance of mental tasks.[183] It provides a unique tool for assessment of neural circuits involved in loss and recovery of function, as well as for measuring the circuits underlying symptoms that are as difficult to study as cognitive changes, fatigue, pain, and sensory disturbances.

### Cerebrospinal Fluid

Cerebrospinal fluid (CSF) is the fluid that circulates around and within the brain and spinal cord. CSF provides a vehicle for removing waste products of cellular metabolism from the nervous system and is believed to be nutritive for both neurons and glial cells and to function as a transport system for biologically active substances such as releasing factors, hormones, neurotransmitters, and metabolites. Sampling this fluid thus provides an index to substances active in the CNS and possibly those involved in MS pathology.

A number of potential CSF disease markers have been reported in MS, including markers that are proposed as distinguishing between different types of MS (Table 2.5). For the most part, these are markers of tissue damage or immune disturbance. None are currently used in routine clinical practice, since they have not proved useful enough to justify serial lumbar punctures.

There has been particular interest in the specificity of oligoclonal bands in MS. Oligoclonal bands are produced by the overrepresentation of particular antibodies that can be visualized when CSF proteins are separated by gel electrophoresis where they appear as separate bands of protein on a gel matrix. Each of the bands contains a single type of antibody produced by a single clone of B cells. Oligoclonal bands are *typical* for the CSF of MS patients, but they are not *exclusive* to MS patients. For example, they are also found in the CSF of patients with other inflammatory status, such as viral brain infections. In MS, however, the particular antigens that elicit each antibody band are unknown.[210] Investigators have recently used molecular approaches such as phage display libraries to probe MS oligoclonal immunoglobulin G (IgG) bands for sequence information related to their antigenic target.[30,48] These are powerful methods that should allow for the identification of antigenic targets for the oligoclonal IgG. A main question, however, is whether the oligoclonal IgG bands represent an immune response directed against the etiologic agent of MS or merely constitute a by-product of immune system activity. In other words, upregulation of the antibody response and the heterogeneous distribution of antibodies into oligoclonal IgG bands could be a result of B-cell hyperactivity rather than an immune response to a specific etiologic pathogen.

## Other Studies

A variety of blood, urine, and mucosal fluid disease markers have been studied in MS, but none of them have provided a reliable disease marker. Again they are either markers of tissue damage (such as S-100) or immune activation (such as neopterin). Blood markers have included matrix metalloproteinases and their tissue inhibitors, circulating adhesion molecules, levels of various cytokines and their receptors, different subpopulations of cells, a variety of antibodies including antiviral and autoreactive antibodies, S-100 levels, and neopterin levels. Urine disease markers have included myelin basic protein-like material, free light chains, neopterin, gliotoxin, and neuron-specific enolase. Mucosal fluid cells and immunoglobulins have also been studied.

## Diagnosis

The diagnosis of MS is based on both clinical parameters, such as medical history and neurological examination, and paraclinical parameters such as MRI, CSF oligoclonal banding, and evoked potentials. There is no MS-specific diagnostic test, and the intermittent nature of the disease and high variability in presenting symptoms make diagnosis difficult (listed in Table 2.2).[163] The presentation of MS can be monosymptomatic or have multifocal signs and symptoms, and many neurodegenerative disorders are similar to MS in their presentation.[184]

The general diagnostic criteria, established in 1965 by a committee sponsored by the National MS Society (the MS Society), state that a diagnosis of "clinically definite" MS (CDMS) requires clinical evidence of two or more white matter lesions on at least two occasions.[195] In 1983, these criteria were expanded by Poser et al. to include the use of paraclinical parameters, and they have since become the standard MS diagnostic criteria (Table 2.6).[168] In July 2000, an international committee met to further revise these criteria, in particular to make MRI information a more integral component and to incorporate diagnostic criteria for primary progressive MS. The results of that meeting, however, were not available at the time of this writing.

The failure of the Poser criteria to incorporate primary progressive MS has recently been addressed by revised criteria that define definite, probable, and possible levels of diagnostic certainty.[209] These criteria are based on clinical findings, CSF abnormalities, brain and spinal cord MRI abnormalities, and evoked potentials. Using these criteria, at least one year of clinical progression must be documented before a diagnosis of primary progressive MS can be made.[209]

MRI reveals neuropathological damage in 70 to 95 percent of people with MS and, because of its sensitivity, is the most helpful paraclinical diagnostic test. However, the use of MRI in MS diagnosis has led to concern that its high sensitivity combined with limited MS specificity leads to misdiagnosis, since other conditions including myelopathy and disseminated encephalomyelitis can cause MRI lesions similar to MS lesions.[69,167] Thus, it is important that imaging be used in combination with clinical data for the diagnosis of MS. Recently, several sets of criteria for the definition of "MRI-definite" MS have been suggested (Table 2.7).[14,69,70,164] Patients with clinically isolated syndromes are particularly difficult to diagnose, and Barkhof et al.[14] and Fazekas[69] have identified criteria that are relevant to such cases.

Although assessment of spinal cord damage using MRI remains behind the development of brain methodology, it can be useful in diagnosing patients suspected of MS, particularly in cases with equivocal or negative brain MRI results.[34,85,128,186] Spinal cord imaging increases the diagnostic sensitivity of MRI and might also enable earlier diagnosis.[128,199]

## Evoked Potentials

When demyelination or sclerosis (scarring) occurs, the conduction of nerve impulses along axons is slowed or interrupted. Impaired conductance is reflected in an increased latency of evoked potentials or an increase in the amount of time that elapses between the presentation of a sensory stimulus and the resulting change in the brain's electrical field. Evoked potentials are measured by placing small electrodes on the head in the region corresponding to the stimuli presented (Table 2.8).

Abnormal evoked responses to different types of stimuli provide clues to the location of plaques or lesions and are useful in detecting "clinically silent" lesions that do not produce easily observable symptoms. However, abnormal evoked responses are not unique to MS. For example, although abnormal visual

**TABLE 2.5** Proposed CSF Disease Markers in MS

| Marker | Description |
| --- | --- |
| **IMMUNE MARKERS** | |
| **Free light chains** | IgG antibodies are composed of light and heavy polypeptide chains. Free light chains are found in patients with chronic infections or inflammatory diseases such as rheumatoid arthritis, but also in healthy individuals particularly following strenuous exercise. |
| **Cytokines and cytokine receptors** | Cytokines are intercellular signaling proteins produced by cells of the immune system and CNS. They are involved in various aspects of disease processes, particularly inflammatory responses. |
| **Oligoclonal bands** | Oligoclonal bands are produced by the overrepresentation of particular antibodies. They are *typical* of the CSF of MS patients, but not *exclusive* to it. |
| **Antiviral antibodies** | Antiviral antibodies are produced by B cells in direct response to an antigen's presence, and certain antiviral antibodies are increased in the CSF of some patients with MS.[194] |
| **Intrathecal immunoglobulin production (IgG, IgM)** | Immunoglobulins are produced by plasma cells and are integral in adaptive immune responses. Polyclonal increases of IgG occur in chronic infection and inflammation. |
| **T cells** | White blood cells responsible for cell-mediated immune responses to antigens, including viral infections. |
| **Adhesion, costimulatory, and other surface molecules** | Upregulated adhesion molecules in blood and CSF indicate sustained potential for inflammation in the CNS throughout the clinical spectrum of MS. |
| **CNS TISSUE MARKERS** | |
| **Myelin basic protein (MBP)** | A major component of myelin, MBP is increased in the CSF of some, but not all, MS patients following a demyelinating episode. |

*continued*

evoked potentials are common in MS, they also occur in compressive lesions of the visual pathway and spinocerebellar degeneration.[184]

Evoked potentials can aid in the localization of lesions, confirm clinically ambiguous lesions, and confirm the organic basis of symptoms.[84] In addition, changes in evoked potentials can be used to measure disease progression and the effectiveness of therapeutic treatment, including treatments designed to improve conduction.[61,155]

**TABLE 2.5** Continued

| Marker | Description |
|---|---|
| **S-100** | S-100 protein is an astroglial-specific protein that binds calcium. When a brain lesion occurs, S-100 is released into both the CSF and the blood.[142] |
| **Neuron specific enolase (NSE)** | As a marker of brain damage, NSE reflects the severity of disease in patients with intracerebral hematoma, subarachnoid hemorrhage, head injury, and certain tumors.[165] |
| **Glial fibrillary acidic protein (GFAP)** | A major constituent of glial filaments in differentiated CNS astrocytes, GFAP has been used for the diagnosis of astrocytic tumors, the study of astrocytic gliosis, and CNS regeneration and transplantation.[62] |
| **Neurofilaments** | Neurofilaments are important for axonal structure, transport, and regeneration. Accumulation of neurofilaments in motor neurons can trigger a neurodegenerative process and may be a key intermediate in the pathway of pathogenesis leading to neuronal loss.[185,230] |
| **Neural cell adhesion molecules** | A modulator of axon outgrowth and cell adhesion that adapts its structure to requirements during development by alternative splicing and posttranslational modification.[60] |
| **Ciliary neurotrophic factor (CNTF)** | CNTF appears to promote remyelination, as well as formation of oligodendroctyes.[132] |

**INFLAMMATORY AND OTHER MARKERS**

| | |
|---|---|
| **Gliotoxin** | Highly cytotoxic for astrocytes and oligodendrocytes, gliotoxin may represent an initial pathogenic factor leading to the neuropathological features of MS, such as blood-brain barrier involvement and demyelination.[139] |
| **Neopterin** | A marker of immune activation, neopterin is increased in CSF of relapsing-remitting patients and correlates with a decrease of *L*-tryptophan, reflecting interferon-gamma-mediated activation of macrophages.[201] |
| **Matrix metalloproteinases** | Matrix metalloproteinases are enzymes that can dissolve the extracellular matrix of the blood-brain barrier.[196] |

**TABLE 2.6** Poser Diagnostic Criteria for MS[a]

| Category | Attacks | Clinical Evidence | Paraclinical Evidence | CSF OB/ IgG | |
|---|---|---|---|---|---|
| **Clinical Diagnosis** | | | | | |
| Definite | 2 | 2 | | | |
| | 2 | 1 | and | 1 | |
| Probable | 2 | 1 | | | |
| | 1 | 2 | | | |
| | 1 | 1 | and | 1 | |
| **Laboratory-Supported Diagnosis** | | | | | |
| Definite | 2 | 1 | or | 1 | + |
| | 1 | 2 | | | + |
| | 1 | 1 | and | 1 | + |
| Probable | 2 | | | | + |

[a]Combinations of various types of evidence are used to diagnose MS under the Poser criteria. More than one combination of clinical and paraclinical evidence can support a diagnosis within a single category. Laboratory-supported diagnosis requires one of two possible immune disturbances in CSF: IgG oligoclonal bands or intrathecal IgG production.

NOTES: *CSF*, Cerebrospinal fluid. *OB*, Oligoclonal bands. *IgG*, Immunoglobulin G. *Clinical evidence* refers to symptoms recorded in medical history or signs observed in neurological examination. *Paraclinical evidence* might include neuroimaging, evoked potentials, CSF oligoclonal banding, or IgG levels.

**TABLE 2.7** MRI Criteria for Definite MS

**Paty et al.[163]**
  • Four or more white matter lesions
  • Lesions >6 mm in diameter
  • Presence of at least one lesion in the periventricular region adjacent to the body of the lateral ventrical, corpus callosum, or infratentorial
  • Ovoid lesions or oval-shaped lesions near the lateral ventricles with the long axis of the lesion 90 degrees to the plane of the lateral ventricle

**Barkhof et al.[14]**
  • At least one gadolinium-enhancing lesion
  • Juxtacortical location (at least one lesion)
  • Periventricular location (at least three lesions)
  • Infratentorial location (at least one lesion)

**Fazekas et al.[69,70]**
  • Three or more T2 hyperintensities
  • At least two of the following lesion characteristics:
        Size >5 mm
        Abutting the ventricular body, infratentorial location

**TABLE 2.8** Evoked Potentials as a Diagnostic Tool in MS

| Evoked Response | Primary Purpose of Test | Stimulus Presented | Location of Recording Electrodes | Frequency of Abnormal Responses (%) | |
|---|---|---|---|---|---|
| | | | | People with Definite MS | People with Probable MS |
| **Visual evoked responses** | Evaluation of optic nerve function | Strobe light flash or reversible checkerboard pattern flash on a computer screen | On the scalp along the vertex and cortex lobes | 85-90 | 58 |
| **Brainstem auditory evoked potentials** | Evaluation of hearing pathways in the brainstem | Series of clicking noises or tone bursts played into earphone | On the scalp along the vertex and on each earlobe | 67 | 41 |
| **Somatosensory evoked responses** | Evaluation of sensory nerve tracts in spinal cord, thalamus, and sensory cortex | Mild electrical stimulus via electrodes on wrists or knees | On the scalp, each wrist (medial nerve), and the knees (peroneal nerve) | 77 | 67 |

The use of evoked potentials as a diagnostic tool has greatly declined since the advent of the MRI, which provides a more comprehensive picture of disease activity. In at least some cases of progressive MS, visual evoked potentials show changes over time where none are detected in MRI scans.[192] In May 2000, the Quality Standards Subcommittee of the American Academy of Neurology concluded that although visual evoked potentials are *probably* useful to identify patients at increased risk of developing clinically definite MS, somatosensory evoked responses are only *possibly* useful for that purpose, and there is insufficient evidence to recommend brainstem auditory evoked potentials as a diagnostic tool.[84]

## Disease Variants: Is MS One Disease or Many?

Although MS is postulated to have an underlying immune-mediated pathogenesis, there is as yet no biologic marker that is disease specific and can be used for diagnostic purposes. Similarly, there is insufficient evidence to allow detection of any putative disease-related infectious agent as a basis for defining the disease. Thus, MS continues to be defined by sets of criteria that have been developed based on clinical and pathologic observations. MS may well be hetero-geneous when viewed from the perspective of genetics, pathogenic mechanisms, clinical phenotypes, and immunopathology. To be considered a truly distinctive variant of MS, any putative distinct disease subtypes defined in one of these categories would have to be correlated with the distinctive features identified in each of the other categories.

Cases classified as MS are recognized where disease distribution is mainly in the spinal cord, hind brain (cerebellum or brainstem), or cerebrum. Different animal models have distinct topographic distributions, some of which seem to have distinct immunopathologies. For example, Theiler's murine encephalomy-elitis virus, the demyelinating disease that afflicts mice, is mainly a spinal cord disease. There is an apparent overrepresentation of specific phenotypes in certain geographic regions. For example, MS that is relatively restricted to the optic nerve and spinal cord is more common in Japan than in other countries.

The Devic's pattern of MS features a predominance of spinal cord and optic nerve involvement. The pathology is considered more destructive than classical MS, and the prognosis is worse. At issue is whether these differences reflect different immunopathogenic mechanisms in a given individual, even when the disease trigger, or initiating event, is not distinct among such individuals. Even in identical twins with MS, the disease course can be markedly different.

## Disease-Modifying Therapies

A number of immunomodulatory agents have been shown in double-blind, placebo-controlled, multicenter Phase III trials to benefit patients with relapsing MS (Table 2.9; see also 1999 review by Rudick[187]).These agents help clinical disease features (they decrease the number of attacks, the severity of attacks, and sustained worsening on neurologic examination) as well as MRI disease features (they decrease the formation of new lesions, the number of contrast-enhancing lesions, the total burden of disease, and brain atrophy). Although all of these drugs have side effects, they are manageable in most patients. The benefit of treatment is sustained for at least several years. It is not yet known whether these agents prevent, reduce, or delay transition from relapsing to progressive MS, but preliminary data suggest that this may be the case. Throughout this report, the term "disease-modifying therapy" is used to distinguish these agents from other medications used to relieve the symptoms of MS that do not alter either the frequency of relapses or the rate of progression.

Beta-interferon (IFN-β) is an anti-inflammatory regulatory cytokine with antiviral, antineoplastic, and immunomodulatory activity. It has a number of effects on the immune system that would be beneficial in MS. For example, it decreases cell migration into the CNS, inhibits T-cell proliferation and expres-sion of cell activation markers, inhibits inducible nitric oxide synthase (the en-zyme that produces nitric oxide, a potentially damaging substance), and enhances

**TABLE 2.9**  Disease-Modifying Therapies for Relapsing MS

| Therapy | Dosing | Major Side Effects |
|---|---|---|
| **CYTOKINE THERAPIES** | | |
| Interferon-β1b (Betaseron) | 250 μg s.c. alternate days | Flu-like symptoms, injection site reactions, menstrual irregularities, decreased white blood cells, elevated liver enzymes |
| Interferon-β1a (Avonex) | 30 μg i.m. once a week | Flu-like symptoms, pain from intramuscular injection |
| Interferon-β1a (Rebif) | 22 μg and 44 μg s.c. three times a week | Flu-like symptoms, injection site reactions, decreased white blood cells, elevated liver enzymes |
| **T-CELL THERAPIES** | | |
| Glatiramer acetate (Copaxone) | 20 mg s.c. daily | Injection site reactions (mild), Immediate postinjection reaction |
| **IMMUNOSUPPRESSIVE THERAPIES** | | |
| Mitoxantrone (Novantrone) | $12 \text{ mg/m}^2$ i.v. once every 3 months | Nausea, hair thinning, menstrual irregularities, infertility, decreased white blood cells, transient discoloration of urine and sclera |

NOTE: i.m. = intramuscular; i.v. = intravenous; s.c. = subcutaneous.

production of the anti-inflammatory cytokine interleukin-10 and of nerve growth factor (which might enhance remyelination and axon repair) (reviewed in 1999 by Rudick[187]). There are two types of recombinant (artificially made) beta-interferon. Beta-interferon-1a (Avonex, Rebif) is a duplicate of human beta-interferon.* Beta-interferon-1b (Betaseron) has three molecular differences from human beta-interferon: it is not glycosylated, there is an amino acid substitution at position 17, and there is no "N-terminal" methionine.[6] The three available beta-interferon therapies are given in different amounts and dosing schedules (Table 2.9). There are well-recognized side effects (most commonly flu-like reactions), which occur maximally during the first weeks or months of therapy. Flu-like reactions can be minimized by initiating therapy with a dose escalation schedule and consistent use of anti-inflammatory premedication during the first few weeks of therapy.

---

*Rebif has been approved for the treatment of relapsing-remitting MS by the European Commission but has not been approved by the Food and Drug Administration in the United States because of the Orphan Drug Act. If tentative approval is received, Rebif could enter the U.S. market in 2003, when the exclusivity periods for Avonex and Betaseron end.

Glatiramer acetate (Copaxone) consists of random polymers of four amino acids, designed to mimic myelin basic protein, an important component of CNS myelin. Glatiramer acetate is believed to work by activating antiinflammatory regulatory T cells, which then migrate into the CNS to inhibit local immune reactions. Glatiramer acetate has an excellent side effect profile. Patients may experience injection site reactions, but they tend to be quite minor. Some 10 to 15 percent of patients experience at least one immediate postinjection reaction characterized by chest tightness, palpitations, flushing, and anxiety within a few minutes of injection. The reaction lasts only minutes and is not dangerous.

Mitoxantrone (Novantrone) is a cytotoxic agent that interferes with DNA synthesis and repair, and suppresses a variety of immune system cells. It also enhances suppressor cell activity. It is given as an intravenous infusion over 5 to 15 minutes, every three months. Mitoxantrone is fairly well tolerated at low doses. In the recent Phase III trial, both the low (5 mg/m$^2$) and high (12 mg/m$^2$) doses showed efficacy, but the high dose gave the best overall results.[111] Mitoxantrone should not be given at a cumulative dose of 140 mg/m$^2$ or higher because of concerns about cardiotoxicity, which also means that this drug can be used for only a few years.

Currently available treatments are highly effective in preventing the type of MS damage that can be visualized using MRI. They are moderately effective in preventing and reducing the severity of relapses, but they are generally disappointing in preventing long-term disability—the most important goal of treatment. This might reflect the timing of treatment, and there has been a recent emphasis on starting therapy at the time MS is first diagnosed. This type of early therapy is likely most effective in delaying or preventing long-term disability, although this effect has not yet been clearly demonstrated through empirical research studies (Richard Rudick, personal communication). Clearly, much remains to be done in the development of therapies for people who suffer from MS.

Two recent studies, the interferon beta-1a (Avonex) prevention study (CHAMPS, Controlled High Risk Subjects Avonex Multiple Sclerosis Prevention) and the interferon beta-1a (Rebif) early treatment (ETOMS, Early Treatment of Multiple Sclerosis) trial, have compared the use of disease-modifying therapy with placebo in patients after their first attack who also have an abnormal brain MRI. These are patients at high risk for MS, but who do not meet current criteria for a definite diagnosis. In both studies, early treatment with a disease-modifying agent significantly delayed onset of a second clinical attack over the two-year study period. Patients who received treatment also showed significantly less MRI disease activity over the next two years. These two trials have led to a reassessment of when disease-modifying therapy should be started. The National MS Society consensus statement endorsed treatment of patients as soon as a definite diagnosis of relapsing MS is made. If new diagnostic criteria are formulated for an MRI-based diagnosis at the time of a first attack, it is likely that the use of disease-modifying therapy will expand to include these early patients.

Beta-interferon and glatiramer acetate have been tested mainly in relapsing MS. It is more controversial whether they benefit progressive MS. Several Phase III trials have examined beta-interferon therapy in patients with secondary progressive MS, with conflicting results. The European Secondary Progressive Study on beta-interferon-1b (Betaseron) showed a significant effect on slowing progression. In contrast, the North American Secondary Progressive beta-interferon-1b study and the European SPECTRIMS beta-interferon-1a (Rebif) study showed no significant effect on progression. These trials did, however, show positive results on secondary outcomes such as relapse rate and MRI disease parameters. The European study, which showed a treatment effect on progression in contrast to the two negative studies, included secondary progressive patients who had a shorter disease duration, were still experiencing relapses, and had contrast-enhancing brain MRI lesions. Considered as a whole, these studies suggest that in the earlier stages of MS, when there is still a significant inflammatory component (reflected in clinical relapses and gadolinium-enhancing lesion activity), beta-interferon may have a positive effect on clinical progression. In the later, non-relapsing, progressive stages of MS, where there appears to be ongoing atrophy relatively independent of contrast-enhancing lesion activity, beta-interferon does not seem to slow progression. The European Phase III trial of Mitoxantrone enrolled both relapsing and secondary progressive MS patients.[111] The drug had a positive effect on progression as indicated by a decrease in the EDSS impairment scale at the end of the study (change of -0.13 compared to +0.23 in the placebo group, p = .038) (for EDSS scale, see Appendix D). An ongoing trial (IMPACT Study) in secondary progressive MS is testing double-dose interferon beta-1a (Avonex) once a week. There have been no major treatment trials in primary progressive and progressive relapsing MS. There currently is an ongoing three-year Phase III trial of glatiramer acetate in primary progressive MS (the Promise trial).

## Treatment Failures

Each of the currently available disease-modifying treatments has shortcomings, including partial efficacy for patients as a group and potential adverse effects. There are four reasons why treatments fail—nonadherence on the patient's part, adverse side effects, production of neutralizing antibodies, and nonresponsive disease (reviewed by Cohen at al., 1999[43]).

Patient adherence is a factor in the efficacy of any medication, but particularly so when a patient's hopes exceed the outcome—which is particularly salient for therapies that are preventive, but not restorative. The primary principles to increase adherence are appropriate selection of patients for treatment, availability of adequate medical support throughout treatment, and perhaps most importantly, patient education before and during treatment. MS patients need to be fully informed that the therapy can prevent relapses and the accumulation of disability, but that it will not improve preexisting manifestations. In addition, some patients are averse to self-injection and will not be persuaded to inject themselves with any medication (unless, perhaps, they are convinced of a substantial and certain benefit, which many MS patients are not).

Health care financing policies vary widely among different countries and even within countries such as the United States and Canada. This will also influence patient adherence. In countries such as France where the costs of MS therapies are fully covered by the state, cost is unlikely to influence adherence, but in countries where patients must assume the full costs of MS disease-modifying therapies themselves, many of them will decide that they cannot afford to pay more than $10,000 (U.S.) annual expense for the modest health benefit they might gain.

Adverse effects are a common reason for discontinuing treatment, but they are generally not serious health threats. The most common side effect of glatiramer acetate is irritation at the injection site, although it is typically mild. The most common side effects of beta-interferon are flu-like symptoms, and these usually resolve after three to six months. (Depression is also a possible side effect and is discussed in greater detail in Chapter 3.) Although only 4 percent of actively treated patients withdrew from beta-interferon clinical trials because of side effects, in clinical practice, 11 percent discontinue within four months of initiating treatment (reviewed in 1999 by Mohr et al.[144]). (The percentage of patients who discontinue treatment because of side effects might, however, decline as physicians become more experienced in managing these side effects.)

Defining nonresponsive disease in individual patients is difficult, because unfortunately patients can continue to experience relapses after initiation of disease-modifying therapy with beta-interferon or glatiramer acetate. Comparison of pre- and post-treatment relapse rates is fraught with problems, and it is often difficult to identify whether an individual patient is responsive to therapy. At a minimum, a patient's level of neurological impairment and disability should remain stable on therapy. Persistent gadolinium-enhancing or T2 lesion accrual should be considered a worrisome feature, even in the absence of clinical evidence of activity or worsening.

Finally, neutralizing antibodies, which can interfere with the effects of interferons, appear in up to 20 percent of patients after two years of beta-interferon treatment. They do not appear to be an issue with glatiramer acetate. Increased neutralizing antibodies appear to be associated with reduced clinical benefit, although there is still some controversy about this point. For example, it is still not known what levels of neutralizing antibodies are clinically significant, how often they persist, and what is the most reliable method of measuring them. More research is needed on testing for neutralizing antibodies in MS patients treated with beta-interferons and how to best use the results to properly manage patient treatment.

## Cost-Effectiveness

Disease-modifying therapies are expensive, costing roughly $8,000 to $10,000 (U.S.) per year.[187] Several studies have indicated that their costs outweigh their benefits, but these analyses have been heavily criticized.[29,177] Forbes and colleagues[73] argued that it is not cost-effective to treat progressive MS patients with interferon beta-1b in Britain and that the money spent on interferon beta-1b would be better spent on other services, such as supportive care and simple interventions to reduce the burden of patients' symptoms. Analyses of cost-effectiveness of medical treatment often use quality-adjusted life-years (QALYs) to measure health benefits (see Box 2.2). The estimated costs of beta-interferon treatment per gain in QALY for relapsing-remitting MS range from 809,000 British pounds ($1,140,000 U.S.)[162] to 2,038,400 British pounds ($2,870,000 U.S.).[152] The estimates are considerably lower in Canada (406,000 to 490,000 Canadian dollars, or $270,000-$330,000 U.S.).[159] For secondary progressive MS, the estimated costs of beta-interferon treatment per gain in QALY range from 874,600 British pounds ($1,230,000 U.S.)[152] to 1,024,000 British pounds ($1,440,000 U.S.).[73] While disease-related expenditures are relatively easy to calculate, the benefits of these expenditures are not so easy to calculate, particu-

---

**BOX 2.2**
**What Are Quality-Adjusted Life-Years?**

Quality-adjusted life-years are a health status measure that includes both quantity and quality of life in a single outcome measure.[21,98] Multiplying life expectancy by a quality-of-life adjustment fraction, or utility, results in a QALY value. Utilities represent the level of quality or value associated with a particular health state, and range in value from 0, representing death, to 1, representing optimal health. Utilities are determined in two ways: by researchers through literature searches for previously conducted utility studies or by direct measurement of utility values based on the assessment of people's values for different levels of health.

The use of QALYs for resource allocation has been widely criticized as discriminatory against the elderly[21] and the disabled[98] by placing less value on extending their lives due to the lower potential for health status improvement. The determination of utility values that accurately reflect the many ways quality of life can be affected is difficult in part because one of the underlying assumptions of QALYs—that the severity of a disease state or disability and the corresponding value represent a fixed quantity—is unlikely to be true. The effect of health status on quality of life depends in large part on an individual's unique perspective.[59] Although the use of QALYs is one of the current standards for such evaluations, it is a crude attempt to express a qualitative, subjective reality in quantitative terms and has been criticized as being of limited value in this respect.[64]

larly in long-term diseases where treatments might slow the progress of disease, but neither cure it nor restore impaired functions.

In addition to the limitations inherent in the use of QALYs, there are other problems with the conclusion that disease-modifying therapies are not cost-effective. The studies done to date have been criticized for using poor economic methodology in interpreting the data.[64,177] In a year 2000 review of immuno-modulatory drugs used to treat MS, the British National Health Service committee on health technology assessment concluded that the cost-effectiveness of these drugs is simply not known.[29] The committee cited a lack of quality clinical trials for each drug, including methodological limitations, poor reporting of data, small sample sizes, short duration, inconsistent treatment regimes and outcome measures, and uncertainty about the clinical significance of reported benefits.[29] The latter criticism might, however, change. New data about these drugs are emerging at such a rapid pace that conclusions about their benefits should be reconsidered as new data from clinical trials become available.

In general, cost-effectiveness analysis should be considered skeptically. Cost-effectiveness is a highly politicized issue in which economic principles are often misapplied.[64] Indeed, the United States health care system often favors economically inefficient delivery of some products—for example, liver transplants—in that health care providers are willing to underwrite additional costs to gain market share. Further, cross-national comparisons have little merit because of differences in national health care systems, as well as other economic and social factors. Finally, although economic analysis reveals important financial trade-offs, all societies hold certain social values that outweigh economic considerations. For many people, the health and well-being of their loved ones and themselves is among the deepest of these values.

## UNDERLYING DISEASE MECHANISMS

Ultimately, the pathogenic mechanisms underlying MS will have to be better understood to design rational therapies.

### Physiology of Myelin and Axons: Normal Function, Demyelination, and Repair

The integrative activity of the nervous system, which underlies motor, sensory, cognitive, and psychological behavior, depends on electrical signaling between neurons. Each neuron encodes its message in the form of action potentials (small all-or-none electrical impulses) that are carried to other neurons via axons, the cable-like fibers that extend from neuron cell bodies. Many axons within the brain and spinal cord are myelinated.

## Myelin Acts as an Insulator

The myelin sheath provides a high-resistance, low-capacitance insulator that increases the reliability and speed of action potentials conducted along axon fibers. Myelin is what makes the white matter of brain white. It is a multilayered sheath formed by the oligodendroglial cells, or oligodendrocytes, that insulate axons (Figure 2.4).[169,173] Each segment of the myelin sheath surrounds the axon in a segmented fashion, with segments (called internodes) periodically interrupted at nodes of Ranvier. The internodal axon is normally surrounded by myelin sheaths whose thicknesses are related to the caliber of the ensheathed axon.[219] In

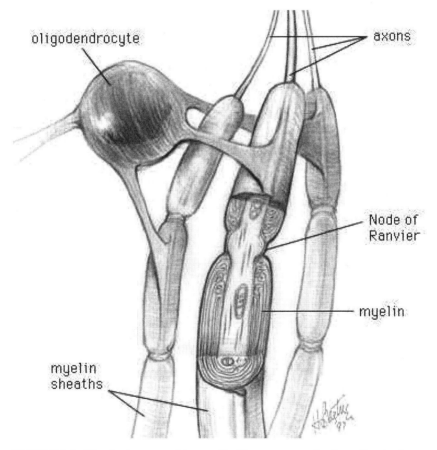

**FIGURE 2.4** Oligodendrocyte making myelin. The processes of a given oligodendrocyte wrap themselves around portions of the surrounding axons. As each process wraps itself around, it forms layers of myelin. Each process thus becomes a segment of the axon's myelin sheath. SOURCE: National Institutes of Health Office of Science Education.

normal myelinated fibers, the action potential does not travel in a continuous manner. On the contrary, it jumps from one node of Ranvier to the next, in a manner known as "saltatory" (derived from the Latin word for "jumping"). Saltatory conduction is a rapid process, with the impulse taking only 20 one-thousandths of a second to jump from one node of Ranvier to the next; as a result, myelinated fibers conduct impulses with a high velocity. Significantly, voltage-dependent sodium channels are clustered at the nodes of Ranvier but are relatively more scarce in the internodal axonal membrane. In contrast, potassium channels, which exist in low density at nodes, are more abundant in the internodal and paranodal axonal membrane, under the myelin sheath.[219] Therefore, loss of the myelin sheath exposes relatively inexcitable axonal membranes; the consequence is that nerve impulses are conducted more slowly or not at all.

### Axonal Conduction Is Impaired in Demyelinated Axons

Following damage to the myelin, conduction velocity is reduced, and conduction slows along the demyelinated axon (Figure 2.5). Studies using evoked potentials to examine human subjects with MS have demonstrated that this slowing of conduction does not, in itself, necessarily produce clinical deficits.[88,96,134] In addition, however, conduction failure can occur in demyelinated axons. When conduction failure occurs, the axon potential is not propagated from one end of the fiber to the other, and information is lost. This produces a clinical deficit. Conduction failure in demyelinated axons is now known to result not only from loss of the insulating myelin, but also from the molecular organization of the axon membrane. Following damage to the myelin, internodal parts of the axon membrane (which had previously been covered by myelin) are uncovered.

### Myelinated Axons Exhibit Complex Molecular Architecture

Prior to the last decade, axonal dysfunction in demyelinating diseases was considered to be due entirely to the loss of the myelin insulation. According to this schema, after the myelin is damaged, there is a "short circuit," and impulse conduction is slowed or fails. It is now known that although the schema described above is partially correct, it is not the whole story. The axon itself exhibits an elegant molecular architecture, and following damage to the myelin, this architecture is disrupted. The molecular architecture of the axon is manifest by the placement of specialized protein molecules, called ion channels, within the membrane of the axon. Sodium channels act as tiny molecular batteries, which produce the depolarization that is necessary for the generation of action potentials. In contrast, potassium channels act as molecular brakes, damping electrical activity. Within myelinated axons, these two types of ion channels have a complementary structure. Sodium channels are clustered in high density in the axon membrane at small gaps in the myelin called nodes of Ranvier, where they support the production of action potentials; they are sparse, however, in the "internodal" parts of the axon membrane beneath the myelin. Their numbers there are too low to support secure conduction, which contributes to conduction failure. Potassium channels, on the other hand, tend to be located in the internodal parts of the axon membrane, beneath the myelin sheath; as a result of this, they are masked by the

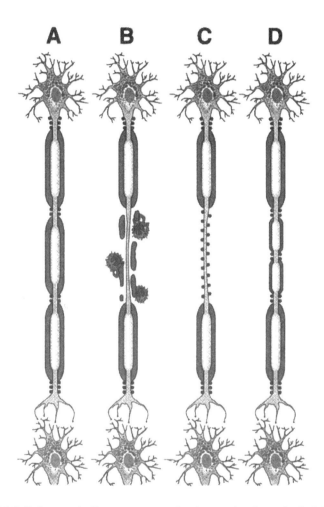

**FIGURE 2.5** Pathogenesis. Current concept of pathogenesis of neurological dysfunction associated with acute multiple sclerosis lesion in relapsing-remitting MS patient. Normal myelinated fibers (A) are demyelinated by inflammatory process (B), which causes conduction block. Na+ channel redistribution (C) and remyelination (D) restore conduction and contribute to clinical remission. SOURCE: Trapp et al.[213] Reprinted with permission of Sage Publications, Inc.

overlying myelin in normal myelinated fibers.[177,181,218] The unmasking of potassium channels by demyelination thus introduces another factor that tends to interfere with the conduction of action potentials.

## Molecular Plasticity in Demyelinated Axons Underlies Restoration of Impulse Conduction

Given that impulse conduction fails in demyelinated axons and that this contributes to clinical deficits, how do remissions occur? It is now clear that demyelinated axons possess a remarkable capability to rebuild themselves at the molecular level. In the weeks following demyelination, demyelinated axons acquire, within regions where myelin has been lost, a density of sodium channels that is high enough to support action potential conduction even in the absence of insulating myelin. The demyelinated nerve fibers insert additional amplifiers (sodium channels) in their membranes so that they are able to conduct action potentials reliably even though there is a short circuit.[23,55,63,74,145]

This is a striking example of neuronal plasticity, in this case at the molecular level. Although this molecular plasticity has been clearly demonstrated in laboratory experiments, a number of important questions remain: How do neurons "know" that their axons have been demyelinated and that there is a need to activate the machinery for synthesis of sodium channels? How do neurons control the synthesis and deployment of sodium channels? What turns on the genes for sodium channels and ensures that the correct types of sodium channels (there are nearly a dozen different types, which are like different types of batteries) are produced following demyelination? Also, how are sodium channels transported and inserted into the correct parts of the axon membrane so that they can function normally? These questions have important therapeutic implications and are currently under study.

## Axonal Degeneration Also Occurs in MS

The presence of axonal degeneration in MS was recognized even in the early descriptions of this disease,[36] but its presence has recently been reemphasized (Figure 2.6).[135,212,219] Axonal transection might be the structural basis for acquisition of permanent (nonremitting) neurological deficits, making it an especially important part of the pathology of MS.[51,119,120] A corollary of this proposition would be that neuroprotective interventions that limit axonal injury should prevent, or at least lessen, the acquisition of new, permanent signs and symptoms in MS. As a step toward the development of neuroprotective strategies in MS, it will be important to delineate the mechanisms that underlie axonal injury in this disorder. Is it a consequence of demyelination? Alternatively, is the axonal damage a by-product of the inflammatory or immune processes involved in triggering demyelination? What is the nature of the "injury cascade" that leads from the initial insult to ultimate degeneration of axons in MS? Understanding the pathogenesis of the process might lead to the development of new therapeutic targets for MS. These questions are being approached in models of other neurological diseases such as trauma and cerebrovascular disease, including stroke, and should be actively pursued in MS research as well.

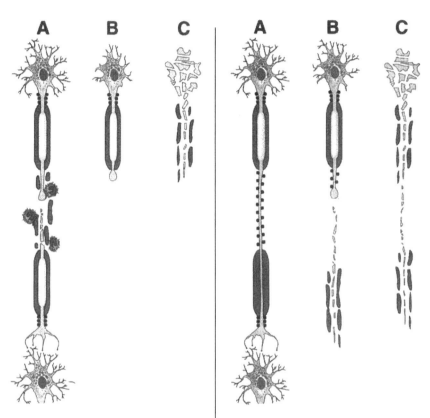

Axonal transection during inflammatory demyelination. According to this schema, axonal transection during (A) is a consistent feature of inflammatory demyelinating lesions. This results in degeneration of the distal axonal segment (B) and irreversible loss of neuronal function. During the relapsing-remitting course of multiple sclerosis (RR-MS), the CNS compensates for axonal destruction.

Axonal degeneration as a result of chronic demyelination. This model posits that axonal viability depends upon oligodendrocyte-derived trophic effect. Chronically demyelinated axons (A) may undergo nerve transection (B) or wallerian degeneration (C), which are caused by lack of myelin trophic support.

**FIGURE 2.6** Axonal transection and degeneration. SOURCE: Trapp et al.[213] Reprinted with permission of Sage Publications, Inc.

## Demyelination and Clinical Signs

MS is defined as a demyelinating disease because the myelin sheaths and their parent cells, the oligodendroglia, are major targets of immune-mediated damage (Figure 2.7).[46,153] The classical lesions are discrete plaques of demyelination, which, depending on disease stage, are associated with varying evidence of inflammation. The clinical signs, which are episodic and are not clinically predictable, are presumably related to the location of the lesions, although clinically "silent" demyelinating lesions also occur. These predominantly white matter lesions occur in multiple brain regions and appear at different times throughout the disease. Common syndromes correlated with lesions in specific areas include visual deficits, weakness and spasticity, eye movement abnormalities, and ataxia (Table 2.10). Lesions are often described as active or chronic, depending on whether there are signs of active inflammation, usually associated with ongoing demyelination, or whether the lesion is stable and does not show signs of inflammatory activity.

### Lesions

**Active Lesions.** Disruption of the blood-brain barrier that normally insulates the brain from pathogenic blood-borne substances is an early event in the development of MS lesions (Figure 2.8).[136] Antigen-specific T cells enter the nervous system, and when they encounter and recognize their specific antigen, a cascade of cytokine expression begins that contributes to the damage of the blood-brain barrier. This can be detected on contrast-enhanced MRI.[136] Examination of active demyelinating lesions in autopsy cases of MS reveals structural and immunopathological abnormalities related to demyelination and abnormalities of oligodendrocytes.[126] The inflammatory response is dominated by lymphocytes and macrophages, but the data on the relative numbers of CD4+ and CD8+ cells are still not settled. A plaque is characterized by loss of myelin sheath and infiltration by macrophages (which show myelin basic protein and myelin-associated glycoprotein immunoreactivities). As the inflammatory responses amplify, macrophages are filled with lipids, myelin damage occurs, and there is apparently some collateral damage to axons. Scattered B cells and plasma cells are also sometimes associated with these lesions.

Immunocytochemical analysis has suggested that there may be leakage of immunoglobulins and complement from vessels at the margins of active plaques. There is evidence for upregulation of a variety of cytokines within MS plaques including various interleukins (IL-1, 2, 4, 6, 10, and 12); beta-interferon; tumor necrosis factor (TNF); and transforming growth factor (TGF). Cytokines are intercellular signaling proteins produced by cells of the immune system and CNS. Their involvement in any disease is complex. They can initiate, sustain, or terminate various aspects of disease processes and are particularly involved in

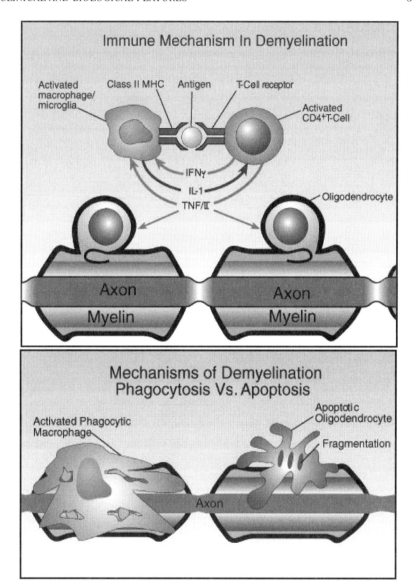

**FIGURE 2.7** Possible mechanisms of demyelination. The mechanisms causing myelin damage are not completely known. Possible mechanisms include a direct toxic effect of tumor necrosis factor (TNF) on myelin (upper panel) or macrophage-mediated damage through either phagocytosis, in which the cell is engulfed and destroyed, or apoptosis, in which cells are induced to self-destruct (lower panel).[136] NOTE: IL = interleukin; MHC = major histocompatibility antigen. SOURCE: Adapted from New Directions in the Management of Multiple Sclerosis. 1994. Berlex Laboratories. Courtesy of John Rose and the Knowledge Weavers, University of Utah.

**TABLE 2.10** Clinical Pathological Correlations in Common Syndromes of MS

| | |
|---|---|
| **Visual deficits** | Often related to the involvement of the optic nerve as occurs in optic neuritis |
| **Eye movement abnormalities** | Frequently associated with plaques involving connections between the brainstem nuclei subserving eye movements |
| **Weakness and spasticity** | One of the consequences of lesions involving the spinal cord or descending motor tracts in the white matter of internal capsule or brainstem |
| **Ataxia** | Usually the result of lesions in cerebellum or its input-output pathways |

inflammatory responses. Specific chemokine receptors are expressed by infiltrating cells in demyelinating MS brain lesions and in CSF. These results imply pathogenic roles for specific chemokine-chemokine receptor interactions in MS and suggest new molecular targets for therapeutic intervention.[163,202]

Some investigators have emphasized that the pattern of pathology suggests a dying-back oligodendrogliopathy (those parts of the cell, such as the most distal process, farthest from the cell body are the most vulnerable).[126] During the active stages of disease, the number of oligodendrocytes can be reduced near the demyelinating foci. Subsequently, there might be partial recruitment of oligodendrocyte precursors that may, in part, repopulate the margins of the plaque and contribute to remyelination.

**Chronic Lesions.** Trapp and colleagues[212] have emphasized that the relapsing-remitting course is intimately related to the inflammatory demyelination and classical plaques, while more chronic progressive forms of the disease are linked to transection, or severing, of axons at sites of inflammation and demyelination. They have shown that severed axons were a consistent component in the lesions of individuals with MS and suggest that the number of these injured axons is correlated to the magnitude of the inflammation within the lesion. Axonal damage might be a pathological correlate of irreversible neurological deficits that occur in patients with progressive MS.[51,212,213,220] In individuals with chronic MS, plaques are often sharply demarcated with scattered lipid-containing macrophages and little evidence of ongoing myelin destruction. Demyelination can be incomplete. The density of axons may be significantly reduced. There is usually astrogliosis within these lesions. It is not clear exactly how the axonal damage that occurs at later stages plays into this complex evolving pathology, but the extent of axonal damage appears to be a critical determinant of whether a person recovers from an attack or not. Lack of recovery from attacks and disease progression are more likely when axons are more severely damaged and repair mechanisms fail.

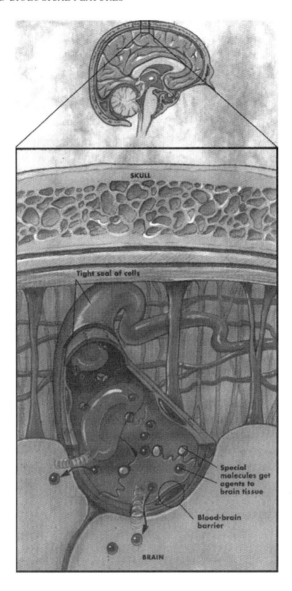

**FIGURE 2. 8** The blood-brain barrier. The tight seal of the cells lining the blood vessels forms a blood-brain barrier that keeps many substances out of the brain. Leaky blood vessels in the body allow many molecules to cross through to other tissues, but the tight construction of the vessels in the head guards against entry of most molecules into the brain. Normally, only certain molecules, for example, blood gases such as oxygen and small nutritional molecules, can cross the blood-brain barrier, but this barrier breaks down when the brain is injured or in certain diseases, such as MS. SOURCE: Reprinted with permission by Lydia Kibiuk/Society for Neuroscience.

A correlation between demyelination and axonal degeneration observed at autopsy is supported by imaging studies, including those that compare the concentrations of N-acetyl aspartate.[119] For example, one study measured the levels of NAA, an amino acid found only in neurons that serves as a biological marker for integrity of the axon and neuronal cell body. The brains of MS patients showed significantly greater side-to-side differences in levels of NAA, indicating decreased neuronal integrity on the side of the brain with lower NAA levels. There was a correlation between this asymmetry in motor function and the asymmetry of NAA concentrations in the internal capsule.[119] Insights into processes that lead to demyelination and axon damage can be obtained by analyzing T1-weighted image hypointensities, proton spectroscopy, MTI, and DTI and by correlating these measures with clinical and pathological findings.

**Gliosis.** Gliosis is a prominent feature of the MS lesion, but it is best regarded as a secondary phenomenon.[146] Whenever the CNS is damaged, it undergoes an injury response, usually called reactive gliosis or glial scarring. The response is broadly the same whatever the source of injury, although the details vary somewhat with different types of pathology.[67] The glial reaction to injury includes recruitment of oligodendrocyte precursor cells, stem cells, microglia, and astrocytes. Formation of the glial scar after CNS injury generally occurs over a period of weeks. Microglia are typically the first cell types to enter the lesion. In the normal brain, they are quiescent with short, branched processes. Following injury, they exhibit various changes, including activation, cell division, and migration to the injury site.[67] During activation, microglia display conspicuous functional plasticity, which involves changes in cell morphology, cell surface receptor expression, and production of growth factors and cytokines, and they become, in general, more macrophage like.[208] Microglia can be either neurotoxic or neurotrophic.

The final glial scar is made up mainly of a meshwork of tightly interwoven astrocyte processes, attached to one another by tight junctions and gap junctions and surrounded by extracellular matrix (reviewed in 1999 by Fawcett and Asher[67]). (Astrocytes are irregularly star-shaped, background structural cells of the nervous system.) Gliosis is usually restricted to the area of demyelination, but it sometimes extends beyond that area. There is no specific way to identify the presence and extent of gliosis in MS lesions through MRI, although the T1 signal might be more sensitive to gliosis than the T2 signal.[24]

The role of astrocytes in gliosis is not completely known.[146] Since there is evidence that glial scars can inhibit both axon growth and myelination, it is clearly important to know what causes them to form, what cells are involved, why they are inhibitory, and how to manipulate them. Finally, although gliosis is generally considered harmful, there is also evidence that the gliotic ensheathment of demyelinated axons might favor the restoration of nerve conduction.[221]

## New Directions for Research on Axons and Myelin

The relapsing-remitting form of MS appears to be related to the demyelination of axons during relapses, followed by the remodeling and remyelination with consequent restoration of conduction that underlies remission. Remyelination is carried out by surviving oligodendrocytes or by the proliferation of progenitor cells that are then stimulated to become oligodendrocytes. Molecular remodeling of demyelinated axons, in terms of their redistributing their sodium channels along the axon, might act as a form of adaptive plasticity; this process may represent a target for future therapies. In contrast, the progressive form of the disease, which appears clinically as an unremitting accumulation of deficits, might reflect the superimposition of axonal injury or degeneration on multiple chronic foci of demyelinated axons. The finding that axonal damage can occur frequently in MS and the suggestion that these lesions contribute to persistent neurological deficits are important issues in MS research.[51,135,212,213,220] Thus, it will be important to understand the mechanisms whereby axons are damaged and to define ways of protecting axons, which may be vulnerable to degeneration, in part due to their proximity to inflammatory and demyelinating foci. It will also be important to search for molecules that promote the regrowth of injured axons to their appropriate targets. Some of the lessons from studies of the repair of spinal cord injury are likely to be relevant here.[81,133] Moreover, because abnormal patterns of ion channels have been found within neurons whose axons are undergoing demyelination,[22] it will be important to understand the factors that influence the regulation of these channels.[219] These lines of research, involving strategies that protect axons from degeneration or promote repair,[81,133] and those agents that can restore conduction in demyelinated axons represent opportunities to restore functions and could have significant implications for therapy.[219] Similarly, future therapeutic approaches might involve replacement of oligodendroglia with pluripotent stem cells (discussed further in Chapter 6). Progenitor cells, those either already present in an individual or provided from another source by injection, can produce myelin in demyelinated foci in experimental animals.[28] Future experimental therapeutics will involve approaches directed at restoring oligodendrocytes to ensheath axonal processes and to induce physiological modeling of axons to restore conduction.

## Immunopathology

The most striking pathology in MS is the immune system's attack and destruction of the body's own myelin sheath, which is why it is believed to be an autoimmune disease, although this has not yet been definitively proven (Box 2.3). The pathogenic trigger that first causes the immune system to attack myelin is unknown, but the immunopathology, or pathological activity of the immune system, that ensues after that initial attack is becoming clearer.

## BOX 2.3
### Autoimmunity and Disease

The immune system defends the body against foreign invaders such as bacteria and viruses. It does so by recognizing that foreign invaders have special markers distinguishing them as "non-self," compared to the body's own tissue (or "self") (Figure 2.9). Normally, the immune system reacts only to non-self invaders, not to its own tissues. Unfortunately, this process is not foolproof. Autoimmunity is an immune response mounted against antigens that are naturally produced within the body, or self-antigens, to cause lasting tissue damage.

In the strictest sense, an autoimmune disease must meet several criteria. First, the disease must be reproduced by transfer of autoantibodies or autoreactive T lymphocytes (T cells) from affected to unaffected individuals. Second, the self-antigen that elicits the immune attack must be identified. Third, this antigen (or a closely related one) should cause a similar disease in an animal model. (Scientifically, it would be best to show that the antigen caused the disease in humans, but it would be unethical to intentionally infect humans, hence, the compromise for evidence in animals). It is now feasible to transfer human genes into animals in an attempt to satisfy these criteria. One of the first so-called transgenic studies that introduced certain human genes into an animal without MS led to the development of a disease resembling MS.[129] Among the newly added genes were those for a specific type of histocompatibility antigen and for a particular type of T-cell receptor that binds to a fragment of a myelin protein (myelin basic protein). This type of study begins to confirm the autoimmune nature of MS.

Human autoimmune diseases, however, are generally classified as such without meeting these three stringent criteria. Circumstantial evidence often is marshaled for classification. For example, patients are classified as having autoimmune disease if they have high levels of autoantibody or autoreactive T cells, or because there is a correlation between the level of immune activity and disease severity. Some examples of autoimmune diseases are listed in Table 2.11.

*Why does the immune system have autoreactive lymphocytes?* During development, the immune system randomly builds a vast repertoire of cells that respond to a multitude of foreign antigens. At the same time, the immune system must weed out those cells that react to self-antigens. Most self-reactive B cells and T cells are removed early during development. Other regulatory mechanisms exist to keep self-reactive lymphocytes unresponsive later on. These are among the normal regulatory mechanisms resulting in immunological tolerance to most self-antigens. Even though there are usually small numbers of autoreactive lymphocytes in a normal adult, most do not cause disease, and some might even serve a (currently unknown) beneficial purpose.[182] With autoimmune disease, however, there are large numbers of autoreactive immune cells. Autoimmune disease thus can be thought of as a failure of normal regulatory mechanisms that guard against autoimmunity.

**What causes a pathological autoimmune response?** The causes of autoimmune response in MS and most other autoimmune diseases are unknown but likely include a combination of genetic susceptibility and exposure to environmental agents. For most autoimmune diseases, the actual genes and environmental agents are unknown. Gender also plays a role because women are disproportionately affected by autoimmune disease. The reasons for the gender difference are also unknown but appear to relate to distinct immune environments in women and men.[224]

**How can genes and environment trigger autoimmune pathology?** Genes control many properties of the immune system. Theoretically, autoimmune disease can occur if any of the genes controlling the immune system's ability to distinguish self from non-self are defective. The genes often suspected of predisposing to autoimmune disease encode proteins, such as histocompatibility antigens, that participate in this complex process of self versus non-self recognition.

Environmental or infectious agents can stimulate pathological autoimmune reactions through at least two possible mechanisms: molecular mimicry, superantigens, and bystander damage (Figure 2.10). Molecular mimicry occurs when a bacterial or viral epitope—the fragment of an antigen that elicits an immune response—is very similar to a self-epitope. This can occur following an infection where an immune cell targeting an epitope on a bacterium subsequently cross-reacts with a self-antigen.[5,46,157,229] Superantigens are proteins from bacteria or retroviruses that lead to widespread activation of T cells. Unlike most antigens, which activate only a specific T cell, superantigens activate approximately one out of every ten T cells.[92] Because of their generic ability to activate so many types of T cells, superantigens may inadvertently activate autoreactive T cells, which then attack self-tissues. In bystander damage, a virus upregulates a nonspecific immune response that then leads to pathology; for example, proinflammatory cytokines might activate Th1 cells or macrophages that contribute to the immunopathology. Once damage occurs, new cellular epitopes become exposed and trigger an immune response in a process called epitope spreading, which can also lead to autoimmune pathology. During an immune response against a particular epitope, the number of lymphocytes that recognize the epitope normally multiplies. Yet, in epitope spreading, the immune response escalates to target other epitopes on the same antigen or on related antigens.[54] In this way, an initially nonpathological autoimmune response expands to produce a pathological response. The underlying basis for epitope spreading in autoimmune diseases is poorly understood.

Another way to produce a pathological autoimmune response is for autoreactive lymphocytes to gain access to a target antigen from which they are ordinarily separated. The brain is one example of an anatomical sanctuary site, because it is protected by the blood-brain barrier of the central nervous system. Normally, T cells that might react against myelin do not pass across this barrier into the central nervous system. In MS, however, T cells become activated, which enables them to penetrate the blood-brain barrier and reach their targets—myelin antigens—thereby generating an autoimmune response.

One of the first pathological processes leading up to MS attacks is thought to be activation of autoreactive T lymphocytes, or T cells, and their migration into the central nervous system.[25,93,116] However, T cells and the inflammatory molecules they secrete are not the only players. Many cells and molecules of the immune system—likely unleashed by T-cell activation—participate in demyeli-

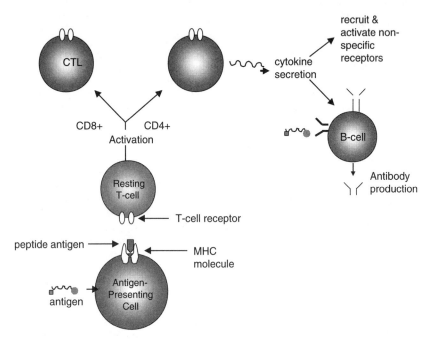

**FIGURE 2.9** Interactions between major cell components of the immune system. This simplified outline shows interactions that occur in response to a foreign antigen. The antigen could be an epitope from a virus particle, bacterium, or other foreign agent. The antigen-presenting cell (APC) ingests the antigen (or in the case of an infecting virus, it may already be within the cell) and processes it into peptide fragments. The major histocompatibility complex (MHC, the cell surface structure characteristic of each individual) presents this target to a resting T cell. Binding of the peptide-MHC complex by the T-cell receptor activates the T cell. In the case of a CD8+ cell, it becomes a cytotoxic T lymphocyte (CTL), which will destroy any cells that have the same peptide-MHC complex on their surfaces. In the case of a CD4+ cell, the activated cell produces and secretes various cytokines that recruit and activate nonspecific effector cells (such as macrophages) or stimulate antigen-bound B cells to produce antibodies. When T and B lymphocytes are activated by a specific antigen, they undergo proliferation, producing more cells with their same antigen specificity. This serves to amplify the immune response against the foreign antigen.

**TABLE 2.11**  Selected Diseases That Are Believed to Be Autoimmune Based

| Disease | Common Symptoms | Proposed Mechanism |
|---|---|---|
| Graves' disease | Hyperthyroidism | Antibodies against the thyrotropin receptor stimulate thyroid function |
| Insulin-dependent diabetes mellitus (Type I diabetes) | Hypoinsulinemia and hyperglycemia | Destruction of insulin-producing cells in pancreas |
| Pemphigoid (various diseases) | Blister formation | Antibodies block adhesion of epidermis to dermis |
| Rheumatoid arthritis | Joint pain and loss of mobility | T-cell-mediated inflammation in the joints |
| Systemic lupus erythematosus | Arthritis, rash, CNS dysfunction, kidney damage | Immune response to numerous cellular antigens, especially DNA |
| Systemic sclerosis (scleroderma) | Thickening of skin; kidney, lung, and gastrointestinal damage | Immune response against topoisomerase I leads to increased formation of collagen in the skin and internal organs |
| Thyroiditis | Hypothyroidism | Destruction of thyroid cells |
| Chronic inflammatory demyelinating polyneuropathy | Weakness and sensory loss | Demyelination of peripheral nerve fibers |
| Guillan-Barré syndrome | Paralysis and loss of reflexes | Demyelination and/or axonal degeneration of peripheral nerve fibers |
| Lambert-Eaton myasthenic syndrome | Muscle weakness | Antibodies against presynaptic calcium channel of the neuromuscular junction (NMJ) disrupt function |
| Myasthenia gravis | Muscle weakness | Antibodies against postsynaptic acetylcholine receptor of the NMJ disrupt function |
| Neuromytonia (Isaac's syndrome) | Muscular twitching, cramps, stiffness, and weakness | Antibodies against potassium channel at the NMJ cause increased muscle activity |
| Rasmussen's encephalitis | Epileptic seizures and neurological dysfunction | Antibodies against subunit of ionotropic glutamate receptor lead to degeneration of one cerebral hemisphere |
| Stiff man syndrome | Axial and limb rigidity; spasms | Antibodies block production of GABA ($\gamma$-aminobutyric acid), an inhibitory neurotransmitter |

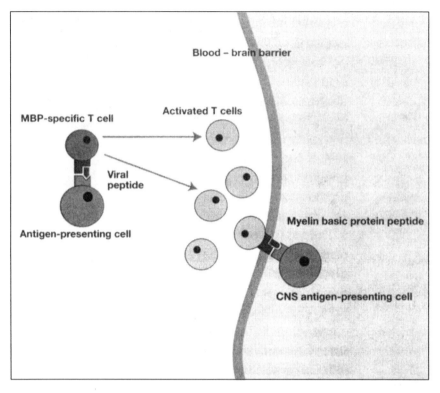

**FIGURE 2.10** Possible mechanism of viral etiology. Although no virus has yet been shown to contribute to the etiology of MS, there are several ways in which this could occur, and one of these is shown in this figure. Activated T cells cross the blood-brain barrier following activation by a microbe with a structural similarity to a component of the myelin sheath. Once inside the brain, these cells attack self-antigens, such as the various myelin proteins that are attacked in MS. NOTE: MBP = myelin basic protein. SOURCE: Steinman and Oldstone, 1997.[206] Reprinted with permission. Adapted from Wucherpfennig and Strominger, 1995.[229]

nation. The entire cascade of immune system events eventually culminates in myelin destruction. The key features of this cascade are not fully understood, including the precise ordering of events, the antigens targeted by T cells, and the contributions of B lymphocytes, or B cells, and other cells of the immune system. Yet, as this section explains, much insight has been gained into the immunopathology of MS. This knowledge has been—and continues to be—fundamental for devising therapies targeted to the immunopathology of MS (Chapter 5).

## T Cells in MS

As much as a century ago, researchers observed that T cells were particularly abundant in MS lesions.[116] Over time, using modern immunologic techniques, they managed to isolate and characterize a particular type of T cell, the autoreactive T cell, from the blood and CSF of MS patients.[225]

These and related findings gave credence to the hypothesis that autoreactive T cells played a dominant role in MS. After all, immunologists have long known that T cells are capable of orchestrating a multifaceted autoimmune attack. However, this was not enough to explain MS pathology. First, elevations in certain types of autoreactive T cells were not unique to MS patients. Second, and more critically, T cells were necessary but not sufficient to cause demyelinating disease in animal models. The transfer of myelin-specific T cells into normal animals initiated only inflammation, not demyelination.[117] This suggested that other immune cells, particularly antibody-producing B cells (Table 2.12) and macrophages, might also play key roles, even if autoreactive T cells launched the process.

**TABLE 2.12** Possible Autoantigens In MS

| | |
|---|---|
| **MYELIN PROTEINS** | |
| Myelin basic protein (MBP) | An important component of the myelin sheath, MBP is located on the cytoplasmic face of the myelin membrane, and constitutes 30-40% of myelin protein by weight. |
| Myelin oligodendrocyte glycoprotein (MOG) | Surface protein on the myelin sheath. |
| Myelin-associated oligodendrocytic basic protein (MOBP) | Structurally similar to MBP, but expressed exclusively in the CNS myelin. Possibly involved in myelin compaction. |
| Proteolipid protein (PLP) | PLP constitutes approximately 50% by weight of myelin protein. PLP spans the myelin membrane, providing increased stability. |
| Myelin-associated glycoprotein (MAG) | The major mediator of axonal-glial contacts essential for the initiation of myelination. |
| **OTHER PROTEINS** | |
| S-100b | Calcium-binding protein associated with astrocytes. |
| Glial fibrillary acidic protein (GFAP) | Major constituent of glial filaments in astrocytes, providing structural stability. Rapidly synthesized in response to CNS trauma or disease. |
| Heat shock proteins | Broad class of stress-responsive proteins that are normal components of the myelin sheath. |
| αB-crystallin | A stress protein that is an immunodominant antigen of CNS myelin in MS patients. |

The prime autoantigen that elicits the autoimmune response in MS is not known. While there are many candidate autoantigens, as yet none is preeminent.

Much MS research focused on myelin basic protein (MBP), located at the inner surface of the myelin membrane. Clinical studies were shaped by research on experimental allergic encephalomyelitis (EAE), the classic animal model of demyelinating disease. In many species, MBP acts as a classical encephalitogenic autoantigen (an antigen capable of serving as the focus of an inflammatory attack in the brain). EAE research further established that in some strains of mice and rats, the autoimmune response to MBP displays two unique features. First, in the initial stages of the immune response in EAE, T cells react only to very small regions of the MBP molecule ("epitope dominance"), even though they later react to many more regions of the molecule ("epitope spreading") (see Box 2.3). Second, the encephalitogenic T cells in EAE use an unusually narrow repertoire of genes for their antigen receptors.[205] (T cells recognize their target antigen by its capacity to bind to specific receptors on their surface membrane, called T-cell receptors [TCRs]). These two features raised hopes for developing immune-based therapies because a more limited range of therapies might succeed in combating MS in early stages.

Unfortunately, these features turned out to be much less prominent in humans with MS. First, human T cells respond to a broader set of MBP epitopes. While there might be a relatively dominant epitope in the central portion of the MBP molecule, there are clearly many other target epitopes along the full sequence of this large polypeptide.[131] Second, MBP-specific T cells use multiple genes for their TCRs, which allows for large variability among individuals.[86] Generally, it appears that the T-cell response against myelin proteins differs greatly between individual patients, a property that suggests the potential need for individually designed immune therapies.

Several research teams have attempted to identify MBP-specific T cells in MS patients.[216,228] Unfortunately, these attempts did not show significant increases in MBP-specific T-cell counts in MS patients compared to healthy blood donors. However, when more definitive assay systems were used, increased frequencies of activated MBP-specific T cells were found in MS patients.[7,20,232] These studies relied on complex methods and were influenced by numerous factors that complicate the interpretation of results. More direct assays, such as those that use binding of oligomeric class II-peptide complexes to specific T cells,[41] might resolve the problem.

To add a further degree of complexity, MBP does not appear to be the only autoantigen in MS: there are a number of additional myelin and nonmyelin proteins that are potential autoantigens in MS. Earlier hypotheses had implicated MBP on the basis of two lines of research. First, studies of EAE had suggested that MBP was indeed the most important, if not the only, encephalitogenic myelin autoantigen. Second, due to its particularly convenient molecular properties, MBP was the only myelin protein available both at high purity and in large quantities.[118] However, thanks to modern biotechnology, even minor myelin proteins are now available in large quantities and can be studied for their encephalitogenic capacity.

Later studies established that many, if not all, myelin proteins are potentially encephalitogenic. Especially interesting among these newly recognized auto-antigens is myelin oligodendrocyte glycoprotein (MOG). In contrast to MBP, which lies on the inside of the myelin sheath, MOG lies on the surface. As one of the few myelin proteins accessible to humoral autoantibodies, MOG is a target for demyelinating immunoglobulins (see next section). In addition, MOG is a very effective autoantigen in rodents and in primates for encephalitogenic T cells.[17] Some studies even demonstrated increased frequencies of MOG-reactive T cells in MS patients.[108,217] These findings clearly warrant general confirmation. It is also important to investigate whether different subtypes of MS, which are distinguished by divergent clinical, genetic, and morphological features, are associated with enhanced T-cell responses against different target autoantigens.[127]

Thus far, research has spotlighted one class of T cells—those with a TCR termed $\alpha\beta$.* $\alpha\beta$ T cells are the major class of immune cells centrally involved in adaptive immune responses against infections and tumors. Much less attention has been given to other T-cell classes ($\gamma\delta$ T cells and NK1 T cells), which may function both as effector cells in autoimmune attacks and as suppressor cells that dampen autoimmune responses.[90,161] There are reports linking the presence of $\gamma\delta$ T cells in the brain (presumably) with the induction of heat shock proteins in MS lesions.[25] Certain members of this broad class of proteins are a normal component of the myelin sheath,[46] yet they are also found outside the CNS as well as in pathogens. The role of heat shock proteins in the development of the MS lesion is unknown, but there are various possibilities. Some of these proteins might act as a target autoantigen, as has been shown in autoimmune diabetes. They might also reflect inflammatory stress inflicted on local CNS cells, or they might be determinants of beneficial anti-inflammatory control mechanisms.[25,42]

Even though the precise pathological roles of T cells and their autoantigens are unresolved, this line of research has generated many approved or emerging therapies. These include vaccination strategies, which use either attenuated myelin-specific T cells[207,33] or peptides representing myelin-specific T-cell receptors[9] as vaccines to strengthen the body's own regulatory responses against pathogenic T cells (reviewed in Zhang et. al., 1998).[233] Also under development are "altered peptide" therapies that use peptide analogues of myelin protein segments to induce autoreactive T cells to produce protective, rather than pathogenic, cytokine mediators.[205] Cytokines, as discussed later, are a functionally diverse set of signaling molecules produced by T cells.

---

*Each ($\alpha$ and $\beta$) refers to a polypeptide chain that forms the T-cell receptor.

## B Cells in MS

B cells (also known as B lymphocytes) have been detected in MS lesions for many years, although less consistently than T cells.[26] While most MS research naturally focused on T cells, evidence also has accumulated for participation by autoreactive B cells. It now appears that both types of lymphocytes actively contribute to MS immunopathology. Autoreactive T cells are thought to launch inflammation and, through their release of cytokines, to stimulate B cells to secrete antibodies that cause demyelination.[93] This is consistent with animal studies finding that EAE can be produced only by injecting myelin-specific T cells in combination with myelin-specific antibodies.[78,123] Without injecting the antibodies, demyelination does not occur.

In MS patients, levels in cerebrospinal fluid of the type of protein known to consist of antibodies (immunoglobulin) are often higher than in healthy people. The increased immunoglobulin is due to production by only a few different clones of B cells that have been induced to proliferate. B cells from the CSF of MS patients have been reported to contain mutations in the DNA sequences that encode antibodies, which is consistent with the notion of an antigen-driven selection of antibodies with high-affinity antigen-binding sites.[170] Such events are commonly observed in immune responses against foreign antigens such as bacterial infections, as well as in humoral autoimmune responses.[171] However, no foreign antigen or autoantigen responsible for the generation of oligoclonal bands in MS has yet been identified.

One recent study using sophisticated immunocytochemistry furnished direct evidence of a pathologic role for autoantibodies. For the first time, MOG-specific antibodies were demonstrated to be bound to myelin debris in active MS lesions.[77] If confirmed and extended to a larger group of patients, this finding would suggest that B-cell-derived autoantibodies might induce myelin destruction. On the other hand, although anti-MOG antibodies are found in the CSF of MS patients, they are also found in CSF of patients with other neurological diseases that are not demyelinating.[103] Thus, despite tantalizing leads, the role of anti-MOG antibodies in MS patients is still unclear.

## Cytokines

Cytokines are soluble proteins produced and released by T cells, macrophages, and certain other cell types. Interferons (IFN- $\alpha$, $\beta$, and $\gamma$), interleukins (including IL- 1, 4, 6, 10, 12, and 13), TGF-b, and the neuropoietic cytokines* (such as ciliary neurotrophic factor and leukemia inhibitory factor) are all different types of cytokines. They generally act as intercellular signaling molecules that regulate

---

*Neuropoietic cytokines are the family of neural growth factors that act on both the nervous and the hematopoietic or immune systems.

and carry out immune functions, but their repertoire is complex. Some function as pro-inflammatory, others as anti-inflammatory agents. Some even have divergent functions during different phases of disease.[32] Cytokines, including the subset known as chemokines (for *chemo*tactic cyto*kines*), also alter the permeability of the blood-brain barrier[105] or act on neural cells.[175] Thus, particular cytokines can initiate, sustain, or terminate inflammatory disease processes. Proinflammatory cytokines and other secretory products of immune cells are proposed in several neurological diseases—including MS—to be toxic to neurons and oligodendrocytes if they are secreted in sufficiently high concentrations over a sustained period of time.[49,82]

In MS, the initial entry of autoreactive T cells into the CNS is thought to trigger the local production of cytokines and chemokines, which in turn begins the inflammatory process and enhances the permeability of the blood-brain barrier.[93] A more permeable blood-brain barrier allows infiltration into the CNS of more immune cells which in turn contribute to the ongoing inflammation. Thus, understanding the roles of cytokines and their temporal sequence of activation is crucial to modifying the course of MS. Much of our present understanding of cytokine action in demyelinating disease comes from studies of animal models, including EAE.

A large body of research is being compiled on the expression and possible function of cytokines as pro- and anti-inflammatory mediators in MS. Some studies have used in situ immunocytochemistry and in situ hybridization to visualize gene expression in lesions, whereas others have relied on the activation of inflammatory cells (T cells, B cells, macrophages) in vitro. Much of the research is comparing material from MS patients with or without treatment with immunomodulatory agents, especially glatiramer acetate and beta-interferon.[93]

Pro-inflammatory cytokines within active MS lesions have been localized to both infiltrating immune cells and glia.[172] Longitudinal studies have linked clinical exacerbation and remission to high and low expression, respectively, of pro-inflammatory cytokines, especially TNF-$\gamma$.[16] For example, secretion of TNF-$\gamma$ and cell adhesion molecules by inflammatory cells is upregulated immediately prior to relapse.[40,179,197] Yet, not all findings could be verified in all patient groups studied.[31,80,178]

Understanding of cytokines and their diverse roles throughout the course of disease, although still incomplete, has nevertheless spawned new treatments. One explanation for the success of glatiramer acetate and beta-interferon relates to their control over cytokine expression: they can induce T cells to switch from a pro-inflammatory phenotype (Th1) to an anti-inflammatory phenotype (Th2).[93] T cells that are switched to an anti-inflammatory phenotype release a variety of cytokines, such as IL-10, that reduce inflammation.

**Immunologically Special Features of the CNS.** CNS tissues were traditionally thought to be exempt from active immune reactivity, but it is now known that the brain is subject to immune surveillance and can be the site of immune responses. Only activated and not resting T cells can cross the blood-brain barrier and interact with local CNS cells. Local glial cells can be stimulated by pro-inflammatory cytokines to express immunologically active molecules, such as the major histocompatability complex (MHC) products, cytokines, and chemo-kines required for local immune responses. Neurons are capable of suppressing immune responses within the CNS. Thus, immune responses are more likely to occur in areas of neuronal degeneration than in intact CNS tissues. Immune reactivity within the CNS must hence be viewed as the balance between the pro-inflammatory signals contributed by activated T cells and other inflammatory cells entering the brain and the anti-inflammatory signals from functional neurons.

## Epidemiology

Epidemiologists define what causes a disease and what puts an individual at risk of getting this disease. They look for correlations such as whether Caucasians are more likely to have MS than Asians or whether residents of one county are more likely to get MS than residents of another. These correlations lead to hypotheses or working models as to which factors actually cause MS and which are only associated with it. These hypotheses or models can then be tested experimentally. Epidemiological studies have limitations, but for a complex disease like MS, they can rule out some factors and highlight others. They are the first step toward finding a biological mechanism for MS, or possibly a cure.

Most epidemiological studies of MS have been observational and retrospective; researchers collected the information (for example, ethnicity, age of onset) from an individual (or from records) that had been diagnosed with MS. Such studies rely on an individual's ability to accurately recall information from years ago, for example, the infections that she or he had before the age of five. Other sources of data, such as death certificates, can contain incorrect information. Despite these shortcomings, a few factors consistently correlate with MS prevalence. Determining how these factors lead to an increased risk of MS has proven more difficult.

The risk of MS increases with increasing distance from the equator. In the United States, this is seen as a gradient of risk, with higher risk in northern regions and a lower risk in the south.[56,114] In Australia, the prevalence of MS increases similarly from lower, subequatorial latitudes to the more southerly latitudes.[89] Studies on migrating populations, although inconclusive, offer tentative support for the hypothesis that environment influences MS risk. Individuals who have moved from a region with one risk level to a region with a higher or lower risk, in general, adopt the risk level of their new home.[56,113] This is especially true for individuals moving from a low-risk to a high-risk area.

Studies carried out in the 1960s and 1970s suggested that this geographical effect had a defined susceptibility period before age 15. Although these data still appear in the MS literature and have led to several hypotheses about the effects of puberty or early dietary effects on MS risk, the sample numbers are too small to support such a tight cutoff.[56,150] A later and larger study assayed the effects of migration by comparing location at birth with location at approximately 24 years of age.[113,114] Although individuals did adopt the risk of their new home, the age values in that study are not precise enough to add to the argument for or against a cutoff. Most recently, a study comparing the prevalence of MS among native-born Australians and Australian immigrants from the United Kingdom (thereby providing a rough control for genetic background) suggests that rather than being established around age 15, environmental risk factors operate over many years and into early adulthood.[89]

Although the migrational studies suggest an environmental correlation with MS, the root cause of this latitude effect is unknown. Differences in diet[150] or sunlight[1,97,121] have been proposed, but neither has been supported by rigorous studies. Alternatively, the geographical distribution of MS could result from the migration either of a viral agent[113] or of individuals (perhaps originally Scandinavians) who carried a pool of susceptible genes.[193]

Ethnicity is another definite risk factor. MS is more prevalent among Caucasians than other groups. In a study of 5,305 U.S. veterans with MS, Caucasian males had twice the risk of MS as African-American males.[114] Other factors can modulate the effect of ethnicity on risk of MS. MS is almost absent among black Africans. African Americans, however, show a low risk of MS; this might be due to genetic mixing with Caucasian Americans or to an environmental effect.[56] MS occurrence among Asians is also quite low. Again, Asian Americans show an intermediate risk for MS between Asians and Caucasian Americans.[137] A discussion of the role of genetics in MS can be found in the next section.

When applied to a complex disorder such as MS, conclusions derived from epidemiologic data of this type must be interpreted cautiously because inapparent explanations may be present. For example, a higher-than-expected incidence of MS observed in South Vietnamese immigrants (a low-risk group) residing in France (a moderate-risk area) superficially suggest a modifying role of the environment on MS. However, this immigrant population was in fact racially mixed and contained substantial numbers of individuals with mixed French and Asian ancestry. Thus, the higher-than-expected MS incidence in these immigrants could have been due to either genetic or environmental factors. Neither factor can be ruled out. A similar argument could explain the incidence of MS in West Indian immigrants residing in Great Britain. On the other hand, the increased incidence of MS observed in Japanese-Americans compared to individuals residing in Japan is not easily explained by racial admixture and does support a role of the environment on MS risk.

As in other autoimmune diseases, women are much more likely to get MS than men, suggesting that hormonal or genetic factors are involved. The ratio of women to men with MS is about 2:1.[57] Among both sexes, the age of onset for

MS ranges between 10 and 59 years,[56] with the highest incidence occurring among individuals in their mid-20s to early 30s, depending on the population examined.[112] Males tend to have a slightly later mean age of onset than females. This results, at least in part, from an increase in the percentage of males with the primary progressive variant. This form of MS has a later onset than other types and affects approximately 15 percent of patients. The ratio of males to females with primary progressive MS is approximately 1:1.

Epidemiological studies have provided conflicting data as to whether an infectious agent (viral or bacterial) either causes or triggers MS. The occurrence of MS epidemics has suggested that an infectious agent might be at work. The two MS epidemics cited most often, one in the Faroe Islands and one in Iceland, were directly preceded by the influx of foreign troops during World War II. Both, however, are open to multiple interpretations. Coincident with the stationing of foreign soldiers, the population of the Faroe Islands received increased medical services[56] and changed its diet.[150] The Icelandic epidemic, on the other hand, began shortly after the arrival of that island's first neurologist.[56] In both cases, the increased prevalence of MS might have resulted from an increased level of detection or a combination of other factors, such as nonspecific immune stimulation resulting from the introduction of a variety of infectious agents into previously unexposed populations. No infectious agent has been associated with either of these MS clusters.

Another area of investigation has explored whether environmental factors contribute to the onset of MS or the probability of MS attacks. Some studies suggest that MS attacks are more likely to occur in the spring and fall than in the winter or summer. Such a finding, if true, suggests that a relationship exists between some viral infections and the risk of exacerbations. Many patients with MS are also at heightened risk for urinary tract, pulmonary, or skin infections, yet the relationship between these potentially preventable infections and the course of MS has never been adequately studied. Additional research in this area is needed.

Perhaps the most clear-cut epidemiologic link to MS attacks is the effect of pregnancy and the postpartum period. Pregnancy is associated with a decrease in the risk for MS attacks, particularly during the third trimester. The postpartum period is, conversely, associated with a significant increase in risk. An immuno-suppressive state in the pregnant mother is created by increased numbers of regulatory T cells (Th2 cells) which, presumably, dampen the autoimmune reaction that produces attacks of MS. The explanation for the increase in attack risk during the postpartum period is less clear but might involve immunostimulation by prolactin, the hormone responsible for milk production.

The absence of supporting evidence does not prove that a virus is *not* connected with the disease. Unrelated individuals (in the case of the adoptee and conjugal studies) may differ in their susceptibilities to infectious agents. Researchers have isolated a variety of viruses from individual MS patients, but to date, no one virus has been isolated from all MS patients examined.[18] It might, however, be the case either that MS is not one single disease or that there are multiple ways to trigger it. Researchers continue to look for causative infectious agents.[18,83] (See section below on infectious causes of MS for further discussion.)

The aggregation of MS in some geographic areas, ethnic populations, or families could be explained by a common environmental exposure, a shared genetic background, or a combination of both environmental and genetic susceptibility. It is likely that in MS, as in other complex disorders, both factors contribute. It is also possible that the relative contributions of environment versus genetics might vary in different situations, depending on the degree to which an individual is genetically susceptible and the specific environmental context. The role of genetic factors in MS is discussed in the next section.

## MS Susceptibility Genes

MS is not considered a genetic disease in the classic sense because it usually occurs sporadically. However, population and family studies are consistent with a principal pathogenic role for genetic risk factors in MS etiology. This genetic component is indicated primarily by the increased relative risk to siblings of affected individuals compared with the general population. Familial aggregation ($\lambda$s) is measured by estimating the ratio of the prevalence (frequency) in siblings versus the population prevalence of the disease. A $\lambda$s of 1 represents no familial clustering of the trait. For MS, the $\lambda$s is estimated to be between 20 (0.02/0.001) and 40 (0.04/0.001).[180] Half-sibling[189] and adoption[58] studies confirm that genetic, and not environmental, factors are responsible for familial aggregation. In addition, twin studies from different populations consistently indicate that a monozygotic twin of an MS patient is at higher risk (25 to 30 percent concordance) for MS than a dizygotic twin (2 to 5 percent),[148,188] providing additional evidence for a significant but complex genetic etiology. Finally, the frequent occurrence of MS in some ethnic populations (particularly those of northern European origin) compared to others (African and Asian groups), irrespective of geographic location, also provides evidence for a complex genetic etiology.[44,156,166] Overall, adoption and family studies suggest that being related to a person with MS is a greater risk factor than living with someone with MS.

A simple genetic model for the inheritance of MS is unlikely to be valid. Such a single-gene hypothesis is at odds with concordance data in twin and family studies and with the observed nonlinear decrease in disease risk as the genetic distance from the relative with MS is increased. It is likely that susceptibility is determined by multiple independent genetic loci (polygenic inheritance), each with a relatively modest contribution to overall risk. It is also possible that there are different genetic causes of susceptibility to MS (genetic heterogeneity). Finally, the genes that contribute to MS susceptibility are likely to be normal, common variants (or alleles) of genes rather than obviously defective mutations.

Most individuals who carry such susceptibility genes would have no obvious deleterious consequences. For example, the DR2 gene (described below) is the most important genetic contributor to MS susceptibility identified to date. Approximately half of patients with MS have this gene, but so do 15 to 20 percent of healthy Caucasians. Thus, only approximately 1 in 250 people who have DR2 develop MS.

The cumulative action of several susceptibility genes, each with weak effects and limited penetrance, is thought to underlie genetic susceptibility to MS. (Penetrance refers to the likelihood that a person carrying an allele will develop specific manifestations caused by that gene.) The effects of individual susceptibility genes may also be influenced by interactions with other genes and by specific environmental exposures. Locus heterogeneity is also likely, meaning that there are different susceptibility genes in different MS patients. The possibility that MS is a heterogeneous disease with different causes or pathological processes adds an additional level of complexity to the analysis. In addition to MS, similar issues are present in other autoimmune diseases such as diabetes mellitus that are genetically complex, and common research tools will be needed to decipher specific disease genes in these different conditions.

**Major Histocompatibility Complex.** The genetic region most clearly associated with MS susceptibility is the major histocompatibility complex (MHC, or HLA [human leukocyte antigen] in humans) locus on the short arm of chromosome 6 (6p21) (Box 2.4). This association has been seen in different population studies that have relied primarily on sporadic patients.[156] Formal genetic linkage to 6p has also been found in several recent whole-genome scans of multiple affected MS families. Many of the MHC genes are extraordinarily variable or polymorphic, reflecting the importance of genetic variation of these critical antigen-presenting molecules in the maintenance of a heterozygous advantage and the need to effectively present a diverse array of antigens if immune homeostasis is to be maintained. Immune homeostasis refers to the capacity of the immune system to respond appropriately to a diverse number of infectious pathogens and tumors without initiating unhealthy responses against self-constituents (auto-

---

**BOX 2.4**
**MHC, HLA, and DR2**

The major histocompatibility complex is a chromosomal region that contains more than 100 genes,[214] many of which make proteins involved in the immune system. It is named for the role it plays in rejecting tissue transplants (*histo-* means tissue). In humans, this region resides on chromosome 6 and is called the human leukocyte antigen gene complex. The terminology is slightly confusing because

*continued*

MHC and HLA also refer to the proteins that some of these genes make. In this report, the term "MHC molecules" is used to indicate the proteins.

The role of the immune system is to differentiate between self and non-self. This allows it to tell the difference between, for example, muscle tissue (self) and an invading virus (non-self) and to respond appropriately. To do this, the immune system relies on several different proteins that specifically bind antigens. This process is analogous to a lock and key. The "lock" is an antibody, a T-cell receptor, or an MHC molecule. The "key" is an antigen, which can be a carbohydrate, lipid, nucleic acid, or protein—anything that binds specifically to a component of the immune system.[15]

This discussion focuses on T-cell receptors and MHC molecules. T-cell receptors sit on the surface of T cells and bind to antigens outside the cell. (In the case of T-cell receptors and MHC molecules, antigens are small protein fragments.) Binding to an antigen signals the T cell either to die, to do nothing, or to become active. The signal context, such as whether the antigen is self or non-self, determines which of these signals is relayed. However the T cell cannot bind the antigen alone. It needs the help of an MHC molecule. MHC molecules sit on the surface of other cells. The MHC molecule, like two outstretched arms, holds onto an antigen and presents it to a T-cell receptor.

There are two major classes of MHC molecules. MHC I molecules, which are expressed on most cell types, present antigens to CD8+ T cells. MHC II molecules, which are expressed on special antigen presenting cells (APCs), present antigens to CD4+ T cells. In humans, there are three main class I molecules, HLA-A, HLA-B, and HLA-C, and three main class II molecules, HLA-DP, HLA-DQ, HLA-DR.

Each arm of the MHC molecule is made up of a separate protein. In the case of MHC I molecules, there is an $\alpha$-chain (A, B, or C) that pairs with the protein $b_2$-microglobulin. An MHC II molecule is made up of an $\alpha$-chain and a $\beta$-chain (for example, DP-$\alpha$ and DP-$\beta$), but the story becomes more complex. Each MHC molecule can bind many but not all of the thousands of antigens that confront the immune system. The immune system relies on diversity among the MHC proteins to help stack the odds in its favor.

The gene for each MHC protein chain comes in different varieties, or alleles. One of the MHC $\beta$-chains has more than 150 alleles.[10] Each of these alleles produces a slightly different protein. The proteins vary just enough that although they all function as MHC proteins, they can bind different antigens. Any one person will have two alleles, at most, for a particular MHC protein (there are two copies of each gene in human cells), but across a population of individuals, this variety becomes more important. For example, in Gambia, West Africa, 25 percent of HLA-B genes are the HLA-B53 allele, compared to less than 1 percent in Europe. HLA-B53 is very effective at presenting an antigen from the parasite that causes malaria to CD8+ T cells. Researchers hypothesize that because HLA-B53 can protect people from the most severe forms of malaria, it is more prevalent in Gambia.[138] Having a particular MHC allele can also be a disadvantage, as researchers have shown in the case of HLA-DR2 and MS. (HLA-DR2 actually designates both a specific DR-a chain allele and a DR-b chain allele.) Scientists still do not understand how HLA-DR2 predisposes individuals to MS, but this might have to do with the MHC molecule's ability to present specific antigens (for example, a fragment of myelin basic protein) to T cells.[129]

immune responses). In Caucasian MS populations of northern European descent, the critical MS-associated genetic region is thought to reside near the class II locus and is comprised of a group of genes with specific polymorphisms (alleles) that tend to occur in certain fixed combinations, termed haplotypes. In molecular terms, the "DR2" haplotype is designated as HLA-DRB1*1501, DQA1*0102, DQB1*0602. DR molecules are comprised of alpha and beta chains (encoded by A and B genes, respectively), and the polymorphisms are predominantly present in the beta chain. Of the more than 100 beta-chain sequence variations identified in humans, only one (1501, also designated as DR2) is associated with MS.

How can the DR2 association with MS be explained? The DR2 molecule itself may have a propensity to bind peptide antigens of myelin and stimulate disease-inducing T cells. DR2 is known to bind with high affinity to a region of MBP (spanning amino acids 89-98) thought to be "immunodominant" in humans. X-ray crystallography of the DR2-MBP peptide complex revealed that the DR2 molecule contains a distinctive hydrophobic pocket in its antigen-binding region, created by a unique alanine residue at the B71 position into which glutamic acid at position 93 of MBP is tightly bound, anchoring the MBP-DR2 complex.[75] In a larger sense, the structure of the antigen-binding domain of DR2 molecules likely facilitates binding of many peptides containing certain amino acid residues, specifically aromatic amino acids. Glatiramer acetate (copolymer 1), a currently available disease-modifying therapy for MS, is a random synthetic protein composed of four amino acids, including tyrosine. The tyrosine residues of processed copolymer peptides likely also bind to the hydrophobic pocket of DR2, perhaps interfering with presentation of this key MBP peptide to encephalitogenic T cells. It is surprising that no data exist on the interaction of DR2 and the response to glatiramer acetate in MS. Another possibility is that the DR2 molecule does not itself predispose to MS but that another nearby gene (perhaps another HLA gene such as DQ) is responsible. DR2 is also linked to other diseases. Besides MS, narcolepsy is the disease most strongly linked to DR2.

**Other MS Susceptibility or Modifier Genes.** In various studies, the HLA region has been estimated to confer somewhere between 10 percent and half of the inheritability of MS. To date, no other genes of major effect have been identified in genomic screens. Several studies appear to demonstrate that a deletion mutation in the CCR5 chemokine receptor gene (a coreceptor for HIV) on chromosome 3 confers a later age of onset or a more benign course of MS; this mutation is also associated with protection against HIV. This is particularly important because the expression of CCR5, which is increased in MS brain lesions, is thought to attract inflammatory cells into tissue. Another locus on chromosome 19q22 near apolipoprotein C1 has been linked to MS in several genomic screens, but the estimated $\lambda s$ is only 1.4. A polymorphism near the gene for myelin basic protein on chromosome 21 was reported to be linked to MS in a family from Finland, but not in other populations. Some studies have suggested linkages or associations with the TCR beta-chain locus on chromosome 7, the immunoglobulin heavy-chain locus on chromosome 14, and a region on chromosome 5, but others have not found similar linkages. The inability to confirm some genetic regions as containing MS susceptibility genes might reflect the small genetic contribution of these putative genes or genetic heterogeneity; alternatively, the original claim might have been spurious.

As noted above, it is likely that an additive model consisting of multiple independent genes, each with small effects, explains the non-MHC genetic contributions to MS. It should be emphasized, however, that the identification of specific genes that have even very minor genetic effects on MS can have an enormous payoff, both in terms of helping to decipher the underlying biology of MS and in pointing to new potential treatments. For example, the genetic studies discussed earlier that identified a role for the CCR5 chemokine receptor suggest that therapies aimed at this receptor could be investigated in people with MS.

## Genetic Heterogeneity in MS

Perhaps the strongest indication that MS is a heterogeneous disorder comes from HLA studies showing an absence of DR2 association in particular ethnic groups or perhaps in some clinical variants. In Japanese patients, one form of MS ("Western type") is characterized by disseminated CNS involvement and is associated with the DR2 haplotype. In contrast, a more restricted form of MS in which optic nerve and/or spinal cord involvement predominate ("Asian MS") is not associated with DR2. Lesions in the non-DR2-associated condition are frequently more severe and necrotizing than in the disseminated form.[109] In one report, the Asian MS form was genetically associated with an HLA gene named DP (the DPB1*0501 allele).[231] Another area of uncertainty is the strength of the association between primary progressive MS (PPMS) and DR2. A number of (relatively) small studies failed to show any association between PPMS and DR2, although a recent larger study from northern Ireland appeared to show an association; it is possible that PPMS represents more than one underlying disorder.

Evidence for genetic heterogeneity is not limited to case-control HLA association studies but is also derived from formal linkage studies. Analysis of the MHC locus in an American multiple affected member MS data set confirmed the significant genetic linkage to this region (lod score of 4.60),* and the specific association with the DR2 allele; however 25 percent of the families that were DR2 negative showed no linkage to the HLA region on 6p21. This indicated most likely the presence of locus heterogeneity in familial MS in Caucasians. A related

---

*Lod scores are based on the *l*ogarithm of the *od*ds of linkage between two genes. A score of 3 or more is considered evidence of a genetic linkage between a known gene (or gene marker) and another unknown gene that underlies a trait (such as MS). That information thus indicates that the trait has a genetic basis and localizes the gene to a specific chromosomal region.

observation in MS-prone Caucasian families is that the phenotypic expression of MS aggregates within families in some cases, suggesting that some clinical manifestations of MS are influenced by an individual's genetic background.

The extent to which distinct clinical forms of MS are associated with different susceptibility genes, as may be the case in EAE (see discussion of animal models), is not known. Also unknown is whether specific genes interact with certain causative agents or triggers. Genetic studies have the potential to answer these questions, particularly when the information is analyzed in combination with epidemiologic, clinical, and neuroimaging data.

## Other Demyelinating Diseases

There are several human and animal diseases of known etiology or pathogenesis that resemble either the clinical or the pathological features of MS (Table 2.13). Animal diseases that resemble MS are discussed under animal models. CNS demyelinating diseases include those mediated by immune responses, infection, and toxins, as well as inherited disorders. Infectious agents can induce direct injury of oligodendrocytes and their myelin membranes, as well as indirect injury via the immune system.

A variety of toxins, such as diphtheria, lysolecithin, cuprizone, and ethidium bromide, have been associated with demyelinating lesions. Many of these toxins induce lysis of the oligodendrocyte, with demyelination as a secondary effect. In addition, nutritional deprivation can be associated with demyelination in the central and peripheral nervous system.

### Immune-Mediated and Virus-Induced CNS Demyelinating Diseases

**ADEM as a Consequence of Vaccination.** Acute disseminated encephalomyelitis (ADEM), also known as post vaccination encephalomyelitis, occurs as a consequence of vaccination with neural antigens. EAE, the most widely used animal model of MS, is the animal counterpart of this human disease. ADEM is characterized pathologically by widespread perivenular inflammation and demyelination. The uniformity of lesions differs from the multi-age lesions found in even the most acute case of MS. Post vaccination immune-mediated damage can also affect the peripheral nervous system.

Since there is no standard laboratory-based test to diagnose the human disorder, the most reliable descriptions of the clinical spectrum of the disease are derived from collections of cases in which epidemiologic and statistical studies support the association of a triggering stimulus and disease. Such criteria are best met by cases associated with immunization with CNS tissue containing vaccines, for example, original Pasteur rabies vaccine. This vaccine complication can occur at all ages. A clinical hallmark of the rabies vaccine-associated form of ADEM is its uniphasic course evolving over days to several weeks.

**TABLE 2.13** CNS Demyelinating Diseases That Resemble MS

| Disease Type | Disease Characteristics |
|---|---|
| **Immune-Mediated Diseases** | |
| Acute disseminated encephalomyelitis (ADEM) | ADEM is characterized pathologically by widespread perivenular inflammation and demyelination. |
| Systemic inflammatory or autoimmune diseases | Multifocal CNS lesions can occur as a component of an array of systemic collagen vascular disorders including systemic lupus eryhemtosus and polyarteritis nodosa. The CNS manifestations may be the presenting feature. The peripheral nervous system is also frequently involved. |
| **Infection-Mediated Disease** | |
| Progressive multifocal leukoencephalitis (PML) | PML is caused by the JC virus, which infects and destroys oligodendrocytes with minimal associated immune response. It typically occurs in immunosuppressed or immunocompromised individuals and is common in AIDS. The disease can feature a subacute progressive or relapsing clinical course. The imaging and pathologic features can be distinguished from classical MS. |
| HTLV-1 myelopathy | HTLV-1 (human T-cell lymphotropic virus type I) infection is sometimes associated with a neurological syndrome called HTLV-1-associated myelopathy/tropical spastic paraparesis (HAM/TSP). Patients with HAM/TSP have a progressive myelopathy, usually with spastic paraparesis, sensory disturbance, bladder dysfunction, and occasionally, optic neuritis. |
| **Inherited Disorders** | |
| Dysmyelinating disorders (leukodystrophies) | These inherited disorders are characterized by specific gene defects that result in either inadequate formation or excess breakdown of myelin. There may be a prominent inflammatory response in the region of myelin breakdown, but this is considered to be secondary to tissue breakdown. To date, therapeutic attempts with immunomodulatory agents in the leukodystrophies, specifically, adrenoleukodystrophy, have been ineffective. |
| **Toxic Disorders** | |
| Toxic optic neuropathy, subacute myelo-optic neuropathy (SMON) | Outbreaks of toxic optic neuropathy and SMON have been described in Cuba and in Japan.[11,12,99] Sporadic cases of toxic optic neuropathy likely account for the disorder tobacco-alcohol amblyopia. Conversely, one need consider whether deficiency syndromes could underlie development of demyelinating syndromes; deficiency of vitamin $B_{12}$, a cofactor in myelin formation, has also been implicated. |

**ADEM as a Consequence of Infection.** ADEM, or postinfectious encephalomyelitis, has been implicated as a consequence of a wide array of viral infections, although for many, the epidemiologic data are not strong enough to support a causal link. Measles virus epidemics have, however, been convincingly linked to ADEM. Postinfectious encephalomyelitis (PIE) is thought to be autoimmune in nature rather than secondary to a direct virus injury for the following reasons: (1) encephalitis appears after the rash clears; (2) there is generally little or no evidence of infectious virus or viral genome in the CNS at the time of the demyelinating disease;[143] and (3) there is evidence of increased reactivity against myelin antigens during the demyelinating disease.[102] Postinfectious encephalomyelitis is generally uniphasic.

Immune system disturbances, which are known to occur following measles virus infection,[104] might underlie the immunopathological response of postinfectious encephalomyelitis. A new direction for studies of PIE involves the possibility of establishing a model for this disease in transgenic mice that express the CD46 measles virus receptor.[158]

Molecular cross-reactivity, or molecular mimicry, has been demonstrated between myelin antigens and an array of viruses. Homologous sequences from viruses have been used to induce EAE (for example, hepatitis virus antigens). The extent of T-cell receptor degeneracy (meaning that the same receptor can respond to a wide sequence of peptides) and T-cell receptor heterogeneity in humans suggests that a wide array of exogenous agents could induce such a disease mechanism. As in MS, the putative infectious trigger could be different in individual MS patients depending on their immunogenetic makeup and the status of their immune system at the time of infection. A remaining challenge in MS is to determine whether any infectious agents detected in the CNS of such cases also persist in the CNS without causing harm or whether they are responsible for generating a pathogenic immune response.

**Recurrent ADEM.** ADEM cases are usually sporadic, and it is sometimes difficult to identify the initiating factor. Relapsing cases of ADEM have been described, especially in younger-age patients. For some cases, characteristic pathologic material has been available. Similarly, the EAE model can be manipulated to produce a relapsing chronic disorder by selecting animals with specific immunogenetic backgrounds and timing their immunizations so that the underlying systemic immune response is amplified or the blood-brain barrier is altered. Such variables could also determine the nature of the response of humans when they are exposed to potential disease-inducing antigens.

**Progressive Multifocal Leukoencephalopathy (PML).** JC virus,* a member of the papovavirus family, is a common pathogen in humans, although the

---

*JC refers to the initials of the individual from whom the virus was isolated in 1970.

primary disease caused by this virus is not characterized. Common symptoms include hemiparesis, aphasia, focal seizures, and visual disturbances. JC virus is thought to reactivate in immunosuppressed hosts, especially individuals with AIDS, producing the opportunistic infection PML. The disease involves a progressive CNS syndrome with symptoms and signs that suggest white matter involvement. Demyelination is usually most prominent in the occipital lobes of the cerebral hemispheres. The histopathology is characterized by the presence of oligodendrocytes with intranuclear inclusion bodies filled with papovavirus infectious particles, indicating that this disease involves a direct, lytic infection of the oligodendrocyte; that is, the oligodendrocyte is broken apart after being infected with the virus. Enlarged astrocytes are also seen, suggesting that the JC virus can transform these cells. Demyelination is a result of the direct oligodendrocyte infection by JC virus. Thus, in PML the immune response is considered to be protective rather than pathogenic.

**Human T-Lymphotropic Virus-1 (HTLV-1).** This retrovirus is common in the tropics as well as Japan, and is usually associated with asymptomatic disease. HTLV-1 infection is infrequently associated with a T-cell leukemia or lymphoma or a neurological syndrome called HTLV-1-associated myelopathy/tropical spastic paraparesis (HAM/TSP). Patients with HAM/TSP have a progressive myelopathy usually with spastic paraparesis, sensory disturbance, bladder dysfunction, and occasionally, optic neuritis. The CSF generally shows a lymphocytic pleocytosis with elevated IgG and oligoclonal IgG bands directed against HTLV-1. Necrotizing lesions with inflammation in the white matter are present in the spinal cord.

HAM/TSP can resemble MS clinically. In fact, a case of HAM/TSP might be diagnosed as MS if it were not for the presence of HTLV-1 antibody and the observation that the HTLV-1 genome can be detected in the CNS.

The pathogenesis of HAM/TSP remains unclear. There are numerous CD8+ T cells that recognize the virus, suggesting that this immune response might foster white matter disease.[20] Infected glial cells are a possible source of inflammatory pathogenic cytokines and might also be the target for these cytolytic T cells.[140] In addition, there is some evidence that molecular mimicry plays a role in disease pathogenesis. Host genetic factors, for example, HLA type, might also be important in determining susceptibility to HAM/TSP after infection.

## Infectious Causes of MS

It has not been proven that MS is caused by an infectious agent, but various data, including the inflammatory nature of the disease, epidemiological studies, and a heightened immune response against several pathogens, suggest an infectious etiology (reviewed in 1998 by Kastrukoff et al.[107]). Demyelinating diseases that clinically and pathologically resemble MS can be caused by viral agents or

**TABLE 2.14**  Koch's Postulate on Causation of Disease by a Pathogen

| Postulate | Limitations |
| --- | --- |
| The pathogen is always present in pathologically affected tissue. | It would be rare to consistently isolate a pathogen from all cases of the disease that it causes because of shortcomings in isolation procedures. |
| The pathogen is not present in tissues from controls. | Pathogens can have a variety of clinical manifestations, from asymptomatic disease to varied diseases. |
| The pathogen can experimentally induce disease. | Host restriction may prevent experimental transmission. |

immunopathological responses (Table 2.14). Infectious agents might be able to cause demyelination either directly, as a result of oligodendrocyte lysis, or indirectly, by means of an immunopathological response. Demyelination mediated by an immunopathological response can occur by a number of mechanisms. For example, the infectious agent can induce a pathogenic cross-reactive immune response (molecular mimicry), or the release of myelin antigens can stimulate an immune response that is directed against white matter antigens and becomes more broad over time (epitope spreading). (See Box 2.3 for a summary of autoimmunity and disease.)

### Identification of MS Pathogens

There are clear limitations to using classical criteria to implicate a pathogen isolated in MS as a causal agent for the disease,[101] as shown in Table 2.14. These issues make it especially difficult to establish the significance of a positive isolation from tissues of a patient with MS.

However, all cases in which an infectious agent causes a disease will clearly not fit standard criteria, and individualization of the requirements is sometimes necessary. Because of these limitations, it is prudent to consider criteria that may be more appropriate and realistic. One could consider the following additional guidelines in analyzing disease causation by a pathogen: consistent transmission or isolation of the pathogen; cure or effective treatment of the disease following elimination of the pathogen; absence of the disease in geographic regions where the pathogen is not present. It may also be appropriate to consider particular molecular signatures related either to the genes of the pathogen or to the transcription expression profile associated with a particular pathogen. Many pathogens have been implicated over the years as etiological agents in MS (Table 2.15).

**TABLE 2.15**  Agents Isolated or Implicated in the Etiology of MS

| | |
|---|---|
| Spirochete | Simian cytomegalovirus |
| Rabies virus | Epstein-Barr virus |
| Scrapie-like agent | Measles virus |
| Parainfluenza virus | HTLV-1 |
| "Carp" agent | MS-associated retrovirus |
| Coronavirus | Human herpesvirus-6 |
| Canine distemper virus | Chlamydia |
| Herpes simplex-1 | |

Some of these claims have been doubted for the following reasons: contamination (for example, spirochete), artifacts of isolation methods (for example, simian cytomegalovirus), and normal flora (for example, herpes simplex-1 [HSV-1]). Although some of these agents are clearly capable of inducing a CNS demyelinating syndrome that resembles MS, it remains uncertain whether particular cases in which a pathogen is isolated represent a rare MS-like case or whether the pathogen may actually be a common cause of MS.

There are various possible explanations of why so many pathogens have been isolated in MS but no single pathogen has been consistently observed. First, there might be a variety of pathogens that can independently cause MS (i.e., the disease is multifactorial), perhaps inducing heterogeneous forms of the disease. Second, MS might not be an infectious disease. The isolations of different pathogens might all be artifactual or related to rare events associated with a particular pathogen. Third, the relationship of the pathogen to MS might be a relatively minor one, possibly through interactions with genetic factors. Finally, the true pathogen might not yet have been identified. Thus far, there is inadequate evidence to either accept or reject suggestions that any particular pathogen is causally related to MS.

A variety of members of the herpes group of viruses (for example, simian cytomegalovirus, Epstein-Barr virus, HSV-1, and human herpesvirus-6 [HHV-6]) have been implicated in the etiology of MS. Members of this group of viruses remain attractive candidates as etiologic agents in MS since they are common pathogens that are known to persist and reactivate from a latent stage (and therefore could trigger the attacks and remissions seen in MS) and in some cases can induce focal demyelination in animals (see discussion of animal models of virus-induced demyelination).

The most recent herpesvirus candidate to generate attention is HHV-6. HHV-6, a common pathogen, is the cause of the childhood disease, roseola (exanthem subitem). This virus is associated with febrile seizures in children,[87] can invade the CNS, and can persist in peripheral blood mononuclear cells and the spinal fluid. In some cases, HHV-6 induces an MS-like disease, which raises the issue of its broader involvement in MS. Some recent studies of HHV-6 have found no[130] or rare[72] evidence of HHV-6 genome in MS CSF (as well as little, if any, evidence of genome from several other members of the herpesvirus group). One recent study reported that there was an increased incidence of HHV-6 (as well as HSV and varicella-zoster virus) genome in CNS tissue from MS cases compared to tissues from controls; however, the differences were not statistically significant (see Sanders[190]). Some investigators have argued that the cell type that is infected by HHV-6 differs in MS CNS compared to controls and, therefore, that the virus plays a role in the pathogenesis of MS.[35] The interpretation of HHV-6 studies may be complicated because HHV-6 infection and the localization of the virus may be altered secondary to inflammation associated with MS or to immunosuppressive treatment of MS patients; therefore, a change in localization of HHV-6 in MS CNS compared to control CNS may be unrelated to any pathogenic role of HHV-6 in MS. Although HHV-6 may not induce the white matter lesions of MS, it remains a possibility that HHV-6 contributes to the demyelination seen in some cases of MS. The recent identification of CD46 as a cellular receptor for HHV-6[191] and the availability of transgenic mice that carry CD46[158] provide an opportunity to develop an experimental model of HHV-6-induced CNS disease pathogenesis.

A recent study found that CSF from MS patients was culture-positive for *Chlamydia pneumoniae* and PCR (polymerase chain reaction)-positive for this agent more commonly than CSF from patients with other neurological disease.[203] In addition, there was evidence of increased antibody against chlamydia in MS CSF, as well as evidence that MS CSF oligoclonal IgG bands were absorbed by chlamydia antigens. This work clearly needs confirmation.

## ANIMAL MODELS OF MS

Members of the public awaiting cures for specific diseases often express impatience with the fact that most research on the biological basis of disease is based on animal studies, complaining that the time and money spent on animal studies would be better invested in clinical trials. However, animal studies are not simply interchangeable with clinical studies. Ultimately, every biologically active substance exerts its effects at the cellular and molecular levels, and the evidence has shown that this is remarkably consistent among mammals, even those as different in body and mind as rats and humans. Thus, animals can serve as models for basic biological processes in humans and can provide information about how drugs work that would not be obtainable in clinical studies.

Animal models in which both spontaneous and induced disease occur have contributed greatly to our knowledge of the pathogenesis of diseases, and in the future, they will be increasingly used to aid in the assessment of various treatment modalities. A variety of animal models have been used to study the pathogenesis and experimental treatment of diseases that share features with MS (Table 2.16).[174]

**TABLE 2.16** Animal Models of MS

| Type of Model | Description |
| --- | --- |
| EAE | Immunization of mice, rats, or primates with myelin proteins (MBP, MOG, PLP) or other autoantigens (PLP). CREAE is a chronic, relapsing type of EAE |
| B-cell models | In contrast to T cells, there is no technology available to routinely clone autoantigen specific B cells. As an alternative approach, B-cell "monoclonal" mice have recently been generated by gene replacement transgenesis |
| Humanized models | Genetic engineering is used to produce animals that express particular human genes hypothesized to be involved in MS |
| Virus-induced demyelinating disease | A variety of viruses can induce CNS demyelination, including Theiler's murine encephalomyelitis virus, mouse hepatitis virus, and herpes simplex virus |

Most of our present knowledge of myelin-specific autoimmunity and, more generally, of immune reactivity within the CNS emanates from experimental animal models. It should, however, be noted that there is a diversity of distinct models, defined by the animal species, the target autoantigen, and the mode of induction. Three basic types of animal models have been developed to understand the disease mechanisms underlying MS: EAE, virus-induced demyelination, and genetically modified animals.

## Experimental Autoimmune Encephalomyelitis (EAE)

EAE models have served, in many respects, as the prototype for current thinking on the pathogenesis of MS. This paralytic disease is characterized by the presence of inflammation and demyelination in the CNS. It is an autoimmune syndrome induced in different susceptible strains and species, generally by intradermal immunization with myelin antigens (natural or synthetic) or by adoptive transfer of T lymphocytes reactive against myelin proteins. The antigens capable of inducing EAE vary depending upon the strain and species of animal, the adjuvants employed, and perhaps also the history of environmental exposures experienced by the animal. EAE should be considered not as a single model but rather as a heterogeneous family of related disorders. Each of the EAE variants reflects different aspects of human MS, and conversely, there is no one EAE model that represents the entire complexity of MS (Table 2.17).

As is the case in MS, susceptibilities to EAE are determined as complex genetic traits. In both disorders, the most evident susceptibility locus resides within the HLA locus. Also in both disorders, locus heterogeneity is extensive (i.e., different loci and genes). Different genes can act at specific stages of the

**TABLE 2.17** Comparison Between Multiple Sclerosis and EAE

|  | MS | EAE |
|---|---|---|
| **Clinical Presentation** | | |
| Relapses and remissions | Present | Present |
| Paralysis | Present | Present |
| Ataxia | Present | Present |
| Visual impairment | Present | Present |
| **Genetics** | | |
| MHC-linked susceptibility | Yes | Yes |
| Females more susceptible | Yes | Yes |
| **Pathology** | | |
| Demyelination | Present | Present |
| Axonal damage | Present | Present |
| T cells reactive to myelin | Present | Present |
| Antibodies to myelin | Present | Present |
| $\alpha$4-integrin, complement | Present | Present |
| TFN-$\alpha$, $\gamma$-IFN | Present | Present |
| **Therapy** | | |
| $\gamma$-IFN, systemic | Worsens | Cures |
| Anti-TNF-$\alpha$, systemic | Worsens | Cures |
| IL-4 transduced T cells | Not done | Cures |
| TNF-$\alpha$ transduced T cells | Not done | Worsens |
| Copaxone (glatiramer acetate) | Improves | Cures |
| Beta-interferon | Improves | Improves |

SOURCE: Larry Steinman, presentation to the committee, November 17, 1999.

EAE or Theiler's murine encephalomyelitis virus (TMEV) disease process, influencing severity, recovery, susceptibility to relapse, remyelination, and other elements of the phenotype. Knowledge of the extensive heterogeneity in disease susceptibility and modifier genes in these MS models should provide targets for study in human MS.

Even within genetically identical littermates, the immune response following immunization with whole myelin is heterogeneous, with different antigenic targets dominating in different individuals. When groups of genetically identical animals are housed in different facilities, the resulting clinical syndromes can be markedly different, presumably reflecting the effects of different individual microenvironments.

Studies of EAE established that the pathogenic agents of the disease are CD4+ T cells, which produce cytokines of the proinflammatory Th1 pattern (IFN-$\gamma$ and TNF-$\alpha$, but no IL-4) upon stimulation. The precursors of these T cells are contained within the normal immune repertoire, but they unfold their pathogenic potential only on activation, by either specific antigens, microbial superantigens, or mitogens.

In EAE induced in the Lewis rat strain (and H-2$^{u}$ mice) by immunization with MBP, the encephalitogenic T cells recognize almost exclusively single, circumscript epitope segments of the MBP in the molecular context of MHC class II (clonal dominance). This dominance can be gradually lost over time, a phenomenon referred to as determinant spreading. Furthermore, in these models, the T-cell receptor for most autoreactive T cells is based on a highly simplified repertoire of structural genes, such as the Vβ8.2 gene for the TCR β-chain. These unusual features of antigen recognition have raised hopes with regard to immuno-specific therapies. Unfortunately, however, they seem to be limited to only a few experimental models. Most EAE models, as well as the human myelin-specific T cells, do not show either striking epitope dominance or T-cell receptor biases.

To date, attempts to identify possible functions of CNS-specific T-cell classes distinct from CD4+ T cells have not led to consistent pictures. Evidence from T-cell transfer models and TCR transgenic mice suggests that CD8+ T cells might help control and limit an ongoing CD4+ dependent EAE process.

**B Cells in EAE.** Most acute EAE models show profuse inflammatory CNS reactions with a conspicuous absence of large-scale demyelination, implying that MS-like demyelination is not caused directly by myelin-specific T cells but must be brought about by other mechanisms. B cells are the best-characterized effectors of this function. Large, confluent inflammatory demyelinated lesions can be produced in rats by transferring encephalitogenic T cells along with a monoclonal antibody against myelin oligodendrocyte glycoprotein. The T cells cause inflammation, thereby opening the blood-brain barrier to the autoantibodies, which enter the CNS where they bind to myelin and destroy it via complement- or phagocyte-dependent mechanisms.[46] "Simple" immunization of rodents with MOG can also produce the same result.[2,53]

In addition to producing humoral autoantibodies, brain-specific B cells target and present myelin antigens to specific T cells. During this presentation process, the B cells may stimulate the activation of specific T cells, with a possible tendency to shift them from Th1 (pro-inflammatory) to Th2 cytokine (anti-inflammatory) profiles.

The roles of autoreactive B cells in the pathogenesis of EAE are incompletely understood, mostly because of technical shortcomings. In contrast to T cells, there is no technology available to routinely clone autoantigen-specific B cells. As an alternative approach, B-cell "monoclonal" mice have recently been generated by gene replacement transgenesis.[124] The germline repertoire of immunoglobulin genes in these mice has been replaced by the mature, rearranged gene encoding a MOG-specific autoantibody. Most, if not all, of the B cells in these mice express immunoglobulin receptors that are autoreactive to MOG. The mice spontaneously produce high titers of anti-MOG autoantibodies in their blood.

**Chronic Relapsing EAE (CREAE).** There is no natural, spontaneous animal model resembling MS. The immunological conditions leading to relapses and remissions of inflammatory demyelinating disease over time are most commonly examined in chronic relapsing versions of EAE. These episodic courses depend on the modes of immunization as well as on genetic factors innate to the host animals. Although the conditions that trigger relapses in CREAE models are not yet well understood, models are expected to provide clues to these essential aspects of MS, especially when refined by the use of suitable transgenic animals.

**Primate EAE.** It has recently been shown that a chronic relapsing EAE in a primate, the common marmoset, is more like MS than other EAE models.[174] This form of EAE, induced in marmosets by immunization with MOG, produces lesions that are almost indistinguishable from fresh, acute human MS plaques.[78] In both the human disease and this animal model, a zone of myelin destruction is seen at the margins of lesions; within the lesions, myelin sheaths are replaced by vesiculated membranous elements. MOG-specific antibodies, thought to be related to the deposition of antigen-specific antibody, are present over the vesiculated myelin. In both settings, oligodendrocytes were spared, and there was some evidence of myelin repair. Axonal pathology, however, was more conspicuous in MS cases than in this animal model. It has been suggested that processes mediated by T-cells initiate the demyelinating lesions and that other effector mechanisms are the principal offenders in damaging the myelin sheath. Mechanisms that initiate the lesion might be immunologically distinct from those that propagate disease. Antibodies might play an important role in these processes.[174] The marmoset EAE model has also confirmed the encephalitogenic potential of autoreactive T-cell clones, whose precursors are preformed in the healthy immune repertoire. At the same time, however, these experiments also show that all T-cell clones are not equally autoaggressive.

### Limitations of MS Animal Models

Experimental animal models of MS are based almost exclusively on the use of rodents, mostly rats and mice. Unfortunately, rodent and human immune systems differ to such a large degree that not all observations made in rodent EAE can be directly translated to human MS.

An important disadvantage of animal models is that they do not necessarily mirror the cellular or molecular pathology of MS. Some types of EAE, for example, produce brisk demyelination, whereas others produce little demyelination. Which is the best model? Since these features of MS are not yet fully understood, it is dificult to know how faithfully any given animal model of MS illustrates the human disease.

In addition, these models are not very tractable for studies on the electrophysiology and biophysics of neuronal function, a serious limitation in a disease such as MS in which symptoms and signs arise from impaired nerve function. Powerful research methods are now available for studying the physiology and biophysics of normal or injured nerve cells. These methods permit neuroscientists to study electrical signaling in both normal and injured neurons, but they require that these nerve cells, with reproducible abnormalities, be reproducibly located, within fractions of a millimeter, in specific parts of the nervous system so that they can be studied. In MS and in most currently available animal models, the pathology is patchy, and the location of demyelinated and injured neurons varies from case to case. For the electrophysiologist who studies neuronal signaling by precisely placing tiny microelectrodes within neurons, studying the physiology of demyelinated or otherwise injured neurons when their location varies from animal to animal is, indeed, a challenge. A model in which focal demyelination, or axonal injury, can be produced at specific locations that are consistent from animal to animal would be a great improvement.

## Virus-Induced Models

Viruses can cause demyelination in several ways, the most straightforward of which is for viruses to lyse, or break open, oligodendrocytes, the myelin-producing cells. In some cases, however, the immune system is also involved. The mechanism by which virus-induced immune-mediated demyelination is carried out is not clear, but roles for molecular mimicry, bystander damage, and superantigen activation of T cells have all been proposed (see Box 2.3).

The best developed models of virus-induced demyelination are those caused by certain strains of TMEV and the mouse hepatitis virus (MHV) (reviewed in Kastrukoff et al.[107]). Probably the most fruitful of the remaining models are those of semliki forest virus (SFV) and herpes simplex virus (HSV) (Table 2.18). The advantages of SFV are its small, simple genome and ease of mutagenesis. Although the HSV genome is large and complex, the wealth of molecular information related to this virus and the ability to manipulate the viral genome make it an attractive model system, as well.

**Theiler's Murine Encephalomyelitis Virus.** The DA strain of TMEV produces an inflammatory demyelinating disease of the spinal cord with lesions that resemble MS. A variety of experimental studies of TMEV-induced demyelination suggest that as in MS, the immune system fosters demyelination. The inflammatory, demyelinating, and multifocal lesions of TMEV infection are mediated at least in part by T cells directed against viral antigens. The inflammatory response directly contributes to tissue damage in this MS-like model, since susceptibility is determined in part by immune response genes and immunosuppression abrogates demyelination.

One to two weeks after inoculation with the DA virus, there is a brisk inflammatory response in the brain with high levels of virus. This is generally a subclinical process since the mouse usually appears normal. After three weeks, the brain pathology virtually disappears, but mice develop a progressive spastic para-

**TABLE 2.18**  Animal Viruses That Induce Demyelination

| Virus | Consequences of Infection in Animals |
|---|---|
| **Theiler's murine ecephalomyelitis virus** | The TO subgroup strains of TMEV produces an inflammatory demyelinating disease of the spinal cord with lesions that resemble MS. A variety of experimental studies of TMEV-induced demyelination suggest that the immune system fosters the white matter disease. |
| **Mouse hepatitis virus** | The many different strains of MHV lead to a plethora of different diseases, including hepatitis, as well respiratory CNS disorders. The presence and extent of demyelination depend on the viral genotype, dosage, and route of inoculation, as well as the strain, age, and immune status of the infected mouse. Virus persists in glial cells of demyelinated mice. |
| **Semliki forest virus** | Experimental infection of mice and rats with specific strains of SFV leads to demyelination; other strains induce an encephalomyelitis. Demyelination depends on the specific strain of virus, the mouse strain, and the immune status of the host.[68] Virus persists in the central nervous system. The role of the immune system in the demyelinating disease remains unclear. |
| **Herpes simplex virus** | Many strains of HSV produce a diffuse encephalitis in mice, but certain virus strains induce an inflammatory demyelinating disease in particular strains. Other strains of mice have multifocal demyelination that can relapse or persist in varied areas of the brain.[106] The role of the immune system in this model is unclear but appears to contribute to the destruction of CNS tissue.[211] |
| **Maedi visna virus** | Maedi visna is found only in sheep. There is no experimental rodent model of maedi visna infection, and therefore one needs to investigate sheep. The absence of markers for the sheep's immune system and of genetically modified sheep with knockouts of different arms of the immune system are clear limitations of the maedi visna model. The pathology of disease varies from an encephalomyelitis to a pure inflammatory demyelination that resembles MS.[37] Virus persists during the disease with a restricted expression in microglial cells. It remains unclear whether demyelination is a result of direct viral lysis or is mediated by the immune response. |
| **Canine distemper virus** | CDV produces a variety of CNS diseases in dogs, including acute and chronic encephalitis and demyelinating disease. Virus persists in the chronic disease and appears to be present in oligodendrocytes in some cases. Work with this model has been limited since dogs are required as the host. The pathogenesis of the demyelinating disease remains unclear. |

paresis associated with an inflammatory demyelinating disease of the spinal cord. Although the titers of DA virus decrease over the first few weeks, virus persists in the central nervous system for the life of the mouse. The persistent virus is said to have a restricted, or incomplete, expression. In other words, viral genome is present, but the levels of infectious virus are low, with relatively little viral capsid protein produced. (The capsid is the protein shell surrounding the viral DNA or RNA and is generally required for viral infectivity.)

Advantages of the TMEV model include the simplicity of its genome, the detailed structural information about the virus, the ease with which it can be genetically manipulated, and finally, the extensive knowledge about the genes and immune system of mice, the natural host of TMEV (see Box 2.5.).

Despite all that is known about TMEV and despite the ease in manipulating this simple virus, the pathogenesis of the demyelinating disease is not yet fully understood. It is clear that viral persistence in the oligodendrocytes and microglia is critical to the development of TMEV-induced demyelination; that is, an ongoing virus infection is always associated with the white matter disease. It is also clear that the immune system contributes to the late demyelinating disease, but exactly how remains poorly understood. Part of the difficulty in dissecting the role of the immune system in the pathogenesis of TMEV (as well as some of the other animal models of virus-induced demyelination) is that it changes over time. Early after infection, the immune system controls the virus infection, but later in

---

**BOX 2.5**
**Advantages of the TMEV Model of**
**Virus-Induced Demyelination**

The following features of TMEV make it an attractive model for studies of virus-induced immune-mediated demyelination:

- **The virus is relatively small and simple**, with only four structural proteins in the infectious particle. The genome is only approximately 8,100 nucleotides in length.
- **A great deal is known about TMEV.** Three strains are completely sequenced. The crystallographic structure of three strains of the virus has been solved, so that the location of every amino acid in the infectious particle is known. The B-cell epitopes that are the targets for neutralizing antibody have been identified and located on the infectious particle. Some of the epitopes on the virus that trigger proliferation of immune CD4+ T cells and some that act as targets for an antivirus cytolytic T-cell response are also known. Some components of the receptor for the virus have been identified.
- **The virus is easily manipulated.** Infectious clones of the virus are available so mutations can be quickly engineered into any region of the genome.
- **There is extensive knowledge about mouse genetics and immunology.** The mouse, which is the natural and experimental host of TMEV, provides a special benefit in studies of the pathogenesis of TMEV-induced demyelinating disease because so much is known about mouse genetics and the immune system. In addition, many genetically engineered mice are available, including those in which specific genes for different components of the immune system have been "knocked out."

the disease, it contributes to the demyelination. In addition, during the disease there appears to be a critical "balance" of the immune response that is necessary for the induction of demyelination: an inadequate immune response early in the disease can lead to the death of the mouse within the first couple of weeks and before the appearance of demyelination, while a very forceful immune response early can lead to clearance of the virus so that no virus persists and white matter disease fails to develop. In other words, viral persistence and demyelination occur only in association with a certain level of the antiviral immune response.

CD4+, as well as CD8+, T cells might be mediators of the late demyelinating disease. DA virus infection induces demyelination in both CD4+ and CD8+ T-cell knockout mice, suggesting that both CD4+ and CD8+ T cells mediate the late demyelinating disease.[149] The targets for these immunopathogenic CD4+ and the CD8+ T cells are unknown. There is some evidence for epitope spreading, in which an increasing number of myelin antigenic epitopes become the target for a CD4+ T-cell response.[141] However, epitope spreading appears to begin after demyelination has become established, so it is unclear how important this mechanism of immunopathology is to DA-induced demyelination, especially early in the white matter disease.

Mouse strains that are resistant to DA-induced demyelinating disease mount an antivirus cytolytic T-cell response and clear the virus. Mouse strains that are susceptible to the late disease do not mount this response, presumably allowing for virus persistence. L*, a small protein synthesized by demyelinating strains of TMEV via alternative translation, is critical for TMEV persistence and demyelination.[38] L* inhibits the antivirus cytolytic T-cell response in susceptible mouse strains through an, as yet, unknown mechanism.[122] Certain cells, for example, oligodendrocytes, may have cell-specific RNA-binding proteins that bind to the viral genome (as well as some nonviral messenger RNAs) and regulate whether L* or the viral capsid proteins are synthesized. The more L* that is synthesized, the more the expression of the virus is restricted.

TMEV induces apoptosis in certain cells, including neurons and macrophages.[100] The relationship between apoptosis and DA-induced demyelination remains an open question.

**Mouse Hepatitis Virus.** There are many different strains of mouse hepatitis virus that lead to a plethora of different diseases, including hepatitis as well as respiratory and CNS disorders. JHM, S, and A59 strains of MHV induce demyelination. The extent of demyelination depends on the virus, including its genotype, dosage, and route of inoculation, as well as on the condition of the infected mouse, including its strain, age, and immune status. Intracerebral inoculation of the JHM strain into weanling mice leads to demyelination in the mice that survive encephalitis. Virus persists in glial cells of demyelinated mice.

At present, there are some notable limitations to MHV pathogenesis studies. MHV has a remarkably large viral genome (32 kb), making this a complex pathogen. A system for efficient and rapid mutagenesis has not yet been perfected, and therefore manipulation of the viral genome is not straightforward.

Investigators initially thought that demyelination occurred as a result of viral lysis of oligodendrocytes independently of the immune system. More recent studies, however, suggested that it does contribute to the demyelination (reviewed in 1996 by Houtman et al.[95]). For example, investigators found that C57BL/6 mice that are immunosuppressed by gamma irradiation before being exposed to the JHM virus develop less severe demyelination. Adoptive transfer of JHM virus-infected splenic T cells to the infected irradiated mice leads to the development of significant demyelination. Other studies in rats showed that transfer of T cells from rats that have JHM virus-induced demyelinating encephalomyelitis leads to the development of experimental allergic encephalomyelitis-like lesions. Studies in CD4+ and CD8+ knockout mice[115] demonstrated that both T-cell types are needed for clearance of the virus; however, CD4+ T cells contribute to central nervous system inflammation and demyelination. A suggestion of the latter study was that the CD4+ T cells influenced the expression of cytokines, specifically the RANTES cytokine, and led to macrophage entry into the CNS; treatment of the infected mice with anti-RANTES antibody resulted in a decrease in macrophage infiltration and demyelination. These studies and conclusions require confirmation.

The committee notes that the following animal models of virus-induced demyelinating disease are particularly likely to yield clues to the pathogenesis of MS:

- *HTLV-1 associated myelopathy.* The HAM/TSP syndrome resembles MS. Because the principles relevant to this human disease might be similar to those in MS, investigating the pathogenesis of this disease could reveal insights into MS pathogenesis. The development of a widely available animal model for HAM/TSP is a high priority.

- *Postinfectious encephalomyelitis.* PIE is of special interest since recurrences following this acute inflammatory white matter disease are so similar to MS attacks that the two diseases are indistinguishable, indicating a close relationship between PIE and MS. The availability of transgenic mice that carry a receptor for measles virus might provide an experimental model for the study of PIE.

- *Theiler's murine encephalomyelitis virus.* The pathological lesions of TMEV are similar to MS plaques; therefore, continuing delineation of the mechanism by which the immune system contributes to the virus-induced demyelination might lead to a better understanding of the pathogenesis of demyelinating disease.

- *Mouse hepatitis virus.* Research on the MHV-induced demyelination model is presently limited by difficulties with site-directed mutagenesis methods. A high priority for research with this virus should be the generation of an infectious MHV cDNA clone and a refinement of mutagenesis techniques.

## Genetically Engineered Models

Molecular genetic manipulation has become one of the most important tools for evaluating gene function in living organisms.[52,79,147] These tools of molecular biology have extended the reach of researchers to a new level of understanding of neurodegeneration mechanisms. The development of animal models for neurodegenerative disorders by means of genetic engineering has revolutionized experimental neurology.[27] The identification and cloning of genes involved in diseases such as Alzheimer's, Huntington's, and amyotropic lateral sclerosis provided the keys to develop mice that overexpress the human genes involved in these diseases (reviewed in 1999 by Brusa[27]). The nonobese diabetic (NOD) mouse is genetically susceptible to diabetes, and transgenic NOD mice have been developed to allow examination of the role of possible autoantigens in the development of diabetes, which like MS involves an inflammatory autoimmune pathology.[227] The NOD mouse has also identified candidate molecules and processes that have influenced research in EAE and MS.[65]

Mutant mice have provided insights into all aspects of biology for generations, but only in the last two decades has it been possible to modify the expression of selected genes, an essential breakthrough for analyzing the role of specific genes in complex processes and diseases such as MS. In addition, identification of the genes that are activated or inactivated in both pathological and repair processes in the CNS will likely reveal new and unexpected targets for uniquely selective disease-modifying therapies in MS.

"Reverse genetics" and "forward genetics" offer contrasting approaches to the analysis of gene function. Forward genetics is an approach to identify genes that are not already implicated in a particular disease or process. Reverse genetics is an approach to identify the role of genes whose involvement in the disease or process being studied is already implicated.

In forward genetics, large numbers of mice are mutagenized (using techniques that mutagenize genes at random); their resulting phenotypes are analyzed to select mutants that exhibit spontaneous MS. The mutated genes in the selected mutants are then positionally cloned and identified. The homologous human clones can also be identified, a task that is becoming vastly simpler as the human genome project nears completion. The advantage of this approach is that the screen is not biased in any way and can reveal genes beyond those already known to be involved in MS. Another advantage of forward genetics is that once a gene is identified in a disease process, one can quickly do a screen for suppressors and enhancers of the phenotype. This will yield the entire biochemical pathway (as opposed to just one step) involved in disease pathogenesis.

One limitation to the forward genetics approach is that only a small percentage of the mutated genes will result in a phenotype relevant to MS. Consequently, large numbers of mutants have to be screened, which is generally expensive, time-consuming, and labor intensive. Yet the rewards—especially for complex diseases and processes that have resisted traditional approaches—are unparalleled.

In reverse genetics, mutant strains of mice that either overexpress or lack specific genes are generated through a variety of techniques. The classic approach to creating transgenic mice is to inject a foreign gene ("transgene") into a fertilized egg, thereby inducing overexpression of the transgene. The egg bearing the transgene is implanted into a host mother. Progeny bearing DNA encoding the transgene are screened, as are the corresponding levels of RNA and protein. This transgene is randomly incorporated into a mouse chromosome and ultimately leads to production of the protein of interest.[27] This approach has been used to transfer human genes (such as those for T-cell receptor, HLA DR2, and CD4) into mice to see if they develop spontaneous MS. One limitation of "knock-in" mice is that genes can be inserted in uneven copy numbers in "replicate" animals or might be integrated into disparate sites in the genome.[226]

Gene expression can also be altered through knockout experiments. Knockout mice, or null mutants, are created using embryonic stem cells and homologous recombination to produce a cell line in which a certain gene has been removed, or ablated. When transferred into an early mouse embryo, these cells can participate in the generation of all cell lineages including germ cells, thereby transmitting their genotype to the next generation. Alternatively, embryonic stem cells can be used to create so-called knock-in mice by inserting a gene into a particular locus.

The transgenic gene-targeting approaches described above all rely on irreversible changes to the genome that are present from the onset of development throughout an animal's life. The function of the gene must be deduced from the phenotype of animals that have been deficient for the product of the disrupted gene throughout development. Yet, many genes play different roles at different stages of development and in different tissues. This presents serious drawbacks (reviewed in 1998 by Gingrich and Roder[79] and in 1999 by Muller[147]). First, an animal with a gene alteration that lethally disrupts development obviously cannot be studied as an adult—even though the gene might play another critical role, for example, in neural repair. This is particularly relevant to MS because many of the genes that regulate embryonic neural development also regulate neural repair in adults. Another limitation of transgenic models is that changes in the regulation of other genes could yield misleading phenotypes, in part because of differences between effects of the gene at different developmental stages, gene redundancy (other genes might also play the role of the missing gene), or adaptive mecha-

nisms that compensate for the missing gene. Even apparently unaltered phenotypes would thus not prove that the gene was not involved in the disease or
process being studied. Another limitation of this approach is that in physiological
responses, gene products tend to be produced in waves, whereas in transgenics,
expression is usually "on" from the time of development.

Alternative approaches in which one gene, or parts of it, can be inactivated or
activated in specific tissues or at specific times ("conditional" and "inducible"
mutants) have recently been developed in this rapidly expanding array of gene-
altering techniques (reviewed in Brusa, 1999;[27] Gingrich and Roder, 1998;[79] and
van der Neut, 1997[215]). This second generation of transgenic technology derives
from the possibility of modulating the suppression of a transgene with external
stimuli, by using a "biological switch" that can turn the foreign gene on and off.

Gene expression patterns in the nervous system are highly regionalized. For
example, the enzymes involved in producing neurotransmitters and their receptors differ from one subpopulation of neurons to another. Other proteins are more
widespread, such as the intermediate filament proteins NF (neurofilament) or
GFAP (glial fibrillary acidic protein), or are ubiquitous, such as N-CAMs (neural
cell adhesion molecules) and integrins.[215] Thus, it would be particularly advanta-
geous to develop tissue-specific mutants for MS research. The development of
inducible systems will become an important tool in the many diverse aspects of
research on the disease mechanisms and possibilities for repair in MS, including
the potential administration of gene therapy.

**Transgenic Mice and Demyelinating Disease.** Transgenic overexpression
of cytokines or gene targets of cytokines in the CNS offers a relatively non-
intrusive mechanism to assess the role of individual cytokines in CNS development, function, and response to insult. A common technique for assessing the
effects of a particular cytokine in EAE is to induce its expression directly in the
CNS. This allows researchers to ask whether expression of the cytokine induces
CNS pathology similar to that seen in MS. Directed expression of transgenes in
the CNS relies on promoters that normally control the expression of CNS-specific
genes. This includes the GFAP gene promoter, which drives expression in astrocytes, as well as the neurofilament promoter (neurons), and the myelin basic
protein promoter (oligodendrocytes). To date, no one has isolated a microglial-
specific promoter.

Only MBP promoters have been used to overexpress gamma-interferon in
the CNS.[47,94,176] Phenotypes of transgenic mice range from a lethal, "jimpy"-like
hypomyelinating mouse,[47]* through progressive demyelinating disease,[94] to mice
with no outward phenotype that nevertheless showed progression from EAE to a

---

*A point mutation in the gene coding for myelin proteolipid protein causes male offspring of jimpy
mice to have little or no myelination. Affected mice develop severe tremors and die prematurely at
approximately 30 days.

chronic demyelinating disease in contrast to control mice that recovered from EAE-induced demyelination.[176] It is of interest that the same laboratory observed both extremes using the same constructs.[13,176] This might be because the transgenes were unevenly integrated at different loci, since levels of expression did not obviously correlate with phenotype in one case.[176] Asymptomatic transgenic mice did, however, show enhanced glial responses to CNS injury,[13] and exacerbated ischemic infarction (Lambertsen et al., unpublished). These asymptomatic mice presumably reflect sub-threshold levels of cytokine. Nevertheless, crossing an asymptomatic MBP promoter-driven gamma-interferon transgenic mouse with MBP or MHC class I mice produced a more extreme jimpy phenotype.[13] This might provide a clue to cytotoxic effects of beta-interferon-$\gamma$ on oligodendrocytes,[3] being perhaps dependent on local interferon-$\gamma$ titers becoming sufficiently high to stimulate MHC I induction.[151] It is not known whether similar mechanisms account for oligodendrocyte pathology in TNF-$\alpha$ and interferon-$\alpha$ transgenic mice.

The IL-3 and IL-12 transgenic mice provide a useful counterpart, there being no obvious suggestion of a direct effect on oligodendrocytes.[39,160] These mice illustrate the potential for direct macrophage and microglial attack on oligodendrocytes, which might occur in TNF-$\alpha$ transgenic mice.[4,33,204] It is not clear from any of these experiments whether activation of immune cells took place within the CNS or following cytokine exit to the periphery. A systemic effect must account for the fact that overexpression of the antiinflammatory cytokine IL-10 protected animals from EAE in two separate preparations.[19,50] The fact that IL-4 transgenic mice did not show similar resistance[19] might reflect insufficient expression within the CNS or strain background differences, given that IL-4 knockout exacerbated disease in another study.[66]

Most recently, a transgenic mouse has been "constructed" that expresses T-cell receptor genes from a human MBP-specific T-cell clone, along with relevant human MHC class II determinants and MBP. Under certain conditions, this "humanized" mouse developed spontaneous EAE that indeed showed inflammation with some demyelination.[129]

**Summary of Genetic Models.** In recent years, there have been many advances in the use of transgenes (including gene knockouts), as well as even more sophisticated models that make use of tissue-specific and time-dependent regulators. These models should facilitate the development of rational therapies and the transfer of knowledge from animal models to the prevention and treatment of human disease.[226] However, although temporally regulated targeting controlled by the administration of an environmental inducer has become feasible with high efficiency for some organs, it remains to be further improved for other tissues, particularly the brain.[147]

New generations of inducible promoters will more faithfully mimic the in vivo kinetics and dynamics of cytokine production. Knock-in mice, in which transgenes are integrated into defined loci through homologous recombination, will likewise overcome the problems of uneven gene copy numbers in replicate animals and disparate sites of integration in the genome.

# REFERENCES

1. Acheson ED. 1977. Epidemiology of multiple sclerosis. *Br Med Bull.*;33:9-14.
2. Adelmann M, Wood J, Benzel I, et al. 1995. The N-terminal domain of the myelin oligodendro-cyte glycoprotein (MOG) induces acute demyelinating experimental autoimmune encephalo-myelitis in the Lewis rat. *J Neuroimmunol.*;63:17-27.
3. Agresti C, D'Urso D, Levi G. 1996. Reversible inhibitory effects of interferon-gamma and tumour necrosis factor-alpha on oligodendroglial lineage cell proliferation and differentiation in vitro. *Eur J Neurosci.*;8:1106-16.
4. Akassoglou K, Bauer J, Kassiotis G, et al. 1998. Oligodendrocyte apoptosis and primary demy-elination induced by local TNF/p55TNF receptor signaling in the central nervous system of transgenic mice: models for multiple sclerosis with primary oligodendrogliopathy. *Am J Pathol.*;153:801-13.
5. Albert LJ, Inman RD. 1999. Molecular mimicry and autoimmunity. *N Engl J Med.*;341:2068-74.
6. Allain H, Schuck S. 1998. Observations on differences between interferons to treat multiple sclerosis. *Journal of Clinical Research*;1:381-392.
7. Allegretta M, Nicklas JA, Sriram S, Albertini RJ. 1990. T cells responsive to myelin basic protein in patients with multiple sclerosis. *Science.*;247:718-21.
8. Amato MP, Ponziani G, Bartolozzi ML, Siracusa G. 1999. A prospective study on the natural history of multiple sclerosis: clues to the conduct and interpretation of clinical trials. *J Neurol Sci.*;168:96-106.
9. Antel JP, Becher B, Owens T. 1996. Immunotherapy for multiple sclerosis: from theory to practice. *Nat Med.*;2:1074-5.
10. Apple RJ, Erlich HA. 1996. HLA class II genes: structure and diversity. Browning M, McMichael A, eds. *HLA and MHC: Genes, Molecules and Function.* Oxford: BIOS Scientific Publishers Limited; 97-109.
11. Arbiser JL, Kraeft SK, van Leeuwen R, et al. 1998. Clioquinol-zinc chelate: a candidate caus-ative agent of subacute myelo-optic neuropathy. *Mol Med.*;4:665-670.
12. Ascherio A. 1997. Antimetabolites and an optic neuropathy epidemic in Cuba. *Am J Clin Nutr.*;65:1092-1093.
13. Baerwald KD, Corbin JG, Popko B. 2000. Major histocompatibility complex heavy chain accumulation in the endoplasmic reticulum of oligodendrocytes results in myelin abnormali-ties. *J Neurosci Res.*;59:160-9.
14. Barkhof F, Filippi M, Miller DH, et al. 1997. Comparison of MRI criteria at first presentation to predict conversion to clinically definite multiple sclerosis. *Brain.*;120 :2059-69.
15. Benjamini E, Leskowitz S. 1991. *Immunology: a Short Course.* NY: Wiley-Liss, Inc.
16. Benveniste EN. 1997. Role of macrophages/microglia in multiple sclerosis and experimental allergic encephalomyelitis. *J Mol Med.*;75:165-73.
17. Bernard CC, Johns TG, Slavin A, et al. 1997. Myelin oligodendrocyte glycoprotein: a novel candidate autoantigen in multiple sclerosis. *J Mol Med.*;75:77-88.
18. Berti R, Jacobson S. 1999. Role of viral infection in the aetiology of multiple sclerosis. Status of current knowledge and therapeutic implications. *CNS Drugs.*;12:1-7.
19. Bettelli E, Das MP, Howard ED, Weiner HL, Sobel RA, Kuchroo VK. 1998. IL-10 is critical in the regulation of autoimmune encephalomyelitis as demonstrated by studies of IL-10- and IL-4-deficient and transgenic mice. *J Immunol.*;161:3299-306.

20. Bieganowska KD, Ausubel LJ, Modabber Y, Slovik E, Messersmith W, Hafler DA. 1997. Direct ex vivo analysis of activated, Fas-sensitive autoreactive T cells in human autoimmune disease. *J Exp Med.*;185:1585-94.
21. Billingham LJ, Abrams KR, Jones DR. 1999. Methods for the analysis of quality-of-life and survival data in health technology assessment. *Health Technol Assess.*;3:1-152.
22. Black JA, Dib-Hajj S, Baker D, Newcombe J, Cuzner ML, Waxman SG. 2000. Sensory neuron specific sodium channel SNS is abnormally expressed in the brains of mice with experimental allergic encephalomyelitis and humans with multiple sclerosis. *Proc Natl Acad Sci U.S.A.*;97:11598-11602.
23. Black JA, Waxman SG, Smith ME. 1987. Macromolecular structure of axonal membrane during acute experimental allergic encephalomyelitis in rat and guinea pig spinal cord. *J Neuropathol Exp Neurol.*;46:167-84.
24. Brex PA, Parker GJ, Leary SM, et al. 2000. Lesion heterogeneity in multiple sclerosis: a study of the relations between appearances on T1 weighted images, T1 relaxation times, and metabolite concentrations. *J Neurol Neurosurg Psychiatry.*;68:627-32.
25. Brosnan CF, Battistini L, Gao YL, Raine CS, Aquino DA. 1996. Heat shock proteins and multiple sclerosis: a review. *J Neuropathol Exp Neurol.*;55:389-402.
26. Brosnan CF, Raine CS. 1996. Mechanisms of immune injury in multiple sclerosis. *Brain Pathol.*;6:243-57.
27. Brusa R. 1999. Genetically modified mice in neuropharmacology. *Pharmacol Res.*;39:405-19.
28. Brustle O, Jones KN, Learish RD, et al. 1999. Embryonic stem cell-derived glial precursors: a source of myelinating transplants. *Science.*;285:754-6.
29. Bryant J, Clegg A, Milne R. 2000. Cost utility of drugs for multiple sclerosis. Systematic review places study in contrast. *BMJ.*;320:1474-5; discussion 1475-6.
30. Burgoon MP, Williamson RA, Owens GP, et al. 1999. Cloning the antibody response in humans with inflammatory CNS disease: isolation of measles virus-specific antibodies from phage display libraries of a subacute sclerosing panencephalitis brain. *J Neuroimmunol.*;94:204-11.
31. Calabresi PA, Tranquill LR, Dambrosia JM, et al. 1997. Increases in soluble VCAM-1 correlate with a decrease in MRI lesions in multiple sclerosis treated with interferon beta-1b. *Ann Neurol.*;41:669-74.
32. Callard R, George AJ, Stark J. 1999. Cytokines, chaos, and complexity. *Immunity.*;11:507-13.
33. Campbell IL, Stalder AK, Akwa Y, Pagenstecher A, Asensio VC. 1998. Transgenic models to study the actions of cytokines in the central nervous system. *Neuroimmunomodulation.*;5:126-35.
34. Campi A, Pontesilli S, Gerevini S, Scotti G. 2000. Comparison of MRI pulse sequences for investigation of lesions of the cervical spinal cord. *Neuroradiology.*;42:669-75.
35. Challoner PB, Smith KT, Parker JD, et al. 1995. Plaque-associated expression of human herpesvirus 6 in multiple sclerosis. *Proc Natl Acad Sci U S A.*;92:7440-4.
36. Charcot M. 1868. Histologie de la sclerose en plaques. *Gaz Hosp.*;141:554-555, 557-558.
37. Chebloune Y, Karr BM, Raghavan R, et al. 1998. Neuroinvasion by ovine lentivirus in infected sheep mediated by inflammatory cells associated with experimental allergic encephalomyelitis. *J Neurovirol.*;4:38-48.
38. Chen HH, Kong WP, Zhang L, Ward PL, Roos RP. 1995. A picornaviral protein synthesized out of frame with the polyprotein plays a key role in a virus-induced immune-mediated demyelinating disease. *Nat Med.*;1:927-31.
39. Chiang CS, Powell HC, Gold LH, Samimi A, Campbell IL. 1996. Macrophage/microglial-mediated primary demyelination and motor disease induced by the central nervous system production of interleukin-3 in transgenic mice. *J Clin Invest.*;97:1512-24.
40. Chofflon M, Juillard C, Juillard P, Gauthier G, Grau GE. 1992. Tumor necrosis factor alpha production as a possible predictor of relapse in patients with multiple sclerosis. *Eur Cytokine Netw.*;3:523-31.

41. Cochran JR, Cameron TO, Stern LJ. 2000. The relationship of MHC-peptide binding and T cell activation probed using chemically defined MHC class II oligomers. *Immunity.*;12:241-50.
42. Cohen IR. 1991. Autoimmunity to chaperonins in the pathogenesis of arthritis and diabetes. *Annu Rev Immunol.*;9:567-89.
43. Cohen JA, Carter JL, Kinkel RP, Schwid SR. 1999. Therapy of relapsing multiple sclerosis. Treatment approaches for nonresponders. *J Neuroimmunol.*;98:29-36.
44. Compston A. 1997. Genetic epidemiology of multiple sclerosis. *J Neurol Neurosurg Psychiatry.*;62:553-61.
45. Confavreux C, Vukusic S, Moreau T, Adeleine P. 2000. Relapses and progression of disability in multiple sclerosis. *N Engl J Med.*;343:1430-1438.
46. Conlon P, Oksenberg JR, Zhang J, Steinman L. 1999. The immunobiology of multiple sclerosis: an autoimmune disease of the central nervous system. *Neurobiol Dis.*;6:149-66.
47. Corbin JG, Kelly D, Rath EM, Baerwald KD, Suzuki K, Popko B. 1996. Targeted CNS expression of interferon-gamma in transgenic mice leads to hypomyelination, reactive gliosis, and abnormal cerebellar development. *Mol Cell Neurosci.*;7:354-70.
48. Cortese I, Tafi R, Grimaldi LM, Martino G, Nicosia A, Cortese R. 1996. Identification of peptides specific for cerebrospinal fluid antibodies in multiple sclerosis by using phage libraries. *Proc Natl Acad Sci U S A.*;93:11063-7.
49. Cotter RL, Burke WJ, Thomas VS, Potter JF, Zheng J, Gendelman HE. 1999. Insights into the neurodegenerative process of Alzheimer's disease: a role for mononuclear phagocyte-associated inflammation and neurotoxicity. *J Leukoc Biol.*;65:416-27.
50. Cua DJ, Groux H, Hinton DR, Stohlman SA, Coffman RL. 1999. Transgenic interleukin 10 prevents induction of experimental autoimmune encephalomyelitis. *J Exp Med.*;189:1005-10.
51. Davie CA, Barker GJ, Webb S, et al. 1995. Persistent functional deficit in multiple sclerosis and autosomal dominant cerebellar ataxia is associated with axon loss . *Brain.*;118 :1583-92.
52. Davies RW, Gallagher EJ, Savioz A. 1994. Reverse genetics of the mouse central nervous system: targeted genetic analysis of neuropeptide function and reverse genetic screens for genes involved in human neurodegenerative disease. *Prog Neurobiol.*;42:319-31.
53. Devaux B, Enderlin F, Wallner B, Smilek DE. 1997. Induction of EAE in mice with recombinant human MOG, and treatment of EAE with a MOG peptide. *J Neuroimmunol.*;75:169-73.
54. Donnenberg AD. 1997. An overview of the immune system: Immunologycial mechanisms in immune deficiency and autoimmunity. Leffell MS, Donnenberg AD, Rose NRE. *Handbook of Human Immunology.* Boca Raton: CRC Press; 47-64.
55. Dugandzija-Novakovic S, Koszowski AG, Levinson SR, Shrager P. 1995. Clustering of Na+ channels and node of Ranvier formation in remyelinating axons. *J Neurosci.*;15:492-503.
56. Ebers GC, Sadovnick AD. Paty DW, Ebers GC, eds. 1997a. *Multiple Sclerosis.* Philadelphia, PA: F.A. Davis Company; 5-28.
57. Ebers GC, Sadovnick AD. 1997b. Susceptibility: Genetics in multiple sclerosis. Paty DW, Ebers GC, eds. *Multiple Sclerosis.* Philadelphia, PA: F.A. Davis Company; 29-47.
58. Ebers GC, Sadovnick AD, Risch NJ. 1995. A genetic basis for familial aggregation in multiple sclerosis. Canadian Collaborative Study Group. *Nature.*;377:150-1.
59. Ellis SJ. 2000. Cost utility of drugs for multiple sclerosis. Analysis goes too far. *BMJ.*;320:1475-6.
60. Elovaara I, Ukkonen M, Leppakynnas M, et al. 2000. Adhesion molecules in multiple sclerosis: relation to subtypes of disease and methylprednisolone therapy. *Arch Neurol.*;57:546-51.
61. Emerson RG. 1998. Evoked potentials in clinical trials for multiple sclerosis. *J Clin Neurophysiol.*;15:109-16.
62. Eng LF, Ghirnikar RS, Lee YL. 2000. Glial fibrillary acidic protein: GFAP-thirty-one years (1969-2000). *Neurochem Res.*;25:1439-51.
63. England JD, Gamboni F, Levinson SR, Finger TE. 1990. Changed distribution of sodium channels along demyelinated axons. *Proc Natl Acad Sci U S A.*;87:6777-80.

64. Evans RW. 1999. Economic malpractice: when methods become an end instead of a means. *Transplantation.*;68:11-2.
65. Eynon EE, Flavell RA. 1999. Walking through the forest of transgenic models of human disease. *Immunol Rev.*;169:5-10.
66. Falcone M, Rajan AJ, Bloom BR, Brosnan CF. 1998. A critical role for IL-4 in regulating disease severity in experimental allergic encephalomyelitis as demonstrated in IL-4-deficient C57BL/6 mice and BALB/c mice. *J Immunol.*;160:4822-30.
67. Fawcett JW, Asher RA. 1999. The glial scar and central nervous system repair. *Brain Res Bull.*;49:377-91.
68. Fazakerley JK, Webb HE. 1987. Semliki Forest virus induced, immune mediated demyelination: the effect of irradiation. *Br J Exp Pathol.*;68:101-13.
69. Fazekas F, Barkhof F, Filippi M, et al. 1999. The contribution of magnetic resonance imaging to the diagnosis of multiple sclerosis. *Neurology.*;53:448-56.
70. Fazekas F, Offenbacher H, Fuchs S, et al. 1988. Criteria for an increased specificity of MRI interpretation in elderly subjects with suspected multiple sclerosis. *Neurology.*;38:1822-5.
71. Filippi M, Rovaris M. 2000. Magnetisation transfer imaging in multiple sclerosis. *J Neurovirol.*;6 Suppl:S115-20.
72. Fillet AM, Lozeron P, Agut H, Lyon-Caen O, Liblau R. 1998. HHV-6 and multiple sclerosis. *Nat Med.*;4:537.
73. Forbes RB, Lees A, Waugh N, Swingler RJ. 1999. Population based cost utility study of interferon beta-1b in secondary progressive multiple sclerosis. *BMJ.*;319:1529-33.
74. Foster RE, Whalen CC, Waxman SG. 1980. Reorganization of the axon membrane in demyelinated peripheral nerve fibers: morphological evidence. *Science.*;210:661-3.
75. Gauthier L, Smith KJ, Pyrdol J, et al. 1998. Expression and crystallization of the complex of HLA-DR2 (DRA, DRB1*1501) and an immunodominant peptide of human myelin basic protein. *Proc Natl Acad Sci U S A.*;95:11828-33.
76. Ge Y, Grossman RI, Udupa JK, et al. 2000. Brain atrophy in relapsing-remitting multiple sclerosis and secondary progressive multiple sclerosis: longitudinal quantitative analysis. *Radiology.*;214:665-70.
77. Genain CP, Cannella B, Hauser SL, Raine CS. 1999. Identification of autoantibodies associated with myelin damage in multiple sclerosis. *Nat Med.*;5:170-5.
78. Genain CP, Nguyen MH, Letvin NL, et al. 1995. Antibody facilitation of multiple sclerosis-like lesions in a nonhuman primate. *J Clin Invest.*;96:2966-74.
79. Gingrich JR, Roder J. 1998. Inducible gene expression in the nervous system of transgenic mice. *Annu Rev Neurosci.*;21:377-405.
80. Giovannoni G, Lai M, Thorpe J, et al. 1997. Longitudinal study of soluble adhesion molecules in multiple sclerosis: correlation with gadolinium enhanced magnetic resonance imaging. *Neurology.*;48:1557-65.
81. Goldberg JL, Barres BA. 1998. Neuronal regeneration: extending axons from bench to brain. *Curr Biol.*;8:R310-2.
82. Gonzalez-Scarano F, Baltuch G. 1999. Microglia as mediators of inflammatory and degenerative diseases. *Annu Rev Neurosci.*;22:219-40.
83. Gonzalez-Scarano F, Rima B. 1999. Infectious etiology in multiple sclerosis: The debate continues. *Trends in Microbiology.*;7:475-7.
84. Gronseth GS, Ashman EJ. 2000. Practice parameter: the usefulness of evoked potentials in identifying clinically silent lesions in patients with suspected multiple sclerosis (an evidence-based review): Report of the Quality Standards Subcommittee of the American Academy of Neurology. *Neurology.*;54:1720-5.
85. Grossman RI, Barkhof F, Filippi M. 2000. Assessment of spinal cord damage in MS using MRI. *J Neurol Sci.*;172:S36-9.

86.  Hafler DA, Saadeh MG, Kuchroo VK, Milford E, Steinman L. 1996. TCR usage in human and experimental demyelinating disease. *Immunol Today.*;17:152-9.
87.  Hall CB, Long CE, Schnabel KC, et al. 1994. Human herpesvirus-6 infection in children. A prospective study of complications and reactivation. *N Engl J Med.*;331:432-8.
88.  Halliday AM, McDonald WI. 1977. Pathophysiology of demyelinating disease. *Brit. Med Bull.*; 33:21-27.
89.  Hammond SR, English DR, McLeod JG. 2000. The age-range of risk of developing multiple sclerosis: evidence from a migrant population in Australia. *Brain.*;123:968-74.
90.  Hayday AC. 2000. [gamma][delta] cells: a right time and a right place for a conserved third way of protection. *Annu Rev Immunol.*;18:975-1026.
91.  Hirsch J, DeLaPaz RL, Relkin NR, et al. 1995. Illusory contours activate specific regions in human visual cortex: evidence from functional magnetic resonance imaging. *Proc Natl Acad Sci U S A.*;92:6469-73.
92.  Ho TW, McKhann GM, Griffin JW. 1998. Human autoimmune neuropathies. *Annu Rev Neurosci.*;21:187-226.
93.  Hohlfeld R. 1999. Therapeutic strategies in multiple sclerosis. I. Immunotherapy. *Philos Trans R Soc Lond B Biol Sci.*;354:1697-710.
94.  Horwitz MS, Evans CF, McGavern DB, Rodriguez M, Oldstone MB. 1997. Primary demyelination in transgenic mice expressing interferon-gamma. *Nat Med.*;3:1037-41.
95.  Houtman JJ, Fleming JO. 1996. Pathogenesis of mouse hepatitis virus-induced demyelination. *J Neurovirol.*;2:361-76.
96.  Hume AL, Waxman SG. 1988. Evoked potentials in suspected multiple sclerosis: diagnostic value and prediction clinical course. *J. Neurol Sci.*;83:191-210.
97.  Hutter CD, Laing P. 1996. Multiple sclerosis: sunlight, diet, immunology and aetiology. *Med Hypotheses.*;46:67-74.
98.  Institute of Medicine. Field MJ, Gold MR, editors. *Summarizing Population Health. Directions for the Development and Application of Population Metrics.* Washington, DC: National Academy Press; 1998.
99.  Ito M, Nishibe Y, Inoue YK. 1998. Isolation of Inoue-Melnick virus from cerebrospinal fluid of patients with epidemic neuropathy in Cuba. *Arch Pathol Lab Med.*;122:520-522.
100. Jelachich ML, Bramlage C, Lipton HL. 1999. Differentiation of M1 myeloid precursor cells into macrophages results in binding and infection by Theiler's murine encephalomyelitis virus and apoptosis. *J Virol.*;73:3227-35.
101. Johnson RT, Gibbs CJ. 1974. Editorial: Koch's postulates and slow infections of the nervous system. *Arch Neurol.*;30:36-8.
102. Johnson RT, Griffin DE, Hirsch RL, et al. 1984. Measles encephalomyelitis—clinical and immunologic studies. *N Engl J Med.*;310:137-41.
103. Karni A, Bakimer-Kleiner R, Abramsky O, Ben-Nun A. 1999. Elevated levels of antibody to myelin oligodendrocyte glycoprotein is not specific for patients with multiple sclerosis. *Arch Neurol.*;56:311-5.
104. Karp CL, Wysocka M, Wahl LM, et al. 1996. Mechanism of suppression of cell-mediated immunity by measles virus. *Science.*;273:228-31.
105. Karpus WJ, Ransohoff RM. 1998. Chemokine regulation of experimental autoimmune encephalomyelitis: temporal and spatial expression patterns govern disease pathogenesis. *J Immunol.*;161:2667-71.
106. Kastrukoff LF, Lau AS, Leung GY, Walker DG, Thomas EE, Walker DG. 1992. Herpes simplex virus type I (HSV I)-induced multifocal central nervous system (CNS) demyelination in mice. *J Neuropathol Exp Neurol.*;51:432-9.
107. Kastrukoff LF, Rice GPA. 1998. Virology. Paty DW, Ebers GC, eds. Multiple Sclerosis. Philadelphia: F.A. Davis Company; 370-402.

108. Kerlero de Rosbo N, Milo R, Lees MB, Burger D, Bernard CC, Ben-Nun A. 1993. Reactivity to myelin antigens in multiple sclerosis. Peripheral blood lymphocytes respond predominantly to myelin oligodendrocyte glycoprotein. *J Clin Invest.*;92:2602-8.

109. Kira J, Kanai T, Nishimura Y, et al. 1996. Western versus Asian types of multiple sclerosis: immunogenetically and clinically distinct disorders. *Ann Neurol.*;40:569-74.

110. Koch-Henriksen N, Bronnum-Hansen H, Stenager E. 1998. Underlying cause of death in Danish patients with multiple sclerosis: results from the Danish Multiple Sclerosis Registry. *J Neurol Neurosurg Psychiatry.*;65:56-9.

111. Krapf H, Morrissey SP, Zenker O, et al. 1999. Mitoxantrone in progressive multiple sclerosis: MRI results of the European phase III trial. *Neurology.*;52:A495.

112. Kurtzke JF. 1997. The Epidemiology of Multiple Sclerosis. Raine CS, McFarland HF, Tourtellotte WWE. *Multiple Sclerosis: Clinical and Pathogenic Basis.* London: Chapman & Hall;91-139.

113. Kurtzke JF. 1997. On the role of veterans in the development of neurology in the United States: a personal reflection. *Neurology.*;49:323-33.

114. Kurtzke JF, Page WF. 1997. Epidemiology of multiple sclerosis in US veterans: VII. Risk factors for MS. *Neurology.*;48:204-13.

115. Lane TE, Liu MT, Chen BP, et al. 2000. A central role for CD4(+) T cells and RANTES in virus-induced central nervous system inflammation and demyelination. *J Virol.*;74:1415-24.

116. Lassmann H. 1999. The pathology of multiple sclerosis and its evolution. *Philos Trans R Soc Lond B Biol Sci.*;354:1635-40.

117. Lassmann H, Brunner C, Bradl M, Linington C. 1988. Experimental allergic encephalomyelitis: the balance between encephalitogenic T lymphocytes and demyelinating antibodies determines size and structure of demyelinated lesions. *Acta Neuropathol (Berl).*;75:566-76.

118. Lassmann H, Wekerle H. Experimental models of multiple sclerosis. Compston A, Ebers GC, Lassmann H, Matthews B, Wekerle H, eds. 1998. *McAlpine's Multiple Sclerosis.* Third ed. London: Churchill Livingston; 409-434.

119. Lee MA, Blamire AM, Pendlebury S, et al. 2000. Axonal injury or loss in the internal capsule and motor impairment in multiple sclerosis. *Arch Neurol.*;57:65-70.

120. Lee M, Reddy H, Johansen-Berg H, et al. 2000. The motor cortex shows adaptive functional changes to brain injury from multiple sclerosis. *Ann Neurol.*;47:606-613.

121. Leibowitz U, Kahana E, Alter M. 1973. When is multiple sclerosis acquired? *Harefuah.*;85:206-08.

122. Lin X, Roos RP, Pease LR, Wettstein P, Rodriguez M. 1999. A Theiler's virus alternatively initiated protein inhibits the generation of H-2K-restricted virus-specific cytotoxicity. *J Immunol.*;162:17-24.

123. Linington C, Bradl M, Lassmann H, Brunner C, Vass K. 1988. Augmentation of demyelination in rat acute allergic encephalomyelitis by circulating mouse monoclonal antibodies directed against a myelin/oligodendrocyte glycoprotein. *Am J Pathol.*;130:443-54.

124. Litzenburger T, Fassler R, Bauer J, et al. 1998. B lymphocytes producing demyelinating autoantibodies: development and function in gene-targeted transgenic mice. *J Exp Med.*;188:169-80.

125. Lublin FD, Reingold SC. 1996. Defining the clinical course of multiple sclerosis: results of an international survey. National Multiple Sclerosis Society (USA) Advisory Committee on Clinical Trials of New Agents in Multiple Sclerosis. *Neurology.*;46:907-11.

126. Lucchinetti CF, Brueck W, Rodriguez M, Lassmann H. 1998. Multiple sclerosis: lessons from neuropathology. *Semin Neurol.*;18:337-49.

127. Lucchinetti CF, Rodriguez M. 1997. The controversy surrounding the pathogenesis of the multiple sclerosis lesion. *Mayo Clin Proc.*;72:665-78.

128. Lycklama a Nijeholt GJ, Uitdehaag BM, Bergers E, Castelijns JA, Polman CH, Barkhof F. 2000. Spinal cord magnetic resonance imaging in suspected multiple sclerosis. *Eur Radiol.*;10:368-76.

129. Madsen LS, Andersson EC, Jansson L, et al. 1999. A humanized model for multiple sclerosis using HLA-DR2 and a human T-cell receptor. *Nat Genet.*;23:343-7.

130. Martin C, Enbom M, Soderstrom M, et al. 1997. Absence of seven human herpesviruses, including HHV-6, by polymerase chain reaction in CSF and blood from patients with multiple sclerosis and optic neuritis. *Acta Neurol Scand.*;95:280-3.

131. Martin R, McFarland HF, McFarlin DE. 1992. Immunological aspects of demyelinating diseases. *Annu Rev Immunol.*;10:153-87.

132. Massaro AR. 1998. Are there indicators of remyelination in blood or CSF of multiple sclerosis patients? *Mult Scler.*;4:228-31.

133. McDonald JW, Liu XZ, Qu Y, et al. 1999. Transplanted embryonic stem cells survive, differentiate and promote recovery in injured rat spinal cord. *Nat Med.*;5:1410-2.

134. McDonald WI. 1977. Acute optic neuritis. *Br J Hosp Med.*;18:42-8.

135. McDonald WI, Miller DH, Barnes D. 1992. The pathological evolution of multiple sclerosis. *Neuropathol Appl Neurobiol.*;18:319-34.

136. McFarland HF. 1998. The lesion in multiple sclerosis: clinical, pathological, and magnetic resonance imaging considerations. *J Neurol Neurosurg Psychiatry.*;64 Suppl 1:S26-30.

137. McFarland HF, Martin R, McFarlin DE. 1997. Genetic Influences in Multiple Sclerosis. Raine CS, McFarland HF, Tourtellott WWE. *Multiple Sclerosis: Clinical and Pathogenetic Basis.* London: Chapman & Hall;205-219.

138. McMichael A. Function of HLA class I restricted T cells. Browning M, McMichael A, eds. 1996. *HLA and MHC: Genes, Molecules and Function.* Oxford: BIOS Scientific Publishers Limited;309-320.

139. Menard A, Amouri R, Dobransky T, et al. 1998. A gliotoxic factor and multiple sclerosis. *J Neurol Sci.*;154:209-21.

140. Mendez E, Kawanishi T, Clemens K, et al. 1997. Astrocyte-specific expression of human T-cell lymphotropic virus type 1 (HTLV-1) Tax: induction of tumor necrosis factor alpha and susceptibility to lysis by CD8+ HTLV-1-specific cytotoxic T cells. *J Virol.*;71:9143-9.

141. Miller SD, Vanderlugt CL, Begolka WS, et al. 1997. Persistent infection with Theiler's virus leads to CNS autoimmunity via epitope spreading. *Nat Med.*;3:1133-6.

142. Missler U, Wandinger KP, Wiesmann M, Kaps M, Wessel K. 1997. Acute exacerbation of multiple sclerosis increases plasma levels of S-100 protein. *Acta Neurol Scand.*;96:142-4.

143. Moench TR, Griffin DE, Obriecht CR, Vaisberg AJ, Johnson RT. 1988. Acute measles in patients with and without neurological involvement: distribution of measles virus antigen and RNA. *J Infect Dis.*;158:433-42.

144. Mohr DC, Dick LP, Russo D, et al. 1999. The psychosocial impact of multiple sclerosis: exploring the patient's perspective. *Health Psychol.*;18:376-82.

145. Moll C, Mourre C, Lazdunski M, Ulrich J. 1991. Increase of sodium channels in demyelinated lesions of multiple sclerosis. *Brain Res.*;556:311-6.

146. Moore GRW. Neuropathology and Pathophysiology of the Multiple Sclerosis Lesion. Paty DW, Ebers GC, eds. 1998. *Multiple Sclerosis.* Philadelphia, PA: F.A. Davis Company;257-327.

147. Muller U. 1999. Ten years of gene targeting: targeted mouse mutants, from vector design to phenotype analysis. *Mech Dev.*;82:3-21.

148. Mumford CJ, Wood NW, Kellar-Wood H, Thorpe JW, Miller DH, Compston DA. 1994. The British Isles survey of multiple sclerosis in twins. *Neurology.*;44:11-5.

149. Murray PD, Pavelko KD, Leibowitz J, Lin X, Rodriguez M. 1998. CD4(+) and CD8(+) T cells make discrete contributions to demyelination and neurologic disease in a viral model of multiple sclerosis. *J Virol.*;72:7320-9.

150. Murrell TG, Harbige LS, Robinson IC. 1991. A review of the aetiology of multiple sclerosis: an ecological approach. *Ann Hum Biol.*;18:95-112.
151. Neumann H, Schmidt H, Cavalie A, Jenne D, Wekerle H. 1997. Major histocompatibility complex (MHC) class I gene expression in single neurons of the central nervous system: differential regulation by interferon (IFN)-gamma and tumor necrosis factor (TNF)-alpha. *J Exp Med.*;185:305-16.
152. Nicolson T, Milne R. 1999. Beta interferons (1a and 1b) in relapsing-remitting and secondary progressive multiple sclerosis. Development and Evaluation Committee Report No. 98. Southampton: Wessex Institute for Health Research and Development.
153. Noseworthy JH. 1999. Progress in determining the causes and treatment of multiple sclerosis. *Nature.*;399:A40-7.
154. Noseworthy JH, Lucchinetti C, Rodriguez M, Weinshenker BG. 2000. Multiple sclerosis. *N Engl J Med.*;343:938-52.
155. O'Connor P, Marchetti P, Lee L, Perera M. 1998. Evoked potential abnormality scores are a useful measure of disease burden in relapsing-remitting multiple sclerosis. *Ann Neurol.*;44:404-7.
156. Oksenberg JR, Seboun E, Hauser SL. 1996. Genetics of demyelinating diseases. *Brain Pathol.*;6:289-302.
157. Oldstone MB. 1998. Molecular mimicry and immune-mediated diseases. *FASEB J.*;12:1255-65.
158. Oldstone MB, Lewicki H, Thomas D, et al. 1999. Measles virus infection in a transgenic model: virus-induced immunosuppression and central nervous system disease. *Cell.*;98:629-40.
159. Otten N. 1998. Comparison of drug treatments for multiple sclerosis. Ottawa: Canadian Coordinating Office for Health Technology Assessment.
160. Pagenstecher A, Lassmann S, Carson MJ, Kincaid CL, Stalder AK, Campbell IL. 2000. Astrocyte-targeted expression of IL-12 induces active cellular immune responses in the central nervous system and modulates experimental allergic encephalomyelitis. *J Immunol.*;164:4481-92.
161. Park SH, Chiu YH, Jayawardena J, Roark J, Kavita U, Bendelac A. 1998. Innate and adaptive functions of the CD1 pathway of antigen presentation. *Semin Immunol.*;10:391-8.
162. Parkin D, Miller P, McNamee P, Thomas S, Jacoby A, Bates D. 1998. A cost-utility analysis of interferon beta for multiple sclerosis. *Health Technol Assess.*;2:iii-54.
163. Paty DW, Hartung H, Ebers GC, et al. 1999. Management of relapsing-remittting multiple sclerosis: diagnosis and treatment guidelines. *European J Neurol.*;6 (suppl):S1-S35.
164. Paty DW, Li DKB. Diagnosis of multiple sclerosis 1998: do we need new diagnostic criteria? Siva et al. eds. 1998. *Frontiers in Multiple Sclerosis.* London: Martin Dunitz;2:47-50.
165. Persson L, Hardemark HG, Gustafsson J, et al. 1987. S-100 protein and neuron-specific enolase in cerebrospinal fluid and serum: markers of cell damage in human central nervous system. *Stroke.*;18:911-8.
166. Poser CM. 1995. Notes on the epidemiology of multiple sclerosis. *J Formos Med Assoc.*;94:300-8.
167. Poser CM. 1997. Misdiagnosis of multiple sclerosis and beta-interferon. *Lancet.*;349:1916.
168. Poser CM, Paty DW, Scheinberg L, et al. 1983. New diagnostic criteria for multiple sclerosis: guidelines for research protocols. *Ann Neurol.*;13:227-31.
169. Prineas JW, Connell F. 1978. The fine structure of chronically active multiple sclerosis plaques. *Neurology.*28:68-75.
170. Qin Y, Duquette P, Zhang Y, Talbot P, Poole R, Antel J. 1998. Clonal expansion and somatic hypermutation of V(H) genes of B cells from cerebrospinal fluid in multiple sclerosis. *J Clin Invest.*;102:1045-50.
171. Radic MZ, Weigert M. 1994. Genetic and structural evidence for antigen selection of anti-DNA antibodies. *Annu Rev Immunol* 1994;12:487-520.
172. Raine CS. 1997. Multiple sclerosis. *Brain Pathology.*;7:1237-1241.

173. Raine CS. 1997. The Norton Lecture: a review of the oligodendrocyte in the multiple sclerosis lesion. *J Neuroimmunol.*; 77:135-52.

174. Raine CS, Cannella B, Hauser SL, Genain CP. 1999. Demyelination in primate autoimmune encephalomyelitis and acute multiple sclerosis lesions: a case for antigen-specific antibody mediation. *Ann Neurol.*;46:144-60.

175. Raivich G, Bohatschek M, Kloss CU, Werner A, Jones LL, Kreutzberg GW. 1999. Neuroglial activation repertoire in the injured brain: graded response, molecular mechanisms and cues to physiological function. *Brain Res Brain Res Rev.*;30:77-105.

176. Renno T, Taupin V, Bourbonniere L, et al. 1998. Interferon-gamma in progression to chronic demyelination and neurological deficit following acute EAE. *Mol Cell Neurosci.*;12:376-89.

177. Richards R, Burls A, Payne N. 2000. Cost utility of drugs for multiple sclerosis. Methods used don't calculate true benefit. *BMJ.*;320:1475; discussion 1475-6.

178. Rieckmann P. 1997. Soluble adhesion molecules (sVCAM-1 and sICAM-1) in cerebrospinal fluid and serum correlate with MRI activity in multiple sclerosis. *Ann Neurol.*;41:236-333.

179. Rieckmann P, Albrecht M, Kitze B, et al. 1995. Tumor necrosis factor-alpha messenger RNA expression in patients with relapsing-remitting multiple sclerosis is associated with disease activity. *Ann Neurol.*;37:82-8.

180. Risch N. 1992. Genetic linkage: interpreting lod scores. *Science.*;255:803-4.

181. Ritchie JM. 1982. Sodium and potassium channels in regenerating and developing mammalian myelinated nerves. *Proc R Soc Lond B Biol Sci.*;215:273-87.

182. Rose NR. Immunologic Diagnosis of Autoimmunity. Leffell MS, Donnenber AD, Rose NRE. 1997. *Handbook of Human Immology.* Boca Raton: CRC Press;111-124.

183. Rosen BR, Buckner RL, Dale AM. 1998. Event-related functional MRI: past, present, and future. *Proc Natl Acad Sci U S A.*;95:773-80.

184. Rosenblum D, Saffir M. 1998. The natural history of multiple sclerosis and its diagnosis. *Phys Med Rehabil Clin N Am.*;9:537-49.

185. Rosengren LE, Karlsson JE, Karlsson JO, Persson LI, Wikkelso C. 1996. Patients with amyotrophic lateral sclerosis and other neurodegenerative diseases have increased levels of neurofilament protein in CSF. *J Neurochem.*;67:2013-8.

186. Rovaris M, Viti B, Ciboddo G, Capra R, Filippi M. 2000. Cervical cord magnetic resonance imaging findings in systemic immune-mediated diseases. *J Neurol Sci.*;176:128-30.

187. Rudick RA. 1999. Disease-modifying drugs for relapsing-remitting multiple sclerosis and future directions for multiple sclerosis therapeutics. *Arch Neurol.*;56:1079-84.

188. Sadovnick AD. 1993. Familial recurrence risks and inheritance of multiple sclerosis. *Curr Opin Neurol Neurosurg.*;6:189-94.

189. Sadovnick AD, Ebers GC, Dyment DA, Risch NJ. 1996. Evidence for genetic basis of multiple sclerosis. The Canadian Collaborative Study Group. *Lancet.*;347:1728-30.

190. Sanders VJ, Felisan S, Waddell A, Tourtellotte WW. 1996. Detection of herpesviridae in postmortem multiple sclerosis brain tissue and controls by polymerase chain reaction. *J Neurovirol.*;2:249-58.

191. Santoro F, Kennedy PE, Locatelli G, Malnati MS, Berger EA, Lusso P. 1999. CD46 is a cellular receptor for human herpesvirus 6. *Cell.*;99:817-27.

192. Sater RA, Rostami AM, Galetta S, Farber RE, Bird SJ. 1999. Serial evoked potential studies and MRI imaging in chronic progressive multiple sclerosis. *J Neurol Sci.*;171:79-83.

193. Sawcer S, Goodfellow PN, Compston A. 1997. The genetic analysis of multiple sclerosis. *Trends Genet.*;13:234-9.

194. Schadlich HJ, Karbe H, Felgenhauer K. 1987. The prevalence of locally-synthesized virus antibodies in various forms of multiple sclerosis. *J Neurol Sci.*;80:343-9.

195. Schumacher GA, Beebe G, Kibler RF, Kurlant LT, Kurtzke JF, McDowell F. 1965. Problems of experimental trials of therapy in multiple sclerosis: Report by the panel on the evaluation of experimental trials of therapy in multiple sclerosis. *Ann NY Acad Med.*;122:552-568.

196. Sellebjerg F, Madsen HO, Jensen CV, Jensen J, Garred P. 2000. CCR5 delta32, matrix metalloproteinase-9 and disease activity in multiple sclerosis. *J Neuroimmunol.*;102:98-106.
197. Sharief MK, Hentges R. 1991. Association between tumor necrosis factor-alpha and disease progression in patients with multiple sclerosis. *N Engl J Med.*;325:467-72.
198. Silver NC, Barker GJ, Miller DH. 1999. Standardization of magnetization transfer imaging for multicenter studies. *Neurology.*;53:S33-9.
199. Simon JH. 2000. The contribution of spinal cord MRI to the diagnosis and differential diagnosis of multiple sclerosis. *J Neurol Sci.*;172:S32-5.
200. Simon JH. 1999. From enhancing lesions to brain atrophy in relapsing MS. *J Neuroimmunol.*;98:7-15.
201. Sorensen PS. 1999. Biological markers in body fluids for activity and progression in multiple sclerosis. *Mult Scler.*;5:287-90.
202. Sorensen TL, Tani M, Jensen J, et al. 1999. Expression of specific chemokines and chemokine receptors in the central nervous system of multiple sclerosis patients. *J Clin Invest.*;103:807-15.
203. Sriram S, Stratton CW, Yao S, et al. 1999. Chlamydia pneumoniae infection of the central nervous system in multiple sclerosis. *Ann Neurol.*;46:6-14.
204. Stalder AK, Carson MJ, Pagenstecher A, et al. 1998. Late-onset chronic inflammatory encephalopathy in immune-competent and severe combined immune-deficient (SCID) mice with astrocyte-targeted expression of tumor necrosis factor. *Am J Pathol.*;153:767-83.
205. Steinman L. 2000. Despite epitope spreading in the pathogenesis of autoimmune disease, highly restricted approaches to immune therapy may still succeed [with a hedge on this bet]. *J Autoimmun.*;14:278-82.
206. Steinman L, Oldstone MB. 1997. More mayhem from molecular mimics. *Nat Med.*;3:1321-2.
207. Stinissen P, Raus J, Zhang J. 1997. Autoimmune pathogenesis of multiple sclerosis: role of autoreactive T lymphocytes and new immunotherapeutic strategies. *Crit Rev Immunol.*;17:33-75.
208. Streit WJ. 2000. Microglial response to brain injury: a brief synopsis. *Toxicol Pathol.*;28:28-30.
209. Thompson AJ, Montalban X, Barkhof F, et al. 2000. Diagnostic criteria for primary progressive multiple sclerosis: a position paper. *Ann Neurol.*;47:831-5.
210. Thompson EJ. 1995. Cerebrospinal fluid. *J Neurol Neurosurg Psychiatry.*;59:349-57.
211. Townsend JJ, Baringer JR. 1979. Morphology of central nervous system disease in immunosuppressed mice after peripheral herpes simplex virus inoculation. Trigeminal root entry zone. *Lab Invest.*;40:178-82.
212. Trapp BD, Peterson J, Ransohoff RM, Rudick RA, Mork S, Bo L. 1998. Axonal transection in the lesions of multiple sclerosis. *New Engl J Med.*;338:278-285.
213. Trapp BD, Ransohoff RM, Fisher E, Rudick RA. 1999. Neurodegeneration in multiple sclerosis: relationship to neurological disability. *The Neuroscientist.*;5:48-57.
214. Trowsdale J. Molecular genetics of HLA class I and class II regions. Browning M, McMichael A, eds. *HLA and MHC: Genes, Molecules and Function.* Oxford: BIOS Scientific Publishers Limited; 1996.
215. Van der Neut R. 1997. Targeted gene disruption: applications in neurobiology. *J Neurosci Methods.*;71:19-27.
216. Vandevyver C, Mertens N, van den Elsen P, Medaer R, Raus J, Zhang J. 1995. Clonal expansion of myelin basic protein-reactive T cells in patients with multiple sclerosis: restricted T cell receptor V gene rearrangements and CDR3 sequence. *Eur J Immunol.*;25:958-68.
217. Wallstrom E, Khademi M, Andersson M, Weissert R, Linington C, Olsson T. 1998. Increased reactivity to myelin oligodendrocyte glycoprotein peptides and epitope mapping in HLA DR2(15)+ multiple sclerosis. *Eur J Immunol.*;28:3329-35.
218. Waxman SG. 1982. Membranes, myelin, and the pathophysiology of multiple sclerosis. *N Engl J Med.*;306:1529-33.

219. Waxman SG. 1998. Demyelinating diseases—new pathological insights, new therapeutic targets. *N Engl J Med.*;338:323-5.
220. Waxman SG. 2000. Multiple sclerosis as a neuronal disease. *Arch Neurol.*;57:22-4.
221. Waxman SG, Black JA, Sontheimer H, Kocsis JD. 1994. Glial cells and axo-glial interactions: implications for demyelinating disorders. *Clin Neurosci.*;2:202-10.
222. Weinshenker BG, Bass B, Rice GP, et al. 1989. The natural history of multiple sclerosis: a geographically based study. I. Clinical course and disability. *Brain.*;112:133-46.
223. Werring DJ, Clark CA, Barker GJ, Thompson AJ, Miller DH. 1999. Diffusion tensor imaging of lesions and normal-appearing white matter in multiple sclerosis. *Neurology.*;52:1626-32.
224. Whitacre CC, Reingold SC, O'Looney PA. 1999. A gender gap in autoimmunity. *Science.*;283:1277-8.
225. Williams KC, Ulvestad E, Hickey WF. 1994. Immunology of multiple sclerosis. *Clin Neurosci.*;2:229-45.
226. Wong FS, Dittel BN, Janeway CA Jr. 1999. Transgenes and knockout mutations in animal models of type 1 diabetes and multiple sclerosis. *Immunol Rev.*;169:93-104.
227. Wong FS, Janeway CA Jr. 1999. Insulin-dependent diabetes mellitus and its animal models. *Curr Opin Immunol.*;11:643-647.
228. Wucherpfennig KW, Hafler DA. 1995. A review of T-cell receptors in multiple sclerosis: clonal expansion and persistence of human T-cells specific for an immunodominant myelin basic protein peptide. *Ann N Y Acad Sci 1995 Jul 7;756:241-58.*;756:241-58.
229. Wucherpfennig KW, Strominger JL. 1995. Molecular mimicry in T cell-mediated autoimmunity: viral peptides activate human T cell clones specific for myelin basic protein. *Cell.*;80:695-705.
230. Xu Z, Cork LC, Griffin JW, Cleveland DW. 1993. Involvement of neurofilaments in motor neuron disease. *J Cell Sci Suppl.*;17:101-8.
231. Yamasaki K, Horiuchi I, Minohara M, et al. 1999. HLA-DPB1*0501-associated opticospinal multiple sclerosis: clinical, neuroimaging and immunogenetic studies. *Brain.*;122:1689-96.
232. Zhang J, Markovic-Plese S, Lacet B, Raus J, Weiner HL, Hafler DA. 1994. Increased frequency of interleukin 2-responsive T cells specific for myelin basic protein and proteolipid protein in peripheral blood and cerebrospinal fluid of patients with multiple sclerosis. *J Exp Med.*;179:973-84.
233. Zhang J, Stinissen P, Medaer R, Truyen L, Raus J. 1998. T-cell vaccination for the treatment of multiple sclerosis. In Zhang J, editor. *Immunotherapy in Neuroimmunologic Diseases.* London, England: Martin Dunitz.

# 3

# Characteristics and Management
of Major Symptoms

The signs and symptoms of multiple sclerosis (MS) are generally related to the most heavily myelinated parts of the central nervous system (CNS), but they are notoriously variable. Some symptoms such as dizziness, tingling sensations on the skin, or visual tracking disturbances are easily forgotten and are often hard for patients to describe. The majority of fleeting cerebral abnormalities seen on magnetic resonance imaging (MRI) cannot be correlated with any symptoms; even chronically demyelinated areas of the optic nerve and spinal cord can be symptom free.[107]

In general, MS patients report mental health as more important than physical impairment and bodily pain in determining their quality of life. This is different from neurologists' beliefs about the most important determinants of health-related quality of life for patients with MS or the beliefs of members of the general public about their own quality of life.[146] Nine of the most prominent symptoms are described in this chapter. They are presented roughly in order of the importance that MS patients assign to them as determinants of overall quality of life, although it should be noted that this ranking is based on a small survey and that individual variability is a prominent feature of all aspects of MS.[146]

## COGNITIVE IMPAIRMENT

Fear of mental change is one of the greatest concerns of MS patients when they learn they have the disease. Cognitive dysfunction is one of the most disabling features of MS and, even when subtle, can begin to limit a person's ability to cope, to stay employed, and to carry out family responsibilities and enjoy life.[140]

Early writers on MS often commented on cognitive and emotional changes, but in the mid-twentieth century, a pattern of denial of these features developed in the medical literature.[143] Just as clinicians passed off the frequent symptoms of pain and fatigue as features of the disease, they also ignored the often seen emotional and cognitive changes (Jock Murray, personal communication). Donald Paty (personal communication) noted that there was a negative reaction to his suggestions in the 1970s that cognitive dysfunction should be a focus of study by the National MS Society. At the time, it was estimated that only 5 percent of MS patients might incur cognitive change, and it was argued that cognitive change was relatively unimportant in MS.[143] By the 1990s, those views had changed, and in 1992, the MS Society and the International Federation of Multiple Sclerosis Societies jointly held a symposium on "Neurobehavioral Disorders in MS: Diagnosis, Underlying Pathology, Natural History and Therapeutics." Cognitive changes are now estimated to occur in about 43 percent of MS cases.[54]

The conviction that cognitive changes must be selectively analyzed and distinguished from other phenomena such as depression and fatigue has emerged only in the last few decades. Standard psychological tests, however, are not very effective in identifying the type of changes that occur in MS. Rao, LaRocca, Fischer, Peyser, and many others have recently made considerable progress in adapting tests that can detect the specific changes seen in this disease,[54,57,130] yet much more remains to be done. Paradoxically, as we are learning to separate and more effectively measure the cognitive changes and the affective changes, this separation has made it possible to learn how they are so often linked (Jock Murray, personal communication).

Cognitive changes in MS generally are not global, but are most often circumscribed to specific processes. Learning, recall of new information, and speed of information processing are affected most often; deficits in visuospatial abilities and executive functions such as reasoning, problem solving, and planning are also common.[54] Performance accuracy is less affected, but it appears affected if timed tests are used.[41] Once cognitive impairment is present, it does not often remit (reviewed in 1999 by Fischer[54]).

Poor memory is a common complaint among MS patients.[3] Depending on sample selection methods and criteria used to define impairment, approximately 20 to 42 percent of MS patients have some deficit in their free recall of recently learned verbal and visual material (reviewed in 1994 by Fischer et al. [56]). Although memory deficits are common, certain processes remain intact. For example, the rate of learning, the likelihood of remembering a specific item based on when it was presented, and the ability to detect semantic characteristics of the material to be learned are preserved in all but the most impaired MS patients. Implicit memory, or the ability to learn new information or skills without explicitly attending to it, is also preserved. Recognition of recently learned information is generally impaired to a much lesser extent than free recall. Impairment of verbal fluency (the ability to rapidly generate words meeting specific phonological or semantic criteria) and, to a lesser extent, confrontation naming (the ability to retrieve the names of objects) are often associated with memory impairment. Decreases in word fluency are common, whereas decreases in verbal comprehension are less common.[4]

A study of 44 MS patients found that on tests of cognitive performance designed to measure planning skills tests the MS group performed on average significantly worse than controls.[8] However, this was due largely to deficits among chronic progressive, as opposed to relapsing-remitting patients. Another caveat is that this was a timed test, so that in addition to planning skills, information processing speed would have influenced performance, which would likely bias the results since this is often affected in MS patients.

## Time Course

The time course of cognitive changes in MS is highly variable, although they appear to occur very early in the disease, often before the onset of other symptoms. Different types of cognitive change can appear in different sequences in different patients, and few studies have documented changes over time in individual patients. In one study, 50 patients were tested early in the disease (on average, 19 months after clinical onset) and again 4.5 years later.[4] Initial tests revealed statistically significant deficits in verbal memory and abstract reasoning relative to controls, with similar results in the follow-up tests. The difference in average scores between patients and controls was about 10 percent. However, the difference in variability was much more striking. The variability in scores for the MS group was consistently greater than for controls, and in 7 out of 15 cases the variance of the MS group was more than twice that of the controls. This suggests that the cognitive performance of many of the MS patients was not measurably affected, whereas others were substantially affected. A simple analysis of group differences is not sufficient to answer this question. This study also illustrates the value of using individual patients as their own controls.

## Association with Other Symptoms

Cognitive and neurological deficits do not appear to develop in parallel, at least not in patients whose disease is still in its early phase.[4] Disease duration is not a good predictor of cognitive function in MS, but disease course influences the likelihood of cognitive impairment. Chronic progressive patients tend to do more poorly on neuropsychological tests than relapsing-remitting patients (reviewed in 2001 by Fischer[55]). Expanded Disability Status Scale (EDSS) scores and specific neurological symptoms are not correlated with cognitive deficits.[8,53,134] The EDSS is shown in Appendix D. Despite this, clinicians consistently overestimate the correlation between physical disablity and cognitive impairment in MS patients.[56]

While some studies report that cognitive function is independent of fatigue,[63,180] others raise the possibility that they might be caused by a disruption of the same neural circuits (see Fischer 2000 for discussion). Depression is generally not strongly related to overall cognitive function. One study of 20 MS patients found that cognitive deficits (attention, visuomotor search, and verbal fluency) were independent of depressive symptoms.[96] Of these, only frontal function impairment was correlated with depression. However, only 4 percent had significant depression scores, and all of these had secondary progressive MS.[53] A cross-sectional study of 24 patients found significant association of cognitive impairment (using tests of abstract verbal and nonverbal memory) with depression, but not with the degree of neurological impairment, specific neurological symptoms, disability, or handicap.[68]

## Neuropathological Correlates

The traditional view that MS is characterized by discrete lesions does not explain the memory and cognitive changes, which would require a more widespread, bilateral change, especially since the complaints often arise early. Recent evidence from the studies of Ian McDonald in Great Britain and Bruce Trapp in the United States indicates that the effects of demyelination and the destruction of axons occur very early in MS and are widespread. Moreover, the process undoubtedly has been going on for a long time before a person experiences the first symptom.

MRI has recently allowed speculation of localization of specific mental changes.[139] Although MRI studies of MS patients have reported correlations between cognitive impairment and total lesion burden (the percentage of the brain that shows lesions on MRI scans), neuroimaging techniques have not reached the point where neuropathological changes can be linked to specific aspects of cognitive impairment (reviewed in 2000 by Rovaris and Filippi[147]). Research on cognitive changes in MS is still in its early stages, and most studies have been relatively small and have not followed changes in individuals. In addition, the application of techniques that allow detection of more specific neuropathological changes, particularly axonal pathology, might provide more useful insights into the causes of cognitive impairment.

## Pathological Laughing and Crying

Pathological laughing and crying is a distinctive type of cognitive change that occurs in a variety of neurological disorders including stroke, amyotropic lateral sclerosis (ALS), Alzheimer's disease, cerebral tumors, and MS. The syndrome is defined as a sudden loss of emotional control—for example, laughing, crying, or both in response to nonspecific, often inconsequential stimuli for no apparent reason. The etiology of pathological laughing and crying is unclear. The cortex and, possibly, prefrontal cortex are thought to be involved. In a study of 152 patients with long-standing disease and significant physical disability (unable to walk without assistance), pathological laughing and crying as distinct from emotional lability affected 10 percent of the patients.[49] (Emotional lability refers to abrupt changes in mood.) A preliminary study indicates that such patients had relatively greater difficulty with speed of information processing than their MS control subjects without pathological laughing and crying.[51]

There have been a number of reviews of euphoria, all suggesting that euphoria is a reflection of organic change. Rabins used pre-MRI studies to show that euphoria was associated with greater brain involvement with MS, particularly in the periventricular areas, but occurred in less than 10 percent of patients.[136] Recent MRI studies indicate that the cognitive and emotional changes are likely to have specific neuroanatomical correlates.

## Management

Initial studies have shown some limited gains by methods of cognitive rehabilitation, and more needs to be known about what approaches would be helpful. Memory failures of MS patients sometimes resemble those found in people with histories of closed-head injury. A study of teaching memory strategies to people with MS found that MS subjects were able to learn the strategies quickly and did not appear to require the lengthy training needed by persons with head injury.[3] Two studies of the effects of amantadine, a medication often prescribed for fatigue, showed either no effect on cognitive function[63] or a modest benefit on processing speed, and that effect was limited to patients who had MS for 7 years or longer.[150] It was recently reported that after a 2-year course of interferon-beta (IFN-β-1a) relapsing MS patients had significantly better cognitive functions than placebo-treated controls.[58] Although assessment of cognitive changes in MS clinical trials is challenging, further tests will be important to clarify this effect.

Until ways of stopping or reducing cognitive change are developed, patients could benefit by any methods that at least help them and provide them with techniques to alleviate the problems. For example, people with memory deficits can use portable tape recorders, daily planners, and computer memory aids to keep track of schedules and review discussions during physician visits or education sessions.

## Research Needs

The revelation of the prevalence of cognitive changes together with the advent of MRI has stimulated a surge of research over the last decade, which has in turn clarified specific needs for further research.

- Research on the underlying pathophysiological changes leading to cognitive and pathological emotional change is needed, because the relationship between pathological changes observed in the disease and the observation of cognitive change is speculative at the present time. Understanding the underlying mechanisms may explain why there isn't a close correlation of cognitive change with disability, disease course, or disease duration.

- Further research on more representative populations of MS patients is necessary to reveal the extent and degree of involvement, and long-term studies are needed on this group (community-based versus clinic populations). Previous studies are on groups that may not be representative.
- We need to know more about the impact of early cognitive changes on the quality of life.[140]
- Further research is needed into the MRI, functional MRI, and PET (positron emission tomography) scan correlates of the cognitive change. We need to understand more about why some patients develop severe cognitive change, others mild or moderate change, and others with long-standing disease have no measurable change.
- Further research is needed into disease-specific neuropsychological tests to better identify early changes in MS, and this should be translated into a standard battery that could be used for the clinic and bedside and as a part of all clinical therapy trials.
- More data are needed to define the temporal course of cognitive changes and would be invaluable in assessing the impact of new agents used in treating MS.
- Better measures of the cognitive changes in MS should be developed, although the need for specific neuropsychological tests for the specific changes noted in MS has been recognized, as developed by Stephen Rao.[139]

## DEPRESSION

### Prevalence and Diagnosis

Depression is the most common mood disorder in MS. Alterations in mood and affective state have long been recognized in MS,[35] although estimates of their prevalence vary widely. Estimates of the prevalence of major depression among MS clinic patients at any one time range from about 15 to 30 percent and from 40 to 60 percent for lifetime prevalence (reviewed in 1995 by Nyenhuis et al.,[126] and in 1997 by Aikens et al.,[1,56]), which is three times that found in the general population. Depression is more prevalent in MS than other neurological disorders, such as Parkinson's disease, in which it is one-half to one-third less prevalent than in MS.[141] However, these estimates might be deceptive because they are typically based on patients attending MS clinics. For example, the estimated prevalence of major depression among stroke patients depends on setting, increasingly linearly from community samples (2 to 4 percent) to primary care settings (5 to 10 percent) to inpatient medical settings (6 to 14 percent).[25] The prevalence of depression among the MS population at large has not been well studied and is probably lower than that among patients attending specialized clinics.

Many studies of depression among MS patients have been plagued by methodological difficulties.[141] Varying diagnostic criteria have been used, including unstandardized tests. Most importantly, factors that affect mood or its assessment are frequently not taken into account. For example, mood can be affected by exacerbations, psychoactive prescription drugs (for example, corticosteroids), and fatigue.

Research on depression in MS is complicated by the fact that validated depression rating scales rely, in part, on evaluations of fatigue and other bodily symptoms that are common in MS, and can occur independently of depression.[126] The Beck Depression Inventory (BDI), which is one of the most widely used depression scales, evaluates depression based on responses to 21 questions, including many that ask about symptoms that overlap with those of MS. For example, subjects are asked whether they get tired more easily than they used to or whether they worry a lot about health problems. Positive answers to such questions from people with MS might have little to do with depressed mood and might simply reflect a realistic appraisal of their condition. Thus, it seems likely that scales such as the BDI would tend to overestimate depression in people with medical conditions that produce certain symptoms. One study that used different scales to measure depression among MS patients found that the apparent prevalence of depression among MS patients varied, depending on the scale used. When only the mood scale was used for the Multiple Depression Inventory (MDI), a self-report depression scale, 18 percent of patients were rated as depressed, in contrast to 31 percent rated with the BDI and 27 percent when the total MDI scale was used.[126] Another study found little difference between the scores of MS patients and healthy controls, except for questions about sexual disinterest for which MS patients exceeded healthy controls.[2] This potential tendency for spurious increase in depression has been noted for other medical conditions and should be carefully evaluated.[23,26]

Although much of the research on depression and MS has focused on the existence of major depressive syndromes, many MS patients suffer from mood alterations that are consistent with depression but do not qualify as major depressive disorder.[76,126]

## Association with Other Symptoms

Depression is not clearly related to the severity or type of disability, type of MS, or duration of symptoms.[52,134] Measures of depression are not related to EDSS values. However, depressive symptoms interfere with daily functioning in medically well individuals as well as in those with chronic disease. Depressed patients tend to function worse in their work, physical, and social roles compared to patients with a variety of medical conditions, including advanced coronary artery disease, arthritis, diabetes, and lung problems.[189] Depression also appears to increase the burden of disability. Smith and Young[162] found that MS patients who met criteria for depression on either the Hospital Anxiety and Depression Scale (HADS) or the Beck Depression Inventory were three times more likely than nondepressed patients to perceive their disability as being greater than their physician did.

Depression is often associated with other neurological symptoms of MS, particularly cognitive impairment, fatigue, and pain, although, as discussed earlier in the section on cognitive impairment, the data on the link between depression and cognitive impairment are inconsistent. These other symptoms can be worsened by depression or can themselves increase depression. For example, depressed MS patients have reduced working memory capacity (reading span),[7] and it is important to establish which causes which or if both are independently caused by the same factors. Both mental fatigue and total fatigue are correlated with depression.[61,93] Depression and disability are significant predictors of fatigue,[93] although as noted above, fatigue is used as an indicator of depression and thus the correlation might be overestimated. Depression has been linked to cognitive impairment in numerous studies, but these have generally been cross-sectional studies in which comparisons are made between different groups of patients tested at a single point in time. Interestingly, the only study that compared depression and cognitive function in individual patients who were tested at times when they were not depressed and during bouts of major depression found no significant correlation between depression and cognitive performance.[154]

While the causes of depression in MS are likely multifactorial, several pathophysiological correlates have been reported. Depression is far less common in patients with lesions that are restricted largely to the spinal cord as opposed to the brain.[136] Measures of brain atrophy, such as enlargement of subarachnoid spaces (sulci, fissures, cisterns) and enlargement of ventricles, are associated with depression in MS patients (reviewed in 2000 by Bakshi et al.).[10] Recent MRI studies have reported that white matter lesions in the frontal and parietal areas of the brain are correlated with depression, suggesting that those lesions might lead to depression by disconnecting the cortical areas in the brain that regulate mood.[10]

## Suicide

As with depression, suicide rates in MS patients are high. The rate of suicide attempts among a group of MS patients who used hospital services in Nova Scotia was three times that of the general population.[59] The suicide rates among Danish women and men with MS are, respectively, 50 and 70 percent greater than those of the general Danish population.[169] It is sobering to note that about one in five patients who ended their lives with Dr. Kevorkian had MS. (He is the assisted-suicide advocate who presided over 47 deaths in the United States from 1990 to 1997.)[43] Risk factors of suicide for men with MS include mental disorders (which includes depression), recent exacerbations, and moderate disability; risk factors for women with MS are not distinct.[168] That study did not include social factors in the analysis of risk factors, but another study reported that people with MS who experience physical decline but have supportive relationships are less likely to commit suicide than those without such relationships.[102]

Depression is generally associated with an increased risk of suicide; about 15 percent of all people with major depression commit suicide.[141] Recognition and treatment of depression thus is an important tool in suicide prevention.[168]

## Treatment

Depression and anxiety among MS patients are often unrecognized and untreated.[50] Although there is a general consensus that depression in MS can often be effectively treated (treatments are listed in Table 3.1), there are few controlled clinical trials of antidepressant treatment in MS. A small double-blind study indicated that desipramine was effective in the treatment of depressive symptoms, although anticholinergic side effects limited the dose that could be given.[155] However, the study did not examine the effect of antidepressant treatment on the functional abilities or perception of disability in these patients. Another study reported that response to pharmacological treatment for depressive symptoms among MS patients was "extremely high," as was the relapse rate after discontinuation of the medication.[156] In that study, conducted in 1996, 51 out of 228 patients (22 percent) received pharmacological treatment for depression. In addition, treatment of depression improves adherence to beta-interferon (IFN-β) therapy (reviewed in 1999 by Walther and Holfeld[185]). Even an eight-week treatment of cognitive behavior therapy administered by telephone has been reported to improve adherence.[117]

Studies conducted in the 1980s reported that as many as 40 percent of MS patients with depression did not receive appropriate treatment (reviewed in 1994 by Fischer et al.[56]). Paradoxically, a survey of MS practitioners suggested that they tend to overestimate the prevalence of major depression in MS.[56] The median estimate made by MS practitioners was that 30 percent of MS patients are depressed at any one time, which is higher than estimates of most studies based on validated depression rating scales.[126]

## Depression as a Side Effect of Interferon Therapy

Based on early clinical trial results, depression is listed as a possible side effect of beta-interferon therapy in MS. However, the data are contradictory (Table 3.2).[185] Patients in the first large, controlled North American clinical trial

**TABLE 3.1** Medications Used to Treat Depression

| Trade Name | Generic Name | Mechanism |
|---|---|---|
| Elavil[153] | Amitriptyline | A tricyclic antidepressant. Amitriptyline is metabolized to nortriptyline, which is an active metabolite. Has significant anticholinergic and sedative effects, with moderate orthostatic hypotension. Has very high ability to block serotonin uptake and moderate activity with respect to norepinephrine uptake. |
| Pamelor[69] | Nortriptyline | A tricyclic antidepressant. Studies suggest that nortriptyline interferes with the transport, release, and storage of catecholamines. Operant conditioning techniques in rats and pigeons suggest that nortriptyline has a combination of stimulant and depressant properties. |
| Paxil[123,153] | Paroxetine | Paxil is a selective serotonin reuptake inhibitor (SSRI), meaning that it blocks serotonin from being reabsorbed into the sender nerve cell. This process increases the amount of serotonin available to be absorbed by the next cell and may help message transmission. |
| Prozac[115,123,153] | Fluoxetine hydrochloride | An SSRI that increases serotonin levels in the midbrain. |
| Tofranil[153] | Imipramine | A tricyclic antidepressant. In MS it is used to treat bladder symptoms, including urinary frequency and incontinence, and also for the management of neurologic pain. |
| Wellbutrin[153] | Bupropion hydrochloride | Mechanism of the antidepressant effect of bupropion is not known. It is a weak blocker of the neuronal uptake of serotonin and norepinephrine; it also inhibits the neuronal reuptake of dopamine to some extent. |
| Zoloft[115,123,153,157] | Sertraline | Zoloft is an SSRI that blocks serotonin from being reabsorbed into the sender nerve cell. This process increases the amount of serotonin available to be absorbed by the next cell and may help transmission of nerve cells. |

**Potential Side Effects**

Dryness of mouth, constipation, increased appetite and weight gain, dizziness, drowsiness, decreased sexual ability, headache, nausea, unusual tiredness or weakness, unpleasant taste, diarrhea, heartburn, increased sweating, vomiting

Dizziness, drowsiness, headache, decreased sexual ability, increased appetite, nausea, unusual tiredness or weakness, unpleasant taste, diarrhea, heartburn, increased sweating, vomiting

Decrease in sexual drive or ability, headache, nausea, problems urinating, decreased or increased appetite, unusual tiredness or weakness, tremor, trouble sleeping, anxiety, agitation, nervousness or restlessness, changes in vision including blurred vision, fast or irregular heartbeat, tingling, burning, or prickly sensations, vomiting

Anxiety, nervousness, insomnia, fatigue, tremor, sweating, gastrointestinal distress, anorexia, diarrhea, dizziness, decreased libido

Dizziness, drowsiness, headache, decreased sexual ability, increased appetite, nausea, unusual tiredness or weakness, unpleasant taste, diarrhea, heartburn, increased sweating, vomiting

Restlessness, agitation, anxiety, insomnia, delusions, hallucinations, psychotic episodes, confusion, paranoia, weight loss

Nausea, diarrhea or loose stools, tremor, trouble sleeping, drowsiness, dry mouth, decreased appetite, weight loss, sweating, anxiety, or decreased sexual drive

**TABLE 3.2** Depression and Beta-Interferon

| Observation | Methods Used to Assess Depression | Study Size[a] | Study Group |
|---|---|---|---|
| Four patients on IFN-β1b attempted and one committed suicide. No patients in the placebo group attempted suicide. | Patient reports | 372 | North American IFN-β clinical trial[174] |
| Depression rates in different dosage groups of beta-interferon-1a were<br>24% on 44 μg<br>21% on 22 μg<br>28% on placebo | Three different rating scales:<br>1. Beck's Hopelessness Scale<br>2. Centre for Epidemiologic Studies' Depression Scale<br>3. General Health Questionnaire | 276 | European IFN-β clinical trial[48] |
| Depression was neither caused nor exacerbated by IFN-β1b. | Three different rating scales:<br>1. Hamilton Depression Rating Scale<br>2. Beck Depression Inventory<br>3. State-Trait Anxiety Inventory<br><br>Patients were interviewed in person at MS clinic by a neuropsychologist | 90 | Borras and coworkers[19] |
| Patients who were depressed before onset of treatment with IFN-β1a became less depressed at initiation of treatment, but returned to pre-treatment levels within 2 months. | Depression-Dejection scale of the Profile of Mood States<br>Patients were interviewed by telephone | 56 | Mohr and coworkers[118] |

[a]In cases where only a subset of patients were analyzed for depression, the numbers reported here are lower than those reported for the full study.

of beta-interferon therapy reported increased symptoms of depression.[174] Four out of 247 patients in the two treatment groups attempted and one committed suicide, but although alarming, this was not statistically significant. In contrast, interferon-treated patients in the comparable European trial showed lower levels of depression than placebo-treated patients, although all were higher than the general population.[133] In contrast to the North American trial which relied only on patients' own assessment of depression, depression among patients in the European trial was measured using three different scales.

Treatment with alpha-interferon is also linked to depression (reviewed in 2000 by Menkes and MacDonald[114] and Trask[178]), although there are conflicting reports.[121] Alpha-interferon does not cross the blood-brain barrier and the mechanisms by which it induces depression is unknown, although it has been proposed that interferon causes decreased serum tryptophan, a serotonin precursor.[114] Decreased serotonin levels are related to the onset of depressed mood.

Other studies have reported varying mood responses to beta-interferon therapy, but the most thorough study indicates that it neither causes nor exacerbates depression in MS patients.[19] At the same time, given the variety of reports of depression and the prevalence of depression among MS patients, potential changes in patients taking beta-interferon therapy should be monitored and treated.

## Conclusions

Despite the consensus that depression is a prevalent and troubling concern among MS patients, much remains unknown about the interaction of affective and neurological symptoms. In 1990, Minden and Schiffer recommended: "More research, using advanced imaging techniques and standardized psychiatric interviews and diagnostic criteria, is needed to clarify connections between depressive symptoms and the neurological disease. Systematic, controlled and appropriate blinded studies that use reliable and valid instruments to detect changes in mood states to assess the efficacy of psychotherapy and pharmacotherapy among depressed MS patients are also important."[116] This recommendation still rings true today. Trask goes so far as to state that "it is almost certain that individuals treated with IFN will experience fatigue and possibly psychiatric side effects such as depression and anxiety."[178]

Although depression is prevalent among MS patients, it is notable that most adapt successfully to the disease. A study that used a variety of standardized scales and interviewing procedures analyzed the psychosocial well-being of 94 people who had lived with MS for more than 10 years on average.[44] The majority, approximately two-thirds, had achieved positive psychosocial adjustment to MS. Another study based on a mailed survey to 125 members of a regional chapter of the MS Society indicated similar results.[47] Based on their responses to a broad spectrum of measures such as family and social relationships, coping strategies, self-esteem, and emotional functioning, most respondents had adapted to MS successfully. At the same time, about 20 percent reported that they felt a need for professional help in coping with depression, compared to more than twice as many (53 percent) who wished for help identifying ways to adapt to their lives with MS. For this sample, help in coping with depression was seen as an important, but not the most important, need.

Depression is one of the more pervasive complications of MS, yet it is frequently unrecognized. Although its cause is unknown, the availability of effective treatment suggests that the more immediate research priority should be aimed at improving patient and physician education. Insofar as understanding the etiology of depression in MS patients can increase the number of people who are effectively treated, this is also a research priority, but the most far-reaching impact will likely come from simply applying available treatments to more people with MS. Because of their frequent contact with people with MS, local MS Society chapters could plan and coordinate services aimed at recognizing and treating depression. Finally, the role of the family should be considered.

## SPASTICITY AND WEAKNESS

Impairments of muscle function are a central feature of MS. They can be manifest in stiffness or involuntary muscle actions as well as in weakness, which limits a muscle's functional capacity. This section focuses on the problems of spasticity, spasms, and weakness. The next major section addresses ataxia and problems of coordination of movement.

Weakness of the limbs is a constant feature of advanced MS and is present in approximately 80 percent of all people with MS (reviewed in Matthews, 1998[107]). Both lower limbs, usually asymmetrically, are most often affected, followed in frequency by weakness in only one lower limb and then weakness in one lower and one upper limb, usually on the same side. Weakness of one arm without leg weakness is uncommon. Motor disability in the limbs is seldom due to weakness alone. Cerebellar ataxia and tremor, particularly in the arms, and loss of postural sense also contribute to weakness. The initial complaint is often of weakness only after exertion, but then it increases gradually until it is a constant presence.

Spasticity is generally defined as a state of increased muscular tone in which abnormal stretch reflexes intensify muscle resistance to passive movements. In clinical practice, the concept of spasticity extends beyond the resistance to passive movement to include a complex disorder of voluntary movement.[107] It is a common symptom of MS. In one survey, 70 percent of 168 MS patients registered with the Northern California Chapter of the MS Society reported that they experienced mild to severe spasticity.[72]

Many MS patients also experience muscle weakness along with spasticity, but it is possible to have spasticity without weakness or to have weakness without spasticity. Spasticity in MS usually affects the legs more than the arms, and it can even offset muscle weakness and aid in standing, walking, and transferring.[86] Spastic paresis, slight or incomplete paralysis due to spasticity, has been cited as the major cause of the loss of ability to work among persons with MS.[60]

The increase in resting muscle tone that characterizes spasticity is also associated with muscle spasms. In the progressive stages of MS, exaggeration of extensor tone can result in *extensor spasms* in which there is forceful activation of leg muscles inducing plantar flexion of the ankle, together with hip and knee joint extension. These spasms are most likely to occur while a patient is lying in bed at night or is awakening in the morning. Spasms can be severe enough to eject a seated patient from a wheelchair. Flexor tone becomes more prominent at later stages of MS and initially causes falling without warning. In *flexor spasms* there is a generalized flexion of muscles at the ankle, knee, and hip, giving rise to limb withdrawal or retraction. Spasms may promote progressive muscle contraction, joint deformities, and ultimately skin damage and breakdown. Both types of spasms may be quite painful, disrupting sleep and adversely affecting activities of daily living.

## Origins of Spasticity and Weakness in Voluntary Movement

Muscle groups normally work together: when one is flexed, its opposing muscle is relaxed. This complementary muscle action depends on the transmission of signals along pathways connecting the brain, motor neurons in the spinal cord, and muscles (Figure 3.1). The CNS damage caused by MS disrupts this

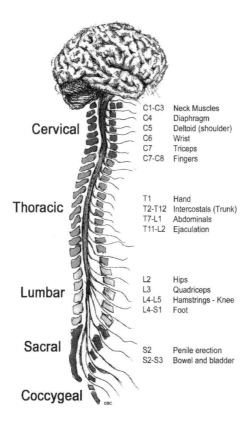

| Cervical | C1-C3 | Neck Muscles |
|---|---|---|
| | C4 | Diaphragm |
| | C5 | Deltoid (shoulder) |
| | C6 | Wrist |
| | C7 | Triceps |
| | C7-C8 | Fingers |
| Thoracic | T1 | Hand |
| | T2-T12 | Intercostals (Trunk) |
| | T7-L1 | Abdominals |
| | T11-L2 | Ejaculation |
| Lumbar | L2 | Hips |
| | L3 | Quadriceps |
| | L4-L5 | Hamstrings - Knee |
| | L4-S1 | Foot |
| Sacral | S2 | Penile erection |
| | S2-S3 | Bowel and bladder |
| Coccygeal | | |

**FIGURE 3.1** Functions controlled by nerves at different levels of the spine. Damage at a particular level of the spine usually impairs functions controlled by all nerves at lower levels. SOURCE: Cheryl Cotman for the Christopher Reeve Paralysis Foundation. Reprinted with permission.

communication, allowing the persistent contraction of the muscle fibers that produces spasticity.

Spasticity is associated with sprouting of descending motor pathways to form new synaptic connections with spinal neurons and with hypersensitivity caused by denervation.[107] Damage to descending motor pathways also causes slowness of movement and weakness. The spinal plaques occurring in many types of spinal MS are associated with a progressive loss of axons and a reduction in diameter or a loss of myelination of residual axons passing through or close to the plaque.[103] There can also be alterations in the numbers and types of excitable sodium membrane channels exposed by the membrane demyelination, further altering the conduction capacity of the damaged axons.

Although the mechanisms leading to spasticity and muscle weakness in MS are not fully understood, knowledge about the mechanisms operating in other conditions may be helpful. For example, the mechanisms related to the spinal cord pathology known to occur in MS may be similar to those in incomplete spinal cord injury. The symptoms of spasticity and weakness in MS can also result from plaques in the supraspinal brain and brainstem, which would suggest a comparison with the results of stroke or intracapsular hemorrhage. However, considerably more is known about the effects of incomplete spinal cord injury. Thus, it is more likely to provide instructive parallels for understanding the pathology and pathophysiology of MS.

## Mechanisms of Spasticity and Spasms

The general features of spasticity in MS appear to resemble those observed in incomplete spinal cord injury, with the added complexities of concurrent hemispheric, visual, and cerebellar lesions. It appears that the effects of the distributed axonal loss and demyelination of the spinal cord are mediated primarily by spinal interneuronal systems that are normally held under tight descending control. These interneuronal controls are mediated by reticulospinal actions, including those provided by monoaminergic fibers, whose actions appear to differ on different classes of neurons. Key features of disruptions of these interneuronal systems are briefly reviewed.

### Increased Stretch Reflex Responsiveness

The group II excitatory interneurons might have special importance in mediating spastic hypertonia, with exaggerated stretch reflex responses in spinal cord injury or MS. These group II interneurons receive strong inhibitory effects from descending monoaminergic pathways, especially $\alpha_2$ norepinephrine (NE) systems.[20,82,124,131] Interruption of these descending pathways releases this interneuron from inhibitory control, providing a strong stretch-evoked excitation. This synapse may be a potential site of action for tizanidine (Zanaflex), an $\alpha_2$ NE agonist used to control spasticity.

There is also recent evidence for disynaptic excitation of motoneurons from group Ia afferents released from both extensor and flexor muscles during locomotion.[6,40] This system is undoubtedly under tight descending control, possibly indirectly, and can greatly amplify the stretch reflexes in both extensor and flexor muscles.

Conversely, group Ia inhibitory interneurons may show reductions in excitability after spinal injury. This change potentially promotes the emergence of unhelpful muscle contraction by limiting the strength of mutual inhibition between agonist-antagonist muscles.[28]

## Special Roles for Free Nerve Ending Mechanoreceptors

Group III (small myelinated) and group IV (small unmyelinated) fibers are known to exert potent reflex actions in spinal cord injury and are likely to be important in MS-induced cord damage as well. Animal models of incomplete spinal cord injury have shown that stretching the extensor muscles to the point where free nerve ending mechanoreceptors are activated produces a sharp inhibition of the same extensors, accompanied by excitation of flexors.[149] This sharp "clasp-knife" inhibition is manifest as a sudden drop in active force and is not causally dependent on the presence of a flexion withdrawal response. The interneurons receiving free nerve ending input are hyperexcitable when spinal cord pathways are interrupted, giving rise to severe extensor inhibition and to concurrent excitation of flexors.

## Exaggerated Flexion Reflexes

Loss of monoaminergic fibers in MS potentially releases flexion reflexes from descending inhibitory controls, giving rise to flexor spasms. Under normal conditions, the interneurons mediating the so-called flexor reflex system are closely regulated by monoaminergic pathways, acting in all probability on 5-$HT_{1b/d}$ (serotonin) receptors, or on $\alpha_2$-adrenergic receptors to depress the excitability of several interneuron pathways. Interruption of this monoaminergic innervation as a result of spinal cord damage (as in MS) releases the capacity of these interneurons to generate "plateau potentials." The plateau potentials in these interneurons may in turn be responsible for the increased responsiveness and the prolonged reflex afterdischarge seen in some flexion responses, especially after long-term spinal cord injury.

## Extensor Spasms

The origins of extensor spasms are presently unclear, and there are no published studies examining their origins in human spinal cord injury or MS. One possible explanation for their occurrence is that the extensor spasm is a fragment of the normal locomotion or standing program in the spinal cord, in which the leg extensors are switched on forcefully to provide weight support during the stance phase of locomotion. Indeed, in intensive study in the cat, Pearson and colleagues demonstrated that the stance phase of fictive locomotion is associated with a switch from force-mediated (Ib) inhibition of extensor muscles to a force-mediated excitation.[112] This switch presumably happens because Ib inhibitory interneurons are gated out during stance, in favor of a parallel group I excitatory pathway. As with the other interneuronal systems discussed above, this excitatory Ib pathway may be under monoaminergic control, which is disrupted in spinal cord injury or MS.

## Treatment of Spasticity

Although little can be done to counter the muscle weakness that occurs in MS, several forms of treatment can be applied to help limit the adverse effects of spasticity. However, treatment plans must be designed to meet individual patient needs and must take into consideration both the benefits and the risks of specific interventions. For some ambulatory patients, for example, treatment of spasticity is less desirable if increased stiffness of the legs facilitates walking by offsetting muscle weakness. Management of spasticity often involves a combination of therapeutic approaches, including control of secondary factors that stimulate spasticity, proper positioning, physiotherapy, and medications. Surgical procedures, such as tendon release, are sometimes used when other interventions are not effective.

Spasticity can be triggered or worsened by a variety of painful or unpleasant stimuli, such as urinary tract infections, fecal impaction, contractures, tight clothing, or ill-fitting footwear. A treatment plan should ensure that these sources of secondary stimulation are eliminated or controlled. Careful attention to balanced and symmetrical positioning when patients are standing, sitting, or lying down is important for preventing fixation in distorted postures induced by spasticity. Proper positioning can help stimulate muscles that are antagonists to those subject to spasticity. Physical therapy helps in maintaining balanced muscle tone, in preventing or treating contractures, and in training muscles in coordinated movement.

Baclofen and tizanidine are the two medications used most often to treat spasticity, with cloazepam and gabapentin usually reserved as secondary medications (Table 3.3). Baclofen, an agonist of $\gamma$-aminobutyric acid-B (GABA B) receptors, reduces presynaptic release of excitatory neurotransmitters and, at higher concentrations, acts postsynaptically to antagonize their actions. Generally given orally, baclofen can also be administered intrathecally through subcutaneous pump to treat more severe spasticity in long-standing MS.[127] Tizanidine stimulates $a_2$-andrenergic receptors in the spinal cord, which inhibits presynaptic release of excitatory amino acids. Tizanidine reduces flexor reflexes and spasms and relieves pain. It appears to reduce muscle strength less than baclofen but may not result in measurably better function (see Kita and Goodkin[92]).

Dantrolene acts within the muscles themselves to produce inhibition of the excitation-contraction coupling process, which leads to reduced muscle strength. Because of its action, it may be better suited for treatment of nonambulatory patients for whom added weakness is less likely to impair mobility. Patients receiving dantrolene should be monitored for liver function because of its potential hepatotoxicity. Benzodiazapines, such as diazepam and clonazepam, act to reduce muscle tone through three mechanisms: suppression of sensory impulses from muscles and skin receptors, postsynaptic potentiation of GABA, and inhibition of excitatory descending pathways. They are generally used in combination with baclofen or other medications.

Intramuscular injections of botulinum A toxin can be helpful, especially for patients with severe localized spasms. The chemical denervation produced by botulinum A toxin can last for up to three months. A study of nine patients with long-standing MS showed reduced spasticity and improved ease of nursing care with no adverse effects.[92,163]

## Recommendations for Further Study of Spasticity in MS

Further research is needed to clarify the mechanisms of spasticity and spasms in MS and to identify opportunities for therapeutic intervention.

- Determine the spectrum of nerve fiber damage in spinal MS and whether this damage involves monoaminergic systems preferentially.
- Determine whether the extensor spasm is a product of the locomotion pattern generator and whether this interneuronal circuitry is under descending monoaminergic control.
- Determine the specific monoamine receptors that influence the stance phase of locomotion and, potentially, the extensor spasms of MS and spinal cord injury (see, for example, Kim et al.[89]).
- Test the possibility that restoration of $5\text{-HT}_{1b/d}$ or $\alpha_2$ NE action in the spinal cord can lead to restoration of flexion reflex interneuronal excitability and a reduction of flexion spasms.
- Determine whether flexor spasms can be reduced by reducing the strength of group III and IV afferent input from muscle to spinal interneurons. For example, group III and IV receptors carry substance P and other peptides and make synapses in lamina I of the cord and in the intermediate nucleus as well. It follows that compounds related perhaps to capsaicin may discharge these transmitters from their afferent terminals and reduce the central actions of these afferents.

**TABLE 3.3** Medications Used to Treat Spasticity

| Trade Name | Generic Name | Mechanism |
|---|---|---|
| Lioresal[64,73,92] | Baclofen | Baclofen is a muscle relaxant and antispasmodic that works by inhibiting the nervous system. Its precise mechanism of action is unknown, although it is thought to inhibit the transmission of impulses between nerve cells. It is administered orally in pill form or via an intrathecal delivery system (a surgically implanted pump). |
| Zanaflex[64,73,92] | Tizanidine | Tizanidine is an $\alpha_2$-adrenergic agonist that reduces spasticity reducing the release of excitatory neurotransmitters and Substance P in the spinal cord. Its greatest effects are on polysynaptic pathways. |
| Klonopin[64] | Clonazepam | Clonazepam is a benzodiazepine and is often prescribed as an anticonvulsant. Benzodiazepines belong to a group of medicines that slow down the central nervous system. |
| Neurontin[37,79] | Gabapentin | Gabapentin is structurally related to the neurotransmitter GABA but it does not interact with GABA receptors. The mechanism by which it exerts its anticonvulsant action is unknown. |
| Botox[64,92] | Botulinum A Toxin | Intramuscular injection typically results in a dose-dependent reduction of hyperactive muscle contraction that lasts for an average of 12.5 weeks and is ultimately reversible. Botox is believed to produce its therapeutic effect by acting selectively on peripheral cholinergic nerve endings to inhibit the release of the neurotransmitter acetylcholine at the neuromuscular junction. |
| Dantrium[64,92] | Dantrolene | Acts directly on skeletal muscle, probably by dissociating the excitation-contraction coupling mechanism as a result of interference with the release of calcium from the sarcoplasmic reticulum. This results in a decreased force of reflex muscle contraction. |

## Potential Side Effects

Drowsiness or unusual tiredness, increased weakness, dizziness or lightheadedness, confusion, unusual constipation, new or unusual bladder symptoms, trouble sleeping, unusual unsteadiness or clumsiness, fainting, hallucinations, severe mood changes, skin rash or itching

Sedation, dry mouth, dizziness, hypotension, vasodilation, constipation, diarrhea, flatulence, nervousness, anxiety, paraesthesia, tremor, seizures, vertigo, agitation, euphoria, stupor, urinary frequency and urgency, back pain, sinusitis, flu-like syndrome

Confusion, depression, double vision or abnormal eye movements, hallucinations, lightheadedness or fainting spells, mood changes, excitability, movement difficulty, muscle cramps, tremors, weakness or tiredness, constipation or diarrhea, difficulty sleeping, headache, nausea, vomiting

Somnolence, ataxia, dizziness, fatigue, nausea, vomiting

Transient weakness in injected or neighboring muscles, skin rash, and flu-like syndrome

Diarrhea, dizziness, drowsiness, weakness, nausea, unusual tiredness, abdominal cramps, blurred or double vision, chills and fever, constipation, frequent urination, headache, loss of appetite, speech difficulties, sleep difficulties, nervousness

## Mechanisms of Muscular Weakness for Voluntary Movement

As with spasticity, the muscle weakness seen in chronic spinal MS probably results from changes in motoneurons and interneuron electrophysiology that are comparable to those observed in incomplete spinal cord injury. These changes result in disruptions of interneuron and motoneuron pathways and in monoaminergic input to spinal motoneurons. Other peripheral changes that may contribute to muscle weakness include muscle wasting, fiber loss, muscle contracture, and joint contractures.

### Loss of Descending Input to Spinal Premotor Interneurons

Communication pathways between the interneurons of the spinal cord and the axons of sensory and motor neurons, which project outside the spinal cord, are essential for generating coordinated muscle commands. Disruption of the axons from corticospinal, rubrospinal, vestibulospinal, and reticulospinal pathways may render these key interneurons less excitable and hence less able to relay motor commands. Loss of descending pathway excitation of key excitatory interneurons can also limit the capacity for other descending or segmental spinal pathways to activate motoneurons and, consequently, to limit voluntary force generation. In addition, some reticulospinal systems control segmental pathways through inhibitory input, and since segmental excitatory and inhibitory systems work in concert to produce normal motor control, disruption of inhibitory input might also contribute to impaired motor function.

### Loss of Monosynaptic Corticospinal and Rubrospinal Projections to Motoneurons

Loss of direct or monosynaptic projections to spinal motoneurons, especially those innervating distal limb musculature, contributes to weakness by limiting a patient's capacity to activate the motoneurons. With fewer axons projecting to the motor neurons, residual descending pathways may have greater difficulty reaching the signal threshold of larger motor neurons, thereby limiting the range of voluntary force that a patient can achieve. In experimental work with monkeys, selective loss of these systems can have a greater effect on fine motor control of digits than on the equally voluntary control of more proximal muscle groups.[98] With the loss of innervation, muscles are also more likely to fatigue because of the associated increase in the sense of effort, both of which are reported frequently by MS patients.

### Loss of Norepinephrine (NE) and Serotonin (5-HT) Input to Spinal Motoneurons.

Damage to spinal pathways projecting from the locus coeruleus (a source of NE projections) and from the raphe nuclei (a source of 5-HT) significantly reduces measurable 5-HT and NE in the spinal cord and alters the response patterns of many spinal interneurons and motoneurons.* Although not documented in humans, animal models of MS, such as experimental autoimmune encephalomyelitis (EAE, see Chapter 2) have shown loss of these monoaminergic fibers.

For motoneurons, loss of monoaminergic input may reduce their excitability by altering their capacity either to develop plateau potentials or to modulate the characteristics of their current-frequency (I-F) relation. (Plateau potentials are sustained depolarizations of neurons that greatly outlast the duration of the initial depolarizing stimulus. The I-F curve is the relation between injected or synaptic current and the resultant firing of the motoneuron.)

Since these monoaminergic effects are not necessarily uniformly distributed throughout a given motoneuron pool, loss of such innervation could differentially affect the recruitment behavior of motoneurons by compressing the range of synaptic current over which motoneurons are recruited and even reversing the recruitment order in some situations (for example, see Powers and Rymer[132]). There are also reductions in motoneuron firing rate, both initially at recruitment and over the full span of rate modulation. These rate reductions (which may result from alterations in the locus and slope of the I-F relation) mean that motoneuron firing rates are no longer well matched to the mechanical twitch properties of the active muscle fibers, rendering the overall muscle contraction less "efficient" (also Gemperline et al.[65]). For a given force level, the higher the level of motoneuronal discharge in the aggregate, the lower the "efficiency" ratio.

### Changes in Muscle Tissue

Observations in patients with spinal cord injuries suggest that patients with severe, long-standing MS may also develop weakness through overt changes in muscle tissue (although, note Tilbery et al.[177]). These changes consist of muscle wasting, shifts in the metabolic properties of muscle fibers (toward glycolytic systems), and a reduction in fatigue resistance. In addition, there may be muscle and joint contractures that are associated with proliferation of connective tissues, shortening of muscle length, loss of muscle fibers, and sometimes joint deformities.

### Recommendations for Further Study of Voluntary Muscle Weakness in MS

Research is needed to clarify the mechanisms producing muscle weakness in MS and to test potential therapies to counter weakness.

---

*The locus coeruleus and raphe nuclei are different points of the motor control relay "stations" in the brain. Neurons projecting from the locus coeruleus transmit their signals largely through norepinephrine; those from the raphe nuclei predominantly use serotonin.

- What is the state of monoaminergic fiber innervation in the spinal cord of chronic MS patients? Is there fiber loss, and if so, is it diffuse or more localized? Is there a disproportionate effect of MS on these nerve fiber types?
- As a screening tool, what happens to force-EMG (electromyocardiogram) relations in paretic muscles of MS patients? Do they shift in such a way as to indicate a reduction in efficiency of muscle activation?
- Determine the recruitment and firing rate properties of motoneurons in patients with muscle weakness associated with MS. Do they suggest that there is a loss of monoaminergic innervation?
- Test whether administration of a 5-HT$_2$ (or $\alpha_2$ NE) agonist improves the performance of motoneurons by increasing their firing rate and normalizing their recruitment patterns. Is this effect associated with recovery of force-EMG relations and a measurable improvement in voluntary force generation?

## ATAXIA AND TREMOR

Ataxia refers to a lack of or reduction in coordination and is invariably associated with tremor, which occurs as an involuntary, rhythmic, oscillatory movement of a body part. These symptoms occur in 75 percent of patients with multiple sclerosis and are most frequently manifested as upper limb intention tremor. They are severely disabling and embarrassing, affecting upper limb function, gait, and in severe cases, balance in standing and sitting. The tremor of multiple sclerosis is frequently just one component of a complex movement disorder that includes dysmetria and other ataxic features, and the underlying mechanisms are poorly understood. Although inflammatory demyelination in different parts of the cerebellum and related areas may produce a distinct tremor, it is nonetheless extremely difficult to classify individual tremors in patients. Tremor remains one of the most difficult symptoms to manage and is associated with a poor outcome in rehabilitation.

### Management of Ataxia

As with spasticity, there are practical components to the management of ataxia, which must be considered prior to other interventions. These include patient education, improving posture and proximal stability during activities, and provision of equipment. The use of weights to dampen tremor have not proved to be very successful, although they may be slightly better if a computer damping device is incorporated. A small exploratory study of therapy input suggested modest benefit.[84] Other treatments involve either drug therapy, which is limited and often not well tolerated, or invasive surgical intervention, which includes thalamotomy and thalamic stimulation.

## Drug Therapy

Few drugs have been evaluated and none adequately. Isoniazid (with pyridoxine) has been shown to be of limited benefit in a number of small studies. It showed some effect in 10 of 13 patients, although this did not translate into improved function, while 4 out of 6 patients showed sufficient benefit that they wished to continue the drug. It is thought to be more useful in postural tremor with an intention component rather than pure intention tremor. Up to 1,200 mg a day in divided doses has been used, increasing gradually from 200 mg twice a day. This drug, which was the first to undergo a randomized controlled trial for the treatment of multiple sclerosis, is not well tolerated and causes gastrointestinal disturbance. There has been even less evaluation of other drugs, including carbamazepine, clonazepam and buspirone. Ethyl alcohol and propranolol have not been found to be useful. A single-blind, cross-sectional study evaluated the role of carbamazepine in cerebellar tremor in 10 patients (7 with MS) and suggested some benefit. More recently, the $5-HT_3$ receptor antagonist, ondansetron, has been evaluated, given by both intravenous and oral routes. Although the I.V. studies looked promising, the more recent placebo-controlled, double-blind parallel group study was negative. Fifty-two patients, the majority of whom had MS, were randomized and the treatment arm received 8 mg per day for one week. Although some benefit in the nine-hole peg test was seen in the treated arm, there was no difference between the groups on the global ataxia rating scale.

## Surgical Intervention

Although thalamotomy of the ventral intermediate nucleus (VIN) has been shown to reduce tremor in Parkinson's disease patients, there has been limited evaluation of its role in tremor relating to MS. In general, it is not as effective in this condition. In selected patients with MS, thalamotomy has been reported to alleviate contralateral limb tremor, initially in about 65 to 96 percent of cases, although in about 20 percent, tremor returns within 12 months. Functional improvement is estimated to occur in only 25 to 75 percent of patients. However, these results are not based on controlled studies, and no prospective study has evaluated the influence of this procedure on overall disability, handicap, and quality of life; nor have side effects been quantified, although they may occur in up to 45 percent of cases. Serious side effects, which include hemiparesis, dysphasia, and dysphagia, occur in up to 10 percent of patients. Experience suggests that optimum results are obtained in patients with relatively stable disease, good mobility, and minimal overall disability status—an extremely small group. Three recent papers have suggested that thalamic stimulation can also alleviate tremor in up to 69 percent of patients in studies involving 13, 5, and 15 patients, respectively.[66,119,191] These were carefully selected patients; for example, the 5 patients reported by Whittle et al. were from an initial group of 17 patients, and no control study has as yet been carried out.[191] Serious side effects were seen in 2 of 15 patients in the study by Montgomery et al.[119] No trial has compared thalamic stimulation versus lesioning, although it is suggested that stimulation is associated with fewer side effects. Other approaches, including extracranial application of brief AC (alternating current) pulsed electromagnetic fields, dynamic systems with multidegree of freedom orthoses, and robotic arms based on virtual reality have not been adequately evaluated.

## Conclusion

Ataxia and its associated tremor remain among the most resistant and disabling symptoms to manage. Current strategies are not evidence based and are of limited benefit.

# BLADDER AND BOWEL DYSFUNCTION

Bladder dysfunction affects up to 90 percent of people with MS at some time during their illness. Bladder dysfunction is the presenting feature in approximately 5 percent of patients, but the incidence increases as the disease progresses. The level of dysfunction relates to the stage of disease, and more than half of patients who cannot walk have bladder complaints (Robert Hamill, personal communication). The symptoms of bladder dysfunction are disruptive to social, vocational, and sexual activities, but they are generally treatable and can be successfully managed (see Table 3.4). Bowel dysfunction is less prevalent than bladder dysfunction in MS, affecting up to 68 percent of patients,[29] but it might be related to bladder dysfunction since people with bladder problems are sometimes reluctant to consume enough fluids, which leads to constipation. Chia et al.[29] found that 52 percent of patients with urinary symptoms also had some degree of bowel dysfunction. The neurological basis for bowel dysfunction in MS is not as clearly defined as it is for the bladder, and treatment options are limited.

## Normal Bladder Control Mechanisms

Neural bladder function control occurs primarily in the sacral spinal cord, as well as the pons, diencephalon, and cerebral cortex in the brain. Activation of the spinal reflex pathway promotes urine retention. Pontine structures ensure that bladder functions are fully integrated. A normal micturition reflex depends on the integrity of the pons and the afferent and efferent pathways active in bladder

**TABLE 3.4** Indications of Bladder Dysfunction

| Type | Definition | Urodynamic Pattern of Dysfunction | Prevalence in Patients with MS and Bladder Dysfunction (%)[a] |
|---|---|---|---|
| Urgency | Urgent need to urinate; causes the bladder to empty at small volumes | Detrusor hyperreflexia, excitability, and spasticity | 85 |
| Frequency | Frequent need to urinate | Detrusor hyperreflexia | 83 |
| Urge Incontinence | Inability to control the bladder, leading to involuntary urination | Detrusor hyperreflexia with or without outlet obstruction, and impaired sphincter contractility | 63 |
| Hesitancy | Difficulty initiating micturition | Detrusor sphincter dyssynergia, and detrusor hyperreflexia with impaired contractility | 49 |
| Interrupted Stream | Difficulty completing micturition | Detrusor sphincter dyssynergia | 43 |
| Sensation of Retention | Inability to completely empty the bladder | Detrusor areflexia | 34 |
| Nocturnal Enuresis | Incontinence during sleep | Detrusor hyperreflexia with impaired sphincter contractility | 14 |

[a]From Betts et al.[16]

function. Activation of the medial aspect of the pons results in detrusor, or bladder muscle, contraction, while activation of the lateral aspect results in urethral sphincter contraction. The ascending afferent pathways to the pontine centers and the descending efferent pathways travel in the anterolateral and lateral columns where demyelinating lesions create dysfunction. Cortical influences permit control of micturition ensuring personal and socially acceptable voiding.

The integrity of central control mechanisms permits bladder filling and maintenance of the filled bladder with little awareness or voluntary participation. Upon reaching normal capacity (350-500 ml), inhibitory pathways provide for suppression of the micturition reflex, activation of sympathetic outflow, and voluntary contraction of the external sphincter. Voiding requires the coordination of a number of control systems such that detrusor muscle activation and relaxation of sphincter mechanisms results in bladder emptying with only a few milliliters of residual urine.

## Patterns of Bladder Dysfunction

Bladder dysfunction in MS results from interruption of the neural control systems, most often in the sacral nerves.[16] As a result, the loss of bladder control is likely to coincide with lower limb spasticity and the diminished ability to respond to urinary urgency by moving to a toilet.

### Detrusor Hyperreflexia

The detrusor is the smooth muscle of the bladder that works in concert with internal and external bladder sphincters to allow normal urination. Micturition occurs when the detrusor muscle contracts while the sphincters relax, expelling urine from the bladder into the urethra.

A spastic or hyperreflexic detrusor muscle is usually secondary to lesions in the spinal cord, leading to increased contractility and decreased capacity of the bladder. Urinary urgency, the most common bladder symptom in MS, is caused primarily by detrusor hyperreflexia. Increased detrusor contractility causes the urge to void to be sensed before the bladder has reached normal capacity, resulting in frequent and urgent voiding of small amounts of urine. When these urges can no longer be controlled, urge incontinence results in the forceful expulsion of urine.

### Detrusor Sphincter Dyssynergia

Detrusor sphincter dyssynergia occurs when detrusor muscle hyperreflexia coincides with outlet obstruction due to contraction of the sphincters or impaired sphincter contractility. It can also coincide with impaired or ineffective detrusor contractility. Detrusor hyperreflexia with outlet obstruction or impaired detrusor contractility often result in hesitancy, retention, or overflow incontinence. Detrusor hyperreflexia with impaired sphincter contractility may result in overflow incontinence or nocturnal enuresis.

### Detrusor Areflexia

Impaired detrusor contractility is another cause of hesitation and retention, which can lead to bladder infections, the reflux of urine from the bladder back into a ureter, and bladder stone formation. Hydronephrosis, the accumulation of urine in the kidney, and renal failure can also occur but are rare in MS.

## Therapy for Bladder Dysfunction

The main goals of treatment are to reduce the frequency of voiding, improve emptying, and decrease incontinence. Detrusor hyperreflexia is most frequently treated through the use of anticholinergic medications, of which several are available (Table 3.5). Although some strategies initially work well for some patients, as the disease progresses, treatment is increasingly less effective. Catheterization is sometimes necessary for patients suffering from retention.

## Future Research in Bladder Dysfunction

Studies of the central and peripheral neurobiological control of micturition will improve our understanding of the roles of the numerous transmitter systems and permit new ideas of drug therapy. Studies of neuroplasticity should be performed to determine the effect of increased lesion load on micturition. Myelin repair and nerve regeneration studies including stem cell biology and the role of neurotrophins in glial and neuronal function and survival might permit repair and restoration of function. Many of these studies will relate directly to spinal cord injury, and joint funding options may be available.

Clinical research into bladder infections and keeping the urine sterile might be surprisingly fruitful, since infections restrict volume and compromise bladder function and pharmacological treatment. Intrathecal therapy to improve bladder function should be further explored. As mentioned above, motor spasticity is also linked with bladder dysfunction, and therapies developed for motor spasticity may improve bladder function. Clinical pathological spinal cord studies in humans are few and would expand our understanding of the relationship of pathology and pathophysiology in MS.

New and emerging technologies could have an impact on bladder dysfunction. Neural stimulators may be helpful in allowing patients to manually stimulate the nerves involved in bladder or sphincter control. The bladder circuit is ideal for developing computer models. Eventually a "bladder-brain" should be able to be developed to be placed in a pouch under the skin like a cardiac pacemaker and provide an integrated computer circuit (servoloop system) for filling and emptying the bladder without any CNS input.

## Normal Bowel Control Mechanisms

Gastrointestinal function, including motility, is controlled primarily by the enteric ganglia, which ensure synchronous contraction of the bowel so that food materials move along the digestive tract. The CNS contributes to bowel function via parasympathetic nervous system (PNS) and sympathetic nervous system (SNS) pathways. The PNS influence occurs via the vagus nerve and the sacral outflow. Vagal input is concentrated in the esophagus, stomach, and proximal small bowel and wanes distally. The SNS influence is via the greater, lesser, and least splanchnic nerves. They are derived from the thoracolumbar outflow and synapse in prevertebral ganglia (coeliac, superior, and inferior mesenteric) before postganglionic sympathetic fibers reach the bowel vasculature and enteric gan-

**TABLE 3.5** Medications Used to Treat Bladder and Bowel Dysfunction

| Trade Name | Generic Name | Indication |
| --- | --- | --- |
| Bentyl[106] | Dicyclomine hydrochloride | Urinary incontinence, gastrointestinal spasms |
| Cytospaz[106] | Hyoscyamine | Bladder spasms |
| DDAVP [90,179] | Desmopressin | Frequent urination |
| Ditropan XL[106] | Oxybutynin chloride; atropine | Overactive bladder, involuntary bladder contractions |
| Hiprex; Mandelamine[87,151] | Methenamine infection | Urinary tract |
| Pro-Banthine[106] | Propantheline bromide | Bladder spasms, cramps |
| Detrol[24] | Tolterodine tartrate | Urinary frequency, urgency, urge incontinence |
| Tofranil[106] | Imipramine | Urinary frequency, fecal incontinence |
| Zostrix[38,39] | Capsaicin | Hyperreflexia |

| Mechanism | Potential Side Effects |
|---|---|
| Cholinergic blocking agent. | Brief euphoria, slight dizziness, feeling of abdominal distention |
| Inhibits the actions of specific neurotransmitters on bladder smooth muscle. | Dry mouth, blurred vision, increased heart rate, dry eyes, headache, nervousness, urinary retention or hesitation, weakness |
| Hormone that works on the kidneys to reduce urine formation. | Runny or stuffy nose, abdominal or stomach cramps, flushing of the skin, headache, nausea, pain in the vulva |
| Relaxes the bladder smooth muscle; increases bladder capacity and delays the initial desire to void. | Dryness, drowsiness, blurred vision, dizziness, abdominal pain, back pain, flu syndrome, hypertension, palpitation, vasodilatation, constipation, diarrhea, flatulence, gastroesophageal reflux, arthritis, insomnia, nervousness, confusion, impaired urination |
| An anti-infective, usually prescribed on a long-term basis for repeated or chronic urinary tract infections. | Nausea, vomiting, skin rash |
| An antispasmodic-anticholinergic medication; it interferes with contractions and spasms. | Constipation, decreased sweating, dryness of mouth, nose, and throat, bloated feeling, blurred vision, difficulty swallowing |
| Acts as a competitive muscarinic receptor antagonist in the bladder to cause increased bladder control. | Dry mouth, headache, dizziness, somnolence, fatigue |
| Has moderate anticholinergic and sedative effects and high orthostatic hypotensive effects; imipramine is biotransformed into its active metabolite, desmethylimipramine (desipramine). | Dizziness, drowsiness, headache, decreased sexual ability, increased appetite, nausea, unusual tiredness or weakness, unpleasant taste, diarrhea, heartburn, increased sweating, vomiting |
| A neurotoxin that, when instilled within the bladder lumen, injures C fibers, producing partial deafferentiation of the bladder and permitting retention of urine. | Transient burning following application, stinging, erythema, cough, respiratory irritation |

glia. Different sympathetic transmitter systems establish "synaptic input" to the vasculature, submucosal plexus, and myenteric plexus. In turn, efferents from the enteric ganglia project to the prevertebral sympathetic ganglia, providing nicotinic input.

## Bowel Dysfunction

Constipation and fecal incontinence are the most common symptoms of bowel dysfunction, with constipation affecting up to 50 percent of people with MS and fecal incontinence affecting approximately 30 percent. Extreme constipation leading to megacolon is a relatively uncommon symptom.

### Constipation

The causes of constipation in MS are not clear. Although symptoms tend to increase in later stages, many people experience constipation throughout the course of the disease. One hypothesis is that constipation in MS is caused by decreased parasympathetic input, although this is considered unlikely since bilateral, strategically placed lesions would have to occur. Another hypothesis is that there is little relationship between constipation in MS and the neurological profile. As mentioned above, the treatment of bladder dysfunction can also contribute to constipation. People with bladder dysfunction are less likely to keep adequately hydrated, and the anticholinergic drugs often used to treat detrusor hyperreflexia can cause constipation since sphincter mechanisms are primarily cholinergic.

### Fecal Incontinence

Fecal incontinence is usually associated with constipation and occurs due to rectal overloading and overflow or when sphincter control and coordination are diminished due to sphincter muscle weakness. Involuntary sphincter relaxation may occur when the rectum is full due to the rectoanal inhibitory reflex, especially in a chronically distended rectum.

## Therapy for Bowel Dysfunction

The main goals of treatment are to enhance gastrointestinal transit and reduce constipation and to prevent or reduce fecal incontinence. Timed evacuation can help with both constipation and fecal incontinence by taking advantage of the gastrocolic reflex, timing bowel movements after food consumption, exercise, or when it is known that a toilet is nearby. Dietary intake can significantly affect constipation. Adequate hydration and dietary fiber promote softer stools. High-fiber foods such as fruits, vegetables, and grains, and supplements such as psyllium and Metamucil increase fecal bulk and decrease gastrointestinal transit time. Fruit juices such as apple and prune juice and dietary supplements such as lactulose stimulate the bowel. Finally, foods such as rice, cheese, and excess protein decrease gastrointestinal transit time and should be avoided.

Medicinal treatments for bowel dysfunction in MS are limited. For constipation, stool softeners and laxatives, as well as smooth muscle stimulants, will decrease transit time. Cisapride, a serotonin receptor agonist, partially restores gastrointestinal motility but may cause cardiac complications secondary to its effects on the potassium channel.† Suppositories and enemas can be used to evacuate the rectum to reduce the risk of incontinence or induce defecation.

Devices used to treat fecal incontinence include the rectal bag and the artificial sphincter. After a surgical procedure called a colostomy, a rectal bag is used to catch feces as it is evacuated through an opening in the abdominal wall. An artificial sphincter can be used to control incontinence, as a last resort. To use the sphincter, the person will compress a pump to divert fluid from an anal cuff to a holding balloon, allowing the sphincter to relax and defecation to occur.

## Research Areas in Bowel Dysfunction

Studies of fundamental neuroscience should parallel those outlined above for the bladder, with the goals of learning more about central control of bowel function, elucidating the local pharmacology of gastrointestinal transit, and identifying the response and plasticity of the central and peripheral neuronal systems to supraspinal central injury. More specifically, examination of the central control of the enteroenteric reflexes and the sacral outflow to the bowel would directly relate to the clinical problems experienced by MS patients. Determining the role of "channels" (for example, potassium and sodium) in neurotransmission and GI transit and developing drugs with 5-HT4 properties, D2 characteristics, or novel agents that target the bowel would be helpful.

Advances are needed in the understanding of human GI motility. These studies should draw on techniques used by gastroenterologists, such as the use of enteric capsules, intraluminal manometers, microminiature strain gauges, digital logging for prolonged recordings, imaging techniques of GI motility, and sphincter electrophysiology to explore the pharmacology of GI function and control. Also, studies of pelvic floor musculature in spinal MS might reveal new data on how to improve the mechanical aspects of sphincter function. As stated above, studies of spinal cord injury would complement studies on patients with spinal MS.

---

†Channels are the pores in cell walls that are opened and closed to permit the passage of specific ions, a key process in all aspects of physiological regulation.

# Visual Disturbances

Visual disturbances resulting from demyelination or inflammation in the optic nerve occur in up to 85 percent of people with MS.[5] These visual disturbances take a variety of forms, including optic neuritis, abnormal eye movements, blurred or double vision, and color distortion. The optic nerve is involved in the first manifestation of disease in about 35 percent of people with MS.[192]

## Optic Neuritis

Optic neuritis (inflammation of the optic nerve) is the most common visual disturbance in MS. In 17 percent of people with MS, optic neuritis was the first evidence of disease, but it can also occur subsequent to other symptoms.[192] Symptoms associated with optic neuritis include rapid vision loss, pain associated with eye movement, dimmed vision, abnormal color vision, altered depth perception, and Uhthoff's phenomenon in which visual loss is associated with increased body temperature.[135]

Optic neuritis usually worsens for three to seven days before gradually improving over the following weeks and months.[192] The prognosis for ultimate recovery of vision following optic neuritis is good, although conduction abnormalities seen by visual evoked potential often persist after recovery.[190] Evidence suggests that recovery from optic neuritis might involve cerebral adaptation to persistently abnormal visual input.

Episodes of optic neuritis are frequently but not always followed by a diagnosis of MS. Estimates of the risk for developing MS within 15 years of an acute bout of optic neuritis range from 45 percent to 80 percent.[135] MRI is the most powerful predictor of whether MS will develop following optic neuritis, as evidenced by the presence and number of lesions in the brain.[135] The Optic Neuritis Treatment Trial is the most extensive study of optic neuritis. This study of 457 subjects with acute optic neuritis found that patients with no initial brain lesions had a 16 percent chance of developing clinically definite MS within the 5-year study period, whereas those with three or more lesions had a 51 percent chance; clinically definite MS developed in 27 percent of all subjects, and probable MS developed in 9 percent.[175]

The Optic Neuritis Study Group found no benefit of oral or intravenous steroid treatment over nontreatment in ultimate visual outcome or in the development of MS. Within five years of their first bout of optic neuritis, 94 percent of all patients had visual acuity of 20/40 or better, although 56 percent reported that their vision had worsened.[175] Patients treated with intravenous methylprednisolone recovered vision more quickly and were half as likely to develop a second event within 2 years, compared to controls and patients treated with oral prednisone.[5,14] However, after two years the protective effect wore off. Further, compared to controls and the I.V. steroid group, the oral steroid group was more likely to have recurrences of optic neuritis within two years.[5] Steroid treatment for optic neuritis did not influence the development of MS. Within five years of treatment there was no significant difference between the number of steroid-treated patients and nontreated patients who developed MS.[175] A small proportion of patients develop progressive visual loss, usually later in the course of the disease. These patients, together with those who fail to recover from an acute episode, might benefit from visual aids.

### Abnormal Eye Movements

Abnormal eye movements result from demyelination of afferent nerve pathways to the eye muscles and occur frequently in MS patients. The type of abnormality depends on the lesion site. The most common visual disturbances are nystagmus, saccadic intrusion, and diplopia.[5,30]

Nystagmus is a back-and-forth eye movement that occurs in 28.5 to 63 percent of people with MS.[5] Nystagmus often results from lesions in the brainstem or cerebellum and can take many forms. It can be jerky or pendular, vertical, horizontal, or circular. Patients with nystagmus sometimes experience dizziness and difficulty reading.[33]

Saccadic intrusion is difficulty in shifting the focus of vision and results in oscillation of the eyes. Smooth pursuit is lost, replaced by a series of saccades. Saccadic intrusion is found in many individuals that do not have MS and is not recommended for routine diagnosis.[113] Other saccadic abnormalities can also occur in MS, including delay in the initiation of saccade, decreased velocity, and oscillation of the eyes following saccade and prior to fixation on the target.[5]

Diplopia, or double vision, is a transient symptom, and estimates of its incidence range from 8 to 22 percent at disease onset and from 29 to 39 percent throughout the course of MS.[33]

Various drugs are used to treat these conditions with moderate results, including baclofen, clonazepam, memantine, scopolamine, gabapentin, and isoniazid for nystagmus, and clonazepam and propranolol for saccadic oscillations (Table 3.6).[30,167] Botulinum toxin injection into extraocular muscles has been shown to decrease the amplitude of nystagmus and improve visual function for about eight weeks in MS patients but is not always well tolerated.[142] Finally, prisms have been shown to stabilize images on the retina and may help MS patients with nystagmus or diplopia.

## FATIGUE

Fatigue, considered the most common symptom in MS, is experienced by 76 to 92 percent of people with the disease.[94,122] Among MS patients, 66 percent report experiencing fatigue on a daily basis,[61] and 33 percent report that fatigue is

**TABLE 3.6** Medications Used to Treat Optic Neuritis and Abnormal Eye Movements[a]

| Trade Name | Generic Name | Mechanism | Potential Side Effects |
|---|---|---|---|
| Solu-Medrol[14,85,125] | Methylprednisolone sodium succinate | Anti-inflammatory corticosteroid often taken intravenously. | Fluid retention, weakness, GI upset, increased intracranial pressure, vertigo, headache, ulcers, hypertension |
| Deltasone[14,135] | Prednisone | Naturally occurring glucocorticoids (hydrocortisone and cortisone), which also have salt-retaining properties, are used as replacement therapy in adrenocortical deficiency states. Their synthetic analogues are primarily used for their potent anti-inflammatory effects in disorders of many organ systems.<br><br>Glucocorticoids cause profound and varied metabolic effects. In addition, they modify the body's immune responses to diverse stimuli. | Fluid retention, muscle weakness, steroid myopathy, loss of muscle mass, osteoporosis, aseptic necrosis of femoral and humeral heads, peptic ulcer, pancreatitis, abdominal distention, impaired wound healing, thin fragile skin, petechiae and ecchymoses, facial erythema, increased sweating, convulsions, vertigo, headache, menstrual irregularities, suppression of growth in children |
| Decadron | Dexamethasone | Decadron is a potent anti-inflammatory synthetic adrenocortical steroid used to reduce inflammation that occurs in MS exacerbations. | Depression, euphoria, hypertension, nausea, anorexia, decreased wound healing, acne, muscle wasting, bone pain, and increased susceptibility to infection |

[a]These are steroid medications used as a symptomatic treatment for acute MS exacerbations, including optic neuritis and abnormal eye movements.

their most troubling symptom.[94] Fatigue affects MS patients of all types and all levels of disability and is not related to patient age, level of neurological impairment, or the EDSS.[94] Assessment of fatigue in MS is complicated by the many potential contributing factors.[176] Antidepressants, beta-blockers, and medications used for spasticity can worsen fatigue, and other problems of MS such as pain, depression, poor sleep, psychological stress, and deconditioning can contribute, as well. For some, fatigue is overwhelming. For others, it is transient, induced by physical activity. It is a particularly pervasive symptom, creating problems for employment, fulfilling family and social roles, getting exercise, and mood—the basic ingredients of life satisfaction.[31]

## Definition and Types of Fatigue

Fatigue can be defined as an overwhelming sense of tiredness, lack of energy, or feeling of exhaustion that is in excess of what might normally be expected.[94] Fatigue can occur as a result of a task or in anticipation of a task. It can be influenced by physical features of the task (such as the length of a run) or by psychological aspects of the task (such as how rewarding it will be) or both. Fatigue can also be interpreted as a sense of effort needed to perform a task, and both physical and mental tasks may result in fatigue. In addition to the sensation or perception of fatigue experienced only by the individual, fatigue may also produce observable changes in behavior, especially as a decrement in performance (for example, a decrease in the ability to process information). Acute fatigue typically resolves after completion of the task. Fatigue that is more chronic and pervasive is frequently associated with illness, stress, and sleep disturbances. Fatigue as a distinct clinical symptom in MS must, however, be distinguished from true muscle weakness, sleepiness or drowsiness, and depression. These conditions can coexist with fatigue but are associated with a different array of conditions that may be amenable to separate treatment.

Attempts to establish a clinical definition of fatigue are complicated by patients' varied uses of the term. Sometimes fatigue is a synonym for other complaints, while at other times the term is applied to a collection of symptoms that occur together. Patients might use the term fatigue to refer to weakness, dizziness, lack of coordination or stamina, feeling "spacey", having poor concentration or cognitive abilities, having "rubber legs", boredom, lack of motivation, malaise, or feeling blue or depressed.

## Causes of Fatigue

The nature of fatigue in MS has yet to be fully characterized, but it is interrelated with physical activity and social engagement.[61,176,182] Plausible mechanisms related to impaired motor function include slowing or alteration of neurotransmitter release and increased nerve conduction times. Measurements of physical fatigue are higher in MS patients with pyramidal tract signs and during relapses.[46] New onset of fatigue may be a sign of impending relapse.[176] Other MS symptoms resulting from impaired motor function, such as spasticity, weakness, and ataxia, may contribute to fatigue by increasing the physical, and psychological, effort required for mobility.[86] Symptoms such as pain and spasticity that interfere with sleep may also be a factor in fatigue. Fatigue is worsened by heat, making physical activity particularly difficult.

One finding across a variety of physical disorders has been that the severity of fatigue rarely correlates well with measures of disease activity (for example, in rheumatoid arthritis or hepatitis C).[71,75] Functioning is often more closely tied, even in physical conditions, to psychological factors and stressors. Although one study concluded that MS-related fatigue is not associated with depression,[95] another suggested that mental fatigue in MS correlates with anxiety and depression but physical fatigue does not.[61,173]

Although one study suggests that MS fatigue might be associated with frontal cortex and basal ganglia dysfunction resulting from demyelination of frontal white matter,[144] other neuroimaging studies have failed to find a significant correlation between fatigue and neuropathology in MS patients.[11,13] Neuroimaging of chronic fatigue syndrome, which has been much more widely studied in this regard than MS, has likewise yielded conflicting results.[99,105] At this stage, reports of fatigue-associated neuropathology in MS should be interpreted cautiously.

## Measurement of Fatigue

Because fatigue is multidimensional, with distinct physical and mental elements, measurement tools must be carefully constructed and carefully used to produce valid, reliable, and meaningful distinctions among the separate elements and differing levels of fatigue. Measurement strategies for fatigue in MS should be closely linked to one or more of the four components of fatigue: behavior, sensation or perception of fatigue, mechanisms of fatigue, and context.

Behavior refers to the physical manifestations of fatigue or a decline in performance, such as making more errors or inability to complete a task. The sensation or perception of fatigue can occur in the absence of any actual physical or mental effort, and it might or might not be in proportion to a particular task. A sense of fatigue can coexist with psychological symptoms (even in the absence of a psychiatric disorder) and with beliefs that result in behaviors—for example, the belief that exertion is harmful and the consequent avoidance of exercise.

The general literature on measurement of mechanisms of fatigue has tended to focus on single causes (for example, infections or psychiatric disorders), a perspective that is difficult to apply to cases where the causes are unknown and possibly many. Physiological mechanisms of fatigue are thought to reflect either peripheral processes operating in the muscles or nerves or central processes operating in the brain. Proposed psychological mechanisms have included beliefs, perceptions, expectations, and symptom amplification. The contextual component of the measurement of fatigue includes an appraisal of the personal, social, occupational, cultural, and physical environment in which the symptom occurs. This component captures the influence of temperature, noise, the family, and stressors on the experience of fatigue.

In studies of MS, various self-report instruments have been used to measure fatigue (summarized in 1998 by Ford and colleagues[61]). These include the Fatigue Severity Scale and the Fatigue Assessment Instrument. Both scales measure the effect of fatigue on functioning. The Fatigue Assessment Instrument measures fatigue severity, whether fatigue is situation specific, the consequences of fatigue, and the response of fatigue symptoms to rest or sleep. Neither scale identifies distinct mental and physical dimensions of fatigue.

In general, the currently available measurement tools, even the most basic ones, require further evaluation. In particular, they must be tested and validated specifically for use by populations with fatigue. Moreover, the "gold standards" that do exist are often poor. Nonetheless, if carefully selected, some of the currently available measurement tools are adequate for clinical trials. These are primarily self-report instruments, such as the SF-36. For most medical conditions, a suitable biological measure or marker of fatigue has not yet been identified.

Disease-specific instruments may offer the advantage of greater sensitivity in detecting change since they incorporate measurements of phenomena more likely to be experienced by persons with a particular condition (for example, swollen joints in rheumatoid arthritis). With these instruments, however, comparability and generalizability are sacrificed.

## Management of Fatigue

Fatigue has a broad impact on functioning for persons with MS. Chapter 4 addresses broader aspects of the management of fatigue in the context of overall strategies for adapting to MS. Noted here are some specific interventions, including medications, that are used in treating fatigue. Exercise programs may help maintain conditioning and improve self-esteem.[129,176] One study suggests that aerobic exercise may be beneficial.[128] Behavior modification therapy may be helpful for identifying strategies to avoid situations that worsen fatigue.

Pharmacological treatment of fatigue has also been tested (see Table 3.7). Amantadine, an antiviral agent, has been shown to improve fatigue compared to a placebo.[95] Pemoline, a CNS stimulant, may also be beneficial, but clinical trials have shown more limited effects than for amantadine.[86,95] Fluoxetine hydrochloride, an antidepressant, may help reduce the components of fatigue attributable to depression.

**TABLE 3.7** Medications Used to Treat Fatigue

| Trade Name | Generic Name | Mechanism | Potential Side Effects |
|---|---|---|---|
| Symmetrel[70,95,115] | Amantadine | Mechanism unknown. An antiviral medication used to prevent or treat certain influenza infections, it is also given as an adjunct for the treatment of Parkinson's disease. | Difficulty concentrating, dizziness, headache, irritability, loss of appetite, nausea, nervousness, purplish red, net-like, blotchy spots on skin, trouble sleeping or nightmares, constipation, dry mouth, vomiting |
| Provigil[104] | Modafinil | Precise mechanism unknown. Has wake-promoting effects similar to amphetamine and methylphenidate. Produces psychoactive and euphoric effects; alterations in mood, perception, and thinking; and feelings typical of other CNS stimulants. | Headache, nervousness, dizziness, depression, anxiety, insomnia, paraesthesia, hypertonia, confusion, emotional lability, ataxia, tremor, diarrhea, dry mouth, anorexia, mouth ulcer, vasodilation, arrhythmia, syncope, urinary retention, abnormal ejaculation |
| Cylert[95,115,171,188] | Pemoline | A CNS stimulant used to treat attention deficit disorder. It is used in MS to relieve certain types of fatigue. Krupp et al.[95] found that treatment with pemoline was no more beneficial than placebo in patients with MS. | Insomnia, elevated heart rate, nervousness, agitation, loss of appetite and weight loss, GI upset, including constipation and diarrhea, hallucinations |
| Prozac[115] | Fluoxetine hydrochloride | A selective serotonin reuptake inhibitor, it increases serotonin levels in the midbrain. | Anxiety, nervousness, insomnia, fatigue, tremor, sweating, GI distress, anorexia, diarrhea, dizziness, decreased libido |

## Recommendations for Further Research

- Studies are needed to gain a better understanding of the phenomenon of fatigue.

- A careful review should be made of the possible tools available to assess each domain of fatigue and to assess the relevance of these tools for MS.

- All studies evaluating physical or mental performance (including trials for treatments such as exercise or cognitive behavioral therapy) should include measures of both perception of effort and actual performance.

- Attempts to elucidate biological markers of fatigue should focus on specific components (for example, perception, mechanism) of fatigue. Possible markers should make clinical and biological sense.

- When objective markers for fatigue are sought, care must be taken to determine that observed alterations are due to fatigue, rather than another confounding process (for example, controlling for affective disorders when performing SPECT [simple photon emission computed tomography] scans of the brain).

- Investigation of biological mechanisms for the perception of fatigue is critical. Given the lack of correlation between perceived fatigue and disease severity in well-recognized diseases, it is crucial to gain a better understanding of perceptual processes.

- Appropriate challenge paradigms should be developed to examine fatigue in MS and other disorders. Asking subjects to perform tasks under more stressful conditions may help identify biological markers of fatigue that are not normally observed under basal conditions.

# SEXUAL DYSFUNCTION

The estimated incidence of sexual dysfunction in MS varies, depending on what source is reviewed. This is not surprising considering the variable nature of the neurologic disorder. Up to 91 percent of men with MS and 72 percent of women have adverse effects on their sexual function, and up to 80 percent of men with MS report erectile dysfunction.[17,67,100,181]

## Desire and Satisfaction

Sexuality has both psychological and physiological components, and both aspects contribute to the level of a person's sexual functioning. However, the incidence of physiological versus psychological sexual dysfunction in men and women with MS is not known. Research addressing this question would be valuable for people living with MS, their partners, and health care providers and also for determining appropriate treatment protocols.

The possibility that the psychological aspects of MS would have a negative impact on sexuality is obvious given the uncertainty of the disorder. Decreased libido has been documented in 22 percent of men with MS[12] in addition to 28 to 60 percent[80] of women; moreover, sexual dysfunction is associated with depression.[109] It has not been determined whether this decrease in libido is related to severity or duration of the disease or is a side effect of medications used. Nor has it been determined whether treatment of depression will improve sexual function. Sixty-four percent of men and 39 percent of women report decreased sexual satisfaction and/or absent sexual activity. Finally, associated marital problems have been noted in 71 percent of MS patients with sexual dysfunction. The relationships of these issues to premorbid psychosexual function are not clearly understood. Furthermore, the impact of MS on performance of sexual activities should be considered. The availability and impact of sexual education and counseling for patients and their partners should also be studied. It is also important to recognize that issues associated with sexuality are different for gay and lesbian populations.[81]

## Sexual Response

One report noted that 58 percent of women and 63 percent of men with MS had problems with anorgasmia.[109] The same study noted that 80 percent of men had erectile dysfunction and 40 percent of women had problems with lubrication, but the study did not provide specific information on the subjects' neurological status.

The arousal and orgasm phases of sexual response are also affected by physiological and psychological issues. Lesions affecting the neurological pathways that control sexual response would affect physiological aspects of sexual response. However, these pathways are not yet well understood (Table 3.8). The intracranial control of sexual arousal is not well defined.[15,148,160] Better documentation of the normal neurologic pathways that control sexual response will be necessary before the physiologic effects of specific neurological lesions on sexual function can be identified. (See Figure 3.1 for location of spinal nerves.)

Cervical cord plaques are thought to affect some 80 percent of patients, intracranial plaques 60 to 90 percent, and sacral cord (lower back) and conus medullaris (lowermost portion of the spinal cord) lesions are thought to occur in up to 63 percent of patients.[101] Thus, some patients will have neurologic lesions affecting the pathways for sexual function whereas others will not. To determine whether there is a physiological reason for altered sexual function, studies that assess the impact of MS on sexual function should provide detailed information regarding the subject's neurological condition. Unfortunately, this is rarely the

**TABLE 3.8** Neurological Pathways That Control Sexual Response in Men and Women

| Sexual Function | Probable Neural Pathway |
|---|---|
| Psychogenic erectile function and lubrication | The spinal pathways are thought to travel in the lateral white columns that synapse on the autonomic motor cells in the lateral gray columns of the lower thoracic and upper lumbar cord.[15,158,160] |
| Reflex erectile function and lubrication | Thought to include sensory transmission via the pudendal nerve to stimulate the sacral parasympathetic nerves. |
| Ejaculation | Both sacral parasympathetic and thoracolumbar sympathetic contributions, in addition to a sacral somatic component. A spinal cord center has been proposed at the twelfth thoracic and first lumbar nerves.[148] |
| Orgasm | Postulated to occur as a reflex response of the autonomic nervous system.[158] |

case. Rather, the information provided is generally limited to the Expanded Disability Status Scale (see Chapter 4 for discussion of the EDSS).[97] Studies published thus far have not found a correlation between level of disability and sexual dysfunction or satisfaction with sexuality.[110]

Some researchers have attempted to link neurological testing with the status of sexual functioning. In men and women with MS, anorgasmia has been correlated with brainstem and pyramidal abnormalities in addition to the total area of plaques on the brain observed via MRI. Betts and colleagues[17] performed posterior tibial and pudendal cortical evoked potentials along with cystometric tests in men with erectile failure and MS. They concluded, as did another group,[91] that the neural lesions associated with impotence are generally above the sacral cord. In addition, men with abnormal pudendal or tibial evoked responses had difficulties with ejaculation and orgasmic dysfunction. One report noted that in women with advanced multiple sclerosis, weakness of the pelvic floor and bladder and bowel dysfunction are correlated with changes in lubrication and orgasmic capacity.[80] However, that report relied on the EDSS and did not provide detailed neurological information regarding women's sexual arousal and the impact of MS.

Another difficulty in the study of sexual function stems from the inaccuracies associated with self-report data.[159] Most importantly, the issues noted in the previous paragraphs should be addressed through the performance of controlled, laboratory-based research to systematically document the physiologic effects of specific neurological dysfunctions associated with MS on sexual function. This should also provide information regarding the incidence of psychological sexual dysfunction affecting persons with MS.

## Treatment of Sexual Dysfunction

Great strides have been made in the treatment of erectile dysfunction, including the availability of vacuum pumps, injection erections, and oral medications (Table 3.9). Most research has evaluated the effect of therapeutic agents on neurogenic erectile dysfunction in general[77,78] or specifically on sexual dysfunction due to spinal cord injury.[42] Only minimal research, however, has concentrated on the amelioration of sexual dysfunction specifically associated with MS. While these results are likely relevant to men with MS, the complex interplay between psychological and physiological issues and sexuality must be considered. As a result, new therapeutic interventions for the remediation of erectile dysfunction should be tested to verify their efficacy in men with MS. Patterns of neurological dysfunction with detailed information about psychosexual functioning should be documented. Furthermore, techniques to treat other sexual dysfunctions in men with MS, including orgasmic dysfunction, should be developed and tested.

Female sexual dysfunction has generally received less attention than male sexual dysfunction, particularly erectile dysfunction. However, the development of oral medications to remediate erection dysfunction has led to a heightened awareness of women's sexuality and associated issues. Sildenafil, a drug previously shown to be safe and effective in the treatment of erectile dysfunction, was recently tested in a small study of 19 women with spinal cord injuries.[161] The results showed that sildenafil can significantly increase the level of subjective sexual arousal in women with neurogenic sexual dysfunction. Further research is needed with a goal of improving the sexual responsiveness and satisfaction of women with MS. Large-scale studies of the use of sildenafil and other new therapeutics to improve female sexual responsiveness should be conducted.

# PAIN

Although multiple sclerosis is not commonly thought of as a painful disease, when MS patients are asked, a surprisingly high proportion report significant pain problems.[32,108,137,170] At the time of their initial presentation, pain is a significant complaint in about one in five patients.[170] Nearly one-half of individuals with MS experience clinically significant pain at some time during the course of the disease. Significantly more women than men report pain.[120] The longer the duration of the disease and the older the patient, the more likely it is that pain will be reported.[32,120] The disconnect between the incidence and severity of the pain and the realization by physicians of its importance to the patient is a major problem for the management of MS.

The reasons for this disconnect are unclear. Physicians and patients tend to focus on weakness, poor coordination, visual impairment, and fatigue, and there

**TABLE 3.9** Medications Used to Treat Erectile Dysfunction

| Trade Name | Generic Name | Mechanism | Potential Side Effects |
|---|---|---|---|
| Viagra[83] | Sildenafil citrate | Causes release of nitric oxide (NO) in the corpus cavernosum during sexual stimulation, which produces smooth muscle relaxation in the corpus cavernosum and allows inflow of blood. | Headache, facial flushing, upset stomach |
| Muse; Prostin VR[78,166] | Alprostadil | A vasodilator that causes blood vessels to expand, increasing blood flow. It is a semisolid suppository pellet that is inserted into the urethra, producing an erection by increasing blood flow. | Burning or aching during erection, erection continuing for more than 4 hours |
| Pavabid[17,184] | Papaverine | A vasodilator that is injected into the penis, producing an erection by increasing blood flow. | Bruising at the injection site, mild burning along the penis, difficulty ejaculating, swelling at the injection site |

is a tendency to underestimate the disability that pain can produce. Another problem is the tremendous variety of pain complaints. Different painful manifestations of MS are seen in different individuals and likely have different underlying mechanisms. Little is known about the mechanism for any of the pain complaints in MS. Some of the pain complaints are transient and accompany the acute attack, whereas others appear relatively late in the course of the disease and are unremitting. There is also an understandable bias toward the belief that if the underlying disease process can be stopped or slowed, the symptom of pain will resolve. Unfortunately, current treatments for MS are of limited impact and the accumulated burden of irreversible damage places the patient at risk for persistent pain.

Among the complaints that often accompany MS are headache and back pain, which are so common in the general population that it would be difficult to establish that MS is the cause (see for example, Rae-Grant et al.[137]). In contrast, painful tonic spasms and tic doloreux in young people are so rarely seen, except in patients with MS, that they probably result directly from the demyelinating process. Optic neuritis is often painful during the acute attack; presumably this is a direct result of the inflammatory process and activation of primary afferent nociceptors.* Sensory changes, such as persistent numbness or tingling of a body part, although not necessarily painful, are experienced by about 80 percent of people with MS.[107]

The sheer variety of pain complaints, their appearance in subsets of MS patients and the fact that the disease is uncommon have been major impediments to clinical therapeutic trials. There are simply too few eligible patients to conduct clinical trials that would have sufficient statistical power to detect a clear therapeutic effect. There have been no controlled clinical trials specifically for pain treatment in multiple sclerosis. This problem and the lack of a good animal model for pain in MS also make it difficult to investigate the pathophysiology of pain in this disease.

Pain complaints in multiple sclerosis can be divided into four broad categories:

1. *Neuropathic pain.* This is chronic and/or recurring pains resulting from the destructive process (i.e., due to abnormal function of damaged neuronal or glial elements). This type of pain is either paroxysmal or static depending on the syndrome. The sensory qualities of these painful conditions clearly identify them as neuropathic.

2. *Acute pain due to the active inflammatory process.* The sensory characteristics of this type of pain are nonspecific, although the pain should temporally track the exacerbations of the underlying demyelinating process.

---

*Nociceptors are neurons that are preferentially sensitive to noxious stimuli or to stimuli that would become noxious if prolonged.

3. *Pain secondary to increased muscle tone.* This includes cramps and spasticity-related muscle pain.

4. *Chronic or recurrent pain of a nonspecific nature* such as neck or back pain, possibly due to increased tone or weakness of muscle. Such syndromes are extremely common in normal individuals, so it is usually difficult to be sure that they are caused by MS.

## Neuropathic Pain Syndromes

### Trigeminal Neuralgia

The occurrence of trigeminal neuralgia in MS patients is well known.[27,120] Trigeminal neuralgia is a unique and easily recognized symptom complex that usually affects the elderly. It consists of brief shock-like (tic-like, or lancinating) pains that often have an electrical quality. The key features are very brief duration of individual shocks (a second or less), pain-free intervals, location in the second and third division of the trigeminal sensory distribution, and the presence of trigger points on the face or in the mouth where light touch will trigger an attack. Although trigeminal neuralgia occurs in less than 3 percent of MS patients, it is much more common and tends to occur at a somewhat younger age in MS patients than in the general population.[27,120] Not surprisingly, there are often associated sensory changes in MS patients with trigeminal neuralgia. Persistent facial pain may occur in MS patients and can have a lancinating component. Persistent (tonic) pain is not seen in idiopathic trigeminal neuralgia.

The same treatment approaches (anticonvulsants and neurolytic lesions) appear to be effective for trigeminal neuralgia whether in the setting of MS or not.[22,88,120] This suggests that MS is a risk factor for trigeminal neuralgia but is insufficient, by itself, to cause the syndrome. One popular theory of idiopathic trigeminal neuralgia is that it represents vascular compression of the central root of the trigeminal ganglion, but this does not explain why trigeminal neuralgia should be overrepresented in MS. It may be that pre-existing demyelination is another risk factor.

In summary, trigeminal neuralgia is an uncommon but severely painful syndrome that occurs significantly more often in MS patients than in the general population. It responds to the usual trigeminal neuralgia therapeutic interventions and appears to share an underlying pathophysiology.

### Painful Tonic Spasms

In contrast to trigeminal neuralgia, painful tonic spasms are rarely observed except in MS.[108] In MS they seem to be relatively common, occurring in between 10 and 20 percent of patients.[183] Their clinical presentation has unique and highly characteristic features. Painful tonic spasms usually occur in the setting of rapid-onset but tonic muscle contractions. Individual spasms are localized to a body part or region. They are brief, rarely lasting more than two minutes, but the pain is usually severe. The painful tonic spasms are often triggered by movement or sensory stimulation, rarely by well-localized and reproducible stimulation of the skin, as in trigeminal neuralgia. Sometimes the pain is accompanied by loss of motor function (i.e., weakness or dysarthria). The location can be anywhere on the body. Fortunately, the syndrome tends to be transient, with a duration of two weeks to two months. Electroencephalogram recordings during painful tonic spasms are normal, suggesting a subcortical origin for the underlying neural discharge.[108] In a recent report with a literature review and five original cases, Spissu and colleagues[165] point out that most patients with painful tonic spasm have at least mild involvement of the pyramidal tract on the side of the pain. In their cases, fMRI studies revealed an acute lesion in the posterior limb of the internal capsule or the cerebral peduncle corresponding somatopically to the affected region.

Although not yet studied in a controlled manner, anticonvulsants such as carbamazepine and gabapentin are reported to provide dramatic relief for many patients with painful tonic spasm in MS.[164]

### Continuous Dysesthetic Pain

This is the most common neuropathic pain in MS.[32,120] It is most often located in the lower extremity and is commonly bilateral. In some cases the trunk and/or upper extremity may be involved. This pain is usually described as burning and is typically most pronounced distally. On exam, patients with this complaint have sensory deficits that overlap the painful regions. All of these patients have a deficit in dorsal column sensory function, and about half have a deficit of pain and/or temperature sensation, presumably due to damage to the spinothalamic tract.[120,183] The association of spinothalamic tract-type deficits and continuous dysesthetic pain is characteristic of central pain syndromes such as poststroke and spinal cord injury pain. These syndromes are notoriously resistant to analgesic treatments.

There have not been any controlled clinical trials of treatments that specifically address this type of pain. There are anecdotal reports that in some patients it responds to tricyclic antidepressants[32,108,120] and anticonvulsants such as gabapentin [79,152] and lamotrigine.[111]

Neuropathic pain can be caused (after nerve injury, for example) by the generation of inappropriate (in some cases, spontaneous) high-frequency bursts of impulses by neurons within the pain pathway. The generation of nerve impulses depends on the activity of specialized proteins called sodium channels, and it is now known that nearly a dozen genes encode distinct sodium channels with different properties, many of which are expressed in sensory neurons.[45] It is well established that following injury to their axons, neurons turn off sodium channel genes that are normally active and turn on others that are normally silent.[45,186] This produces an abnormal ensemble of sodium channels whose electrical activity can cause less activity.[36] Evidence is beginning to emerge suggesting that similar changes in sodium channel expression can occur in neurons whose axons are subjected to inflammation[172] or demyelination.[18] The identification and characterization of the abnormal ensemble of sodium channel(s) is a promising area for research, that may provide a basis for new pharmacological treatments.

### Acute Radicular Pain

Acute radicular pain has been reported as a presenting symptom in MS.[138] In several patients there was a report of trauma preceding the onset of the pain. However, in most, there was no obvious trauma. In 2 of 11 patients, there was an MRI-demonstrated plaque at the appropriate site. The quality of the pain, its duration, or its response to treatment was not reported.

### Muscle Spasms and Cramps

This problem is mentioned in most large series of pain complaints in MS. This type of pain can be seen in people without any underlying neurological condition but is often present in association with upper motor neuron damage and accompanies spasticity. There are numerous treatment strategies for spasticity, none totally satisfactory. A recently published small controlled study of 20 patients demonstrated a significant benefit of gabapentin for symptoms of spasticity, including painful spasms.[37]

This type of pain may also be responsive to cannabinoids. In a retrospective, uncontrolled study of 112 MS patients in the United States and the United Kingdom, Consroe and colleagues[34] reported that smoking cannabis relieved a variety of pain complaints. More than 90 percent of patients reported improvement in muscle pain, leg pain, and spasticity. A similar percentage reported improvement in their tremor. This report takes on added significance in view of studies in a mouse model of MS (chronic relapsing EAE), which demonstrated significant improvement in tremor and spasticity with a synthetic CB1 receptor agonist.* This evidence warrants controlled clinical trials.

---

*The CB1 receptor is the primary cannabinoid receptor in the brain and can be stimulated by a variety of agonists, including THC.

## Acute Pain Due to the Inflammatory Process

### Optic Neuritis

This type of pain is most clear-cut when MS is heralded by optic neuritis. In such cases, pain often accompanies the attack. The pain is aching and exacerbated by eye movements. The reported response to glucocorticoids supports the general feeling that this type of pain represents activation of dural nociceptors by the inflammatory process.[32] In other situations such as headache and back pain, the association of pain with an acute inflammatory attack is less clear.

### Headache

Headaches are such a common occurrence in the general population that it is difficult to prove that MS can cause them. Nonetheless, the weight of evidence suggests that it can. In a prospective study, Rolak and Brown[145] found an overall incidence of headache of 52 percent, which is much higher than in the general population. Both tension-type and migraine headaches were common and there was no characteristic "MS headache." Furthermore, they were not able to establish a higher incidence of headache in correlation with clinical exacerbations based on other symptomatology. In contrast, in a retrospective study of 1,113 MS patients, Freedman and Gray reported 44 patients in whom an attack or exacerbation were heralded by a migraine attack.[62] Although their definition of migraine was somewhat loose, 27 of these patients had no prior history of migraine. Headache accompanying attacks seems to be more common in children (Stephen Hauser, personal communication). It is of interest in this regard that Haas et al.[74] reported a 16-year-old girl who presented with a severe headache and internuclear ophthalmoplegia but little else neurologically. On imaging, her sole abnormality was in the region of the midbrain periaqueductal gray, an area implicated in migraine pathogenesis.[187] Subsequent clinical course and the presence of oligoclonal bands in her cerebrospinal fluid established the diagnosis of MS in this case.

In summary, there seems to be some evidence that headache is a common complaint in MS and may be a direct consequence of disease activity.

## Pain Due to Increased Muscle Tone

In any neurological condition characterized by spasticity (i.e., upper motor neuron disease), patients are at risk for muscle pain due to spasm. Spasticity is common in MS, especially over time as the lesion burden increases. Spasticity is most likely to involve the legs. MS patients frequently report leg spasms and cramps.[32,120] This type of pain improves if spasticity can be controlled with standard medications such as baclofen, dantrolene, benzodiazepines, and most recently gabapentin.[37]

## Back Pain

Back pain is common in MS.[32,120] It is described as aching, usually in the lower back, and is exacerbated by prolonged sitting or standing and the abnormal gait. The most common cause appears to be musculoskeletal. This type of pain, as in patients who are neurologically intact, has two common musculoskeletal causes: degenerative disease around the disks, foramina, and facet joints, and myofascial pain due to disuse and spasticity. This type of pain responds to physical therapy, trigger point injections with stretching, anti-inflammatory agents, and analgesics. In addition, especially in patients treated with glucocorticoids, there is the possibility of vertebral compression fractures secondary to osteoporosis. Urinary tract infection in patients with bladder dysfunction is also a consideration in some patients with subacute back pain.

## Summary

Pain is a frequent accompaniment of MS, and for a small group of MS patients, pain is the worst aspect of the disease.[137] Despite treatment, many MS patients have ongoing pain. Pain may be due to inflammatory disease activity, in which case it is usually transient and may respond to glucocorticoids. In other cases, the accumulating burden of CNS damage may lead to irreversible lesions that cause neuropathic pain. The neuropathic pain syndromes are of two types: paroxysmal and constant. Paroxysmal phenomena (trigeminal neuralgia and painful tonic spasms) are recurrent and appear to respond well to anticonvulsant medications. Constant dysesthetic pains vary in intensity and appear to be resistant to currently available treatments. However, the committee did not find any satisfying data on this point. Another set of pain types are of musculoskeletal origin: back pain, probably related to weakness, disuse, and immobilization, and limb pains that are apparently due to increased muscle tone and take the form of spasms and cramps. The former seem to respond to aggressive physical therapy, whereas spasm-related pains improve with the treatment of spasticity. Finally, there is the controversial issue of headache, which seems to have an increased incidence in MS patients but no characteristic pattern and no established relationship to disease activity.

## Research Recommendations

Attention should be paid to evaluating pain in future clinical trials. Pain relates to both pathophysiology and quality of life, and should be considered in future clinical trials.

Multicenter clinical trials are essential to evaluate currently available treatments, especially for the constant dysesthetic pain that is currently the most refractory of the multiple pain syndromes accompanying MS. Cannabinoids might be particularly promising for patients with spasticity but should also be evaluated for other nonparoxysmal pain complaints.

To establish whether acute disease activity is associated with pain, an effort should be made to correlate new-onset clinical signs, MRI with gadolinium, and pain location, quality, and time course. Response to anti-inflammatory agents could be studied as well.

Continued efforts should be made to understand the pathophysiology of a neuropathic pain, including the continuous dysesthetic pain that occurs in patients with demyelinating diseases such as MS. Efforts to understand abnormal expression of ion channels in demyelinated neurons appear promising. The extensive literature on spinal cord injury and pain offers a number of models that could be extended to this type of study so that it can address demyelinating lesions (for example, Brewer and Yezierski, 1998[21]). In addition, although it is difficult to assess continuous pain in animals, the mouse models for inflammatory demyelination offer an area where parallel human and animal work could progress.

### Lesion Location

A specific attempt should be made to identify patients with new-onset continuous dysesthetic pain for functional imaging in a concerted effort to locate the relevant pathology. In these patients, quantitative sensory testing should be carried out, especially to assess spinothalamic tract function (heat, heat pain, cold, cold pain). In addition, examination should look for signs of a hyperpathic state (summation, sensory radiation, pain with light mechanical stimulation [allodynia]). With these data in hand, it might be possible to move closer to determining whether the animal model mirrors the human pain problem.

### Studies on Nervous System Inflammation and Pain

It appears likely that inflammation per se can lead to abnormal hyperexcitability of pain-signaling neurons. By understanding the underlying molecular mechanisms, it may become possible to devise better interventions.

## REFERENCES

1.  Aikens JE, Fischer JS, Namey M, Rudick RA. 1997. A replicated prospective investigation of life stress, coping, and depressive symptoms in multiple sclerosis. *J Behav Med.*;20:433-45.

2. Aikens JE, Reinecke MA, Pliskin NH, et al. 1999. Assessing depressive symptoms in multiple sclerosis: is it necessary to omit items from the original Beck Depression Inventory? *J Behav Med.*;22:127-42.

3. Allen DN, Goldstein G, Heyman RA, Rondinelli T. 1998. Teaching memory strategies to persons with multiple sclerosis. *J Rehabil Res Dev.*;35:405-410.

4. Amato MP, Ponziani G, Pracucci G, Bracco L, Siracusa G, Amaducci L. 1995. Cognitive impairment in early-onset multiple sclerosis. Pattern, predictors, and impact on everyday life in a 4-year follow-up. *Arch Neurol.*;52:168-72.

5. Anderson D, Cox T. Visual Signs and Symptons. Paty DW, Ebers GC, eds. 1998. *Multiple Sclerosis*. Philadelphia, PA: F.A. Davis Company;229-256.

6. Angel MJ, Guertin P, Jimenez T, McCrea DA. 1996. Group I extensor afferents evoke di-synaptic EPSPs in cat hindlimb extensor motorneurones during fictive locomotion. *J Physiol (Lond).*;494:851-61.

7. Arnett PA, Higginson CI, Voss WD, et al. 1999. Depressed mood in multiple sclerosis: relationship to capacity-demanding memory and attentional functioning. *Neuropsychology.*;13:434-46.

8. Arnett PA, Rao SM, Grafman J, et al. 1997. Executive functions in multiple sclerosis: an analysis of temporal ordering, semantic encoding, and planning abilities. *Neuropsychology.*;11:535-44.

9. Baker D, Pryce G, Croxford JL, et al. 2000. Cannabinoids control spasticity and tremor in a multiple sclerosis model. *Nature.*;404:84-7.

10. Bakshi R, Czarnecki D, Shaikh ZA, et al. 2000. Brain MRI lesions and atrophy are related to depression in multiple sclerosis. *Neuroreport.*;11:1153-8.

11. Bakshi R, Miletich RS, Henschel K, et al. 1999. Fatigue in multiple sclerosis: cross-sectional correlation with brain MRI findings in 71 patients. *Neurology.*;53:1151-3.

12. Barak Y, Achiron A, Elizur A, Gabbay U, Noy S, Sarova-Pinhas I. 1996. Sexual dysfunction in relapsing-remitting multiple sclerosis: magnetic resonance imaging, clinical, and psychological correlates. *J Psychiatry Neurosci.*;21:255-8.

13. Baron W, Metz B, Bansal R, Hoekstra D, de Vries H. 2000. PDGF and FGF-2 signaling in oligodendrocyte progenitor cells: regulation of proliferation and differentiation by multiple intracellular signaling pathways. *Mol Cell Neurosci.*;15:314-29.

14. Beck RW, Cleary PA, Anderson MM Jr, et al. 1992. A randomized, controlled trial of corticosteroids in the treatment of acute optic neuritis. The Optic Neuritis Study Group. *N Engl J Med.*;326:581-8.

15. Bennett CJ, Seager SW, Vasher EA, McGuire EJ. 1988. Sexual dysfunction and electro-ejaculation in men with spinal cord injury: review. *J Urol.*;139:453-7.

16. Betts CD, D'Mellow MT, Fowler CJ. 1993. Urinary symptoms and the neurological features of bladder dysfunction in multiple sclerosis. *J Neurol Neurosurg Psychiatry.*;56:245-50.

17. Betts CD, Jones SJ, Fowler CG, Fowler CJ. 1994. Erectile dysfunction in multiple sclerosis. Associated neurological and neurophysiological deficits, and treatment of the condition. *Brain.*;117:1303-10.

18. Black JA, Fjell J, Dib-Hajj S, et al. 1999. Abnormal expression of SNS/PN3 sodium channel in cerebellar Purkinje cells following loss of myelin in the taiep rat. *Neuroreport.*;10:913-8.

19. Borras C, Rio J, Porcel J, Barrios M, Tintore M, Montalban X. 1999. Emotional state of patients with relapsing-remitting MS treated with interferon beta-1b. *Neurology.*;52:1636-9.

20. Bras H, Cavallari P, Jankowska E, McCrea DA. 1989. Comparison of effects of monoamines on transmission in spinal pathways from group I and II muscle afferents in the cat. *Exp Brain Res.*;76:27-37.

21. Brewer KL, Yezierski RP. 1998. Effects of adrenal medullary transplants on pain-related behaviors following excitotoxic spinal cord inujury. *Brain Research.*;798:83-92.

22. Brisman R. 1987. Trigeminal neuralgia and multiple sclerosis. *Archives of Neurology.*;44:379-81.
23. Brown-DeGagne AM, McGlone J, Santor DA. 1998. Somatic complaints disproportionately contribute to Beck Depression Inventory estimates of depression severity in individuals with multiple chemical sensitivity. *J Occup Environ Med.*;40:862-9.
24. Brynne N, Stahl MM, Hallen B, et al. 1997. Pharmacokinetics and pharmacodynamics of tolterodine in man: a new drug for the treatment of urinary bladder overactivity. *Int J Clin Pharmacol Ther.*;35:287-95.
25. Burvill PW, Johnson GA, Jamrozik KD, Anderson CS, Stewart-Wynne EG, Chakera TMH. 1995. Prevalence of depression after stroke: The Perth Community Stroke Study. *Br J Psychiatry.*;166:320-7.
26. Cavanaugh SA. 1994. Depression in medically ill: Critical issues in diagnostic assessment. *Psychosomatics.*;36:48-49.
27. Chakravorty BG. 1966. Association of trigeminal neuralgia with multiple sclerosis. *Arch Neurol.*;14:95-9.
28. Chen D, Theiss RD, Ebersole K, Miller JF, Rymer WZ, Heckman CJ. 2001. Spinal interneurons that receive input from muscle afferents are differentially modulated by dorsolateral descending systems. *J Neurophys.*;85:1005-8
29. Chia YW, Fowler CJ, Kamm MA, Henry MM, Lemieux MC, Swash M. 1995. Prevalence of bowel dysfunction in patients with multiple sclerosis and bladder dysfunction. *J Neurol.*;242:105-8.
30. Clanet MG, Azais-Vuillemin C. 1997. What is new in the symptomatic management of multiple sclerosis? Thompson AJ, Polman C, Hohlfeld R, eds. *Multiple Sclerosis: Clinical Challenges and Controversies.*
31. Clayton DK, Rogers S, Stuifbergen A. 1999. Answers to unasked questions: writing in the margins. *Res Nurs Health.*;22:512-22.
32. Clifford DB, Trotter JL. 1984. Pain in multiple sclerosis. *Arch Neurol.*;41:1270-2.
33. Compston A, Ebers GC, Lassman H, McDonald WI, Matthews B, Wekerle H, eds. 1998. McAlpine's Multiple Sclerosis. Third Edition ed. New York: Churchill Livingstone.
34. Consroe P, Musty R, Rein J, Tillery W, Pertwee R. 1997. The perceived effects of smoked cannabis on patients with multiple sclerosis. *Eur Neurol.*;38:44-8.
35. Cottrell SS, Wilson SAK. 1926. The affective symptomatology of disseminated sclerosis. *J. Neurol. Psychopathol.*;7:1-30.
36. Cummins TR, Waxman SG. 1997. Downregulation of tetrodotoxin-resistant sodium currents and upregulation of a rapidly repriming tetrodotoxin-sensitive sodium current in small spinal sensory neurons after nerve injury. *J Neurosci.*;17:3503-14.
37. Cutter NC, Scott DD, Johnson JC, Whiteneck G. 2000. Gabapentin effect on spasticity in multiple sclerosis: a placebo-controlled, randomized trial. *Arch Phys Med Rehabil.*;81:164-9.
38. De Ridder D, Chandiramani V, Dasgupta P, Van Poppel H, Baert L, Fowler CJ. 1997. Intravesical capsaicin as a treatment for refractory detrusor hyperreflexia: a dual center study with long-term followup. *J Urol.*;158:2087-92.
39. De Seze M, Wiart L, Joseph PA, Dosque JP, Mazaux JM, Barat M. 1998. Capsaicin and neurogenic detrusor hyperreflexia: a double-blind placebo-controlled study in 20 patients with spinal cord lesions. *Neurourol Urodyn.*;17:513-23.
40. Degtyarenko AM, Simon ES, Norden-Krichmar T, Burke RE. 1998. Modulation of oligosynaptic cutaneous and muscle afferent reflex pathways during fictive locomotion and scratching in the cat. *J Neurophysiol.*;79:447-63.
41. Demaree HA, DeLuca J, Gaudino EA, Diamond BJ. 1999. Speed of information processing as a key deficit in multiple sclerosis: implications for rehabilitation. *J Neurol Neurosurg Psychiatry.*;67:661-3.

42. Derry FA, Dinsmore WW, Fraser M, et al. 1998. Efficacy and safety of oral sildenafil (Viagra) in men with erectile dysfunction caused by spinal cord injury. *Neurology.*;51:1629-33.
43. Detroit Free Press. March 3, 1997. 47 People, 1 Wish: The Individuals Who Chose the Same Final Act. *Detroit Free Press.*:(NWS);8A.
44. Devins GM, Seland TP, Klein G, Edworthy SM, Saary MJ. 1993. Stability and determinants of psychosocial well-being in multiple sclerosis. *Rehabilitation Psychology.*;38.
45. Dib-Hajj S, Black JA, Felts P, Waxman SG. 1996. Down-regulation of transcripts for Na channel alpha-SNS in spinal sensory neurons following axotomy. *Proc Natl Acad Sci U S A.*;93:14950-4.
46. Djaldetti R, Ziv I, Achiron A, Melamed E. 1996. Fatigue in multiple sclerosis compared with chronic fatigue syndrome: A quantitative assessment. *Neurology.*;46:632-5.
47. Eklund V-A, MacDonald ML. 1991. Description of persons with multiple sclerosis, with an emphasis on what is needed from psychologists. *Professional Psychology: Research and Practice.*;22:277-284.
48. European Study Group on Interferon beta-1b in Secondary Progressive MS. 1998. Placebo-controlled multicentre randomised trial of interferon beta-1b in treatment of secondary progressive multiple sclerosis. European Study Group on interferon beta-1b in secondary progressive MS. *Lancet.*;352:1491-7.
49. Feinstein A. 1997. Multiple sclerosis, depression, and suicide. *BMJ.*;315:691-2.
50. Feinstein A, O'Connor P, Gray. T, Feinstein K. 1999. The effects of anxiety on psychiatric morbidity in patients with multiple sclerosis. *Multiple Sclerosis.*;5:323-326.
51. Feinstein A, O'Connor P, Gray T, Feinstein K. 1999. Pathological laughing and crying in multiple sclerosis: A preliminary report suggesting a role for the prefrontal cortex. *Multiple Sclerosis.*;5:69-73.
52. Feinstein A, Ron M. 1998. A longitudinal study of psychosis due to a general medical (neurological) condition: establishing predictive and construct validity. *J Neuropsychiatry Clin Neurosci.*;10:448-52.
53. Filippi M, Alberoni M, Martinelli V, et al. 1994. Influence of clinical variables on neuropsychological performance in multiple sclerosis. *Eur Neurol.*;34:324-8.
54. Fischer JS. 1999. Assessment of neuropsychological function. Rudick RA, Goodkin DE, Editors. *Multiple Sclerosis Therapeutics.* London, UK: Martin Dunitz Ltd.;31-47.
55. Fischer JS. Cognitive impairment in multiple sclerosis. Cook SD. *Handbook of Multiple Sclerosis.* 3rd ed. New York: Marcel Dekker, Inc.; In Press;Vol. 53:233-252.
56. Fischer JS, Foley FW, Aikens JE, Ericson GD, Rao SM, Shindell S. 1994. What do we really know about cognitive dysfunction, affective disorders, and stress in multiple sclerosis? A practitioner's guide. *J Neuro Rehab.*;8:141-164.
57. Fischer JS, LaRocca NG, Miller DM, Ritvo PG, Andrews H, Paty D. 1999. Recent developments in the assessment of quality of life in multiple sclerosis (MS). *Multiple Sclerosis.*;5:251-9.
58. Fischer JS, Priore RL, Jacobs LD, et al. 2000. Neuropsychological effects of interferon beta-1a in relapsing multiple sclerosis. Multiple Sclerosis Collaborative Research Group. *Ann Neurol.*;48:885-92.
59. Fisk JD, Morehouse SA, Brown MG, Skedgel C, Murray TJ. 1998. Hospital-based psychiatric service utilization and morbidity in multiple sclerosis. *Can J Neurol Sci.*;25:230-5.
60. Ford HL, Johnson MH. 1995. Telling your patient he/she has multiple sclerosis. *Postgrad Med J.*;71:449-52.
61. Ford H, Trigwell P, Johnson M. 1998. The nature of fatigue in multiple sclerosis. *J Psychosom Res.*;45:33-8.
62. Freedman MS, Gray TA. 1989. Vascular headache: a presenting symptom of multiple sclerosis. *Can J Neurol Sci Feb.*;16:63-6.

63. Geisler MW, Sliwinski M, Coyle PK, Masur DM, Doscher C, Krupp LB. 1996. The effects of amantadine and pemoline on cognitive functioning in multiple sclerosis. *Arch Neurol.*;53:185-8.
64. Gelber D, Jozefczyk P. 1999. Therapeutics in the Management of Spasticity. *Neurorehabilitation and Neural Repair.*;13:5-14.
65. Gemperline JJ, Allen S, Walk D, Rymer WZ. 1995. Characteristics of motor unit discharge in subjects with hemiparesis. *Muscle Nerve.*;18:1101-14.
66. Geny C, Nguyen JP, Pollin B, et al. 1996. Improvement of severe postural cerebellar tremor in multiple sclerosis by chronic thalamic stimulation. *Mov Disord.*;11:489-94.
67. Ghezzi A, Malvestiti GM, Baldini S, Zaffaroni M, Zibetti A. 1995. Erectile impotence in multiple sclerosis: a neurophysiological study. *J Neurol.*;242:123-6.
68. Gilchrist AC, Creed FH. 1994. Depression, cognitive impairment and social stress in multiple sclerosis. *J Psychosom Res.*;38:193-201.
69. Gill D, Hatcher S. 2000. Antidepressants for depression in people with physical illness (Cochrane Review). *Cochrane Database Syst Rev.*;4.
70. Giovannoni G, Miller DH. 1999. Multiple sclerosis and its treatment. *J R Coll Physicians Lond.*;33:315-22.
71. Goh J, Coughlan B, Quinn J, O'Keane JC, Crowe J. 1999. Fatigue does not correlate with the degree of hepatitis or the presence of autoimmune disorders in chronic hepatitis C infection. *Eur J Gastroenterol Hepatol.*;11:833-8.
72. Goodin DS. 1999. Survey of multiple sclerosis in northern California. Northern California MS Study Group. *Mult Scler.*;5:78-88.
73. Groves L, Shellenberger MK, Davis CS. 1998. Tizanidine treatment of spasticity: a meta-analysis of controlled, double-blind, comparative studies with baclofen and diazepam. *Adv Ther.*;15:241-51.
74. Haas DC, Kent PF, Friedman DI. 1993. Headache caused by a single lesion of multiple sclerosis in the periaqueductal gray area. *Headache Sep.*;33:452-5.
75. Hagen KB, Smedstad LM, Uhlig T, Kvien TK. 1999. The responsiveness of health status measures in patients with rheumatoid arthritis: comparison of disease-specific and generic instruments. *J Rheumatol.*;26:1474-80.
76. Hainsworth MA. 1994. Living with multiple sclerosis: the experience of chronic sorrow. *J Neurosci Nurs.*;26:237-40.
77. Heller L, Keren O, Aloni R, Davidoff G. 1992. An open trial of vacuum penile tumescence: constriction therapy for neurological impotence. *Paraplegia.*;30:550-3.
78. Hirsch IH, Smith RL, Chancellor MB, Bagley DH, Carsello J, Staas WE Jr. 1994. Use of intracavernous injection of prostaglandin E1 for neuropathic erectile dysfunction. *Paraplegia.*;32:661-4.
79. Houtchens MD, Richert JR, Sami A, Rose JW. 1997. Open label gabapentin treatment for pain in multiple sclerosis. *Mult Scler.*;3:250-3.
80. Hulter BM, Lundberg PO. 1995. Sexual function in women with advanced multiple sclerosis. *J Neurol Neurosurg Psychiatry.*;59:83-6.
81. Institute of Medicine. Solarz AL, ed.. *Lesbian Health: Current Assessment and Directions for the Future.* Washington, D.C.: National Academy Press; 1999.
82. Jankowska E, Hammar I, Chojnicka B, Heden CH. 2000. Effects of monoamines on interneurons in four spinal reflex pathways from group I and/or group II muscle afferents. *Eur J Neurosci.*;12:701-14.
83. Jarow JP, Burnett AL, Geringer AM. 1999. Clinical efficacy of sildenafil citrate based on etiology and response to prior treatment. *J Urol.*;162:722-5.
84. Jones L, Lewis Y, Harrison J, Wiles C. 1996. The effectiveness of occupational therapy and physiotherapy in multiple sclerosis patients with ataxia of upper limb and trunk. *Clin Rehab.*;10:277-82.

85. Kapoor R, Miller DH, Jones SJ, et al. 1998. Effects of intravenous methylprednisolone on outcome in MRI-based prognostic subgroups in acute optic neuritis. *Neurology.*;50:230-7.
86. Kesselring J, Thompson AJ. 1997. Spasticity, ataxia and fatigue in multiple sclerosis. *Baillieres Clin Neurol.*;6:429-45.
87. Kevorkian CG, Merritt JL, Ilstrup DM. 1984. Methenamine mandelate with acidification: an effective urinary antiseptic in patients with neurogenic bladder. *Mayo Clin Proc.*;59:523-9.
88. Khan OA. 1998. Gabapentin relieves trigeminal neuralgia in multiple sclerosis patients. *Neurology.*;51:611-4.
89. Kim D, Adipudi V, Shibayama M, et al. 1999. Direct agonists for serotonin receptors enhance locomotor function in rats that received neural transplants after neonatal spinal transection. *J Neurosci.*;19:6213-24.
90. Kinn AC, Larsson PO. 1990. Desmopressin: a new principle for symptomatic treatment of urgency and incontinence in patients with multiple sclerosis. *Scand J Urol Nephrol.*;24:109-12.
91. Kirkeby HJ, Poulsen EU, Petersen T, Dorup J. 1988. Erectile dysfunction in multiple sclerosis. *Neurology.*;38:1366-71.
92. Kita M, Goodkin DE. 2000. Drugs used to treat spasticity. *Drugs.*;59:487-95.
93. Kroencke DC, Lynch SG, Denney DR. 2000. Fatigue in multiple sclerosis: relationship to depression, disability, and disease pattern. *Mult Scler.*;6:131-6.
94. Krupp LB, Alvarez LA, LaRocca NG, Scheinberg LC. 1988. Fatigue in multiple sclerosis. *Arch Neurol.*;45:435-7.
95. Krupp LB, Coyle PK, Doscher C, et al. 1995. Fatigue therapy in multiple sclerosis: results of a double-blind, randomized, parallel trial of amantadine, pemoline, and placebo. *Neurology.*;45:1956-61.
96. Krupp LB, Sliwinski M, Masur DM, Friedberg F, Coyle PK. 1994. Cognitive functioning and depression in patients with chronic fatigue syndrome and multiple sclerosis. *Arch Neurol.*;51:705-10.
97. Kurtzke JF. 1983. Rating neurologic impairment in multiple sclerosis: an expanded disability status scale (EDSS). *Neurology.*;33:1444-52.
98. Kuypers HGJM. 1973. Desmedt J, ed. *New Developments in Electromyography and Clinical Neurophysiology.* Basel: Karger;36-68.
99. Lange G, Wang S, DeLuca J, Natelson BH. 1998. Neuroimaging in chronic fatigue syndrome. *Am J Med.*;105:50S-53S.
100. Lilius HG, Valtonen EJ, Wikstrom J. 1976. Sexual problems in patients suffering from multiple sclerosis. *J Chronic Dis.*;29:643-7.
101. Litwiller SE, Frohman EM, Zimmern PE. 1999. Multiple sclerosis and the urologist. *J Urol.*;161:743-57.
102. Long DD, Miller BJ. 1991. Suicidal tendency and multiple sclerosis. *Health Soc Work.*;16:104-9.
103. Lovas G, Szilagyi N, Majtenyi K, Palkovits M, Komoly S. 2000. Axonal changes in chronic demyelinated cervical spinal cord plaques. *Brain.*;123 :308-17.
104. Lyons TJ, French J. 1991. Modafinil: the unique properties of a new stimulant. *Aviat Space Environ Med.*;62:432-5.
105. Mainero C, Faroni J, Gasperini C, et al. 1999. Fatigue and magnetic resonance imaging activity in multiple sclerosis. *J Neurol.*;246:454-8.
106. Malone DC, Okano GJ. 1999. Treatment of urge incontinence in Veterans Affairs medical centers. *Clin Ther.*;21:867-77.
107. Matthews B. 1998. Symptoms and signs of multiple sclerosis. Compston A, Ebers GC, Lassman H, McDonald WI, Matthews B, Wekerle H. *McAlpine's Multiple Sclerosis.* 3 ed. London: Churchill Livingstone;:145-190.
108. Matthews WB. 1975. Paroxysmal symptoms in multiple sclerosis. *J Neurol Neurosurg Psychiatry.*;38:619-23.

109. Mattson D, Petrie M, Srivastava DK, McDermott M. 1995. Multiple sclerosis. Sexual dysfunction and its response to medications. *Arch Neurol.*;52:862-8.
110. McCabe MP, McDonald E, Deeks AA, Vowels LM, Cobain MJ. 1996. The Impact of multiple sclerosis on sexuality and relationships. *Journal of Sex Research.*;33:241-248.
111. McCleane GJ. 1998. Lamotrigine can reduce neurogenic pain associated with multiple sclerosis. *Clin J Pain.*;14:269-70.
112. McCrea DA, Shefchyk SJ, Stephens MJ, Pearson KG. 1995. Disynaptic group I excitation of synergist ankle extensor motoneurones during fictive locomotion in the cat. *J Physiol (Lond).*;487:527-39.
113. Meienberg O, Muri R, Rabineau PA. 1986. Clinical and oculographic examinations of saccadic eye movements in the diagnosis of multiple sclerosis. *Arch Neurol.*;43:438-43.
114. Menkes DB, MacDonald JA. 2000. Interferons, serotonin and neurotoxicity. *Psychol Med.*;30:259-68.
115. Metz LM, Patten SB, McGowan D. 1999. Symptomatic therapies of multiple sclerosis. *Biomed Pharmacother.*;53:371-9.
116. Minden SL, Schiffer RB. 1990. Affective disorders in multiple sclerosis. Review and recommendations for clinical research. *Arch Neurol.*;47:98-104.
117. Mohr DC, Likosky W, Bertagnolli A, et al. 2000. Telephone-administered cognitive-behavioral therapy for the treatment of depressive symptoms in multiple sclerosis. *J Consult Clin Psychol.*;68:356-61.
118. Mohr DC, Likosky W, Dwyer P, Van Der Wende J, Boudewyn AC, Goodkin DE. 1999. Course of depression during the initiation of interferon beta-1a treatment for multiple sclerosis. *Arch Neurol.*;56:1263-5.
119. Montgomery EB Jr, Baker KB, Kinkel RP, Barnett G. 1999. Chronic thalamic stimulation for the tremor of multiple sclerosis. *Neurology.*;53:625-8.
120. Moulin DE, Foley KM, Ebers GC. 1988. Pain syndromes in multiple sclerosis. *Neurology.*;38:1830-4.
121. Mulder RT, Ang M, Chapman B, Ross A, Stevens IF, Edgar C. 2000. Interferon treatment is not associated with a worsening of psychiatric symptoms in patients with hepatitis C. *J Gastroenterol Hepatol.*;15:300-3.
122. Multiple Sclerosis Council for Clinical Practice Guidelines. 1998. Fatigue and Multiple Sclerosis: Evidence-based management for fatigue in multiple sclerosis. Paralyzed Veterans of America.
123. Nahas Z, Arlinghaus KA, Kotrla KJ, Clearman RR, George MS. 1998. Rapid response of emotional incontinence to selective serotonin reuptake inhibitors. *J Neuropsychiatry Clin Neurosci.*;10:453-5.
124. Noga BR, Bras H, Jankowska E. 1992. Transmission from group II muscle afferents is depressed by stimulation of locus coeruleus/subcoeruleus, Kolliker-Fuse and raphe nuclei in the cat. *Exp Brain Res.*;88:502-16.
125. Noseworthy JH. 1993. Clinical trials in multiple sclerosis. *Curr Opin Neurol Neurosurg.*;6:209-15.
126. Nyenhuis DL, Rao SM, Zajecka JM, Luchetta T, Bernardin L, Garron DC. 1995. Mood disturbance versus other symptoms of depression in multiple sclerosis. *J Int Neuropsychol Soc.*;1:291-6.
127. Ordia JI, Fischer E, Adamski E, Spatz EL. 1996. Chronic intrathecal delivery of baclofen by a programmable pump for the treatment of severe spasticity. *J Neurosurg.*;85:452-7.
128. Petajan JH, Gappmaier E, White AT, Spencer MK, Mino L, Hicks RW. 1996. Impact of aerobic training on fitness and quality of life in multiple sclerosis. *Ann Neurol.*;39:432-41.
129. Petajan JH, White AT. 1999. Recommendations for physical activity in patients with multiple sclerosis. *Sports Med.*;27:179-91.
130. Peyser JM, Rao SM, LaRocca NG, Kaplan E. 1990. Guidelines for neuropsychological research in multiple sclerosis. *Arch Neurol.*;47:94-7.

131. Pohjasvaara T, Leppavuori A, Siira I, Vataja R, Kaste M, Erkinjuntti T. 1998. Frequency and clinical determinants of poststroke depression. *Stroke.*;29:2311-7.
132. Powers RK, Rymer WZ. 1988. Effects of acute dorsal spinal hemisection on motoneuron discharge in the medial gastrocnemius of the decerebrate cat. *J Neurophysiol.*;59:1540-56.
133. PRISMS (Prevention of Relapses and Disability by Interferon beta-1a Subcutaneously in Multiple Sclerosis) Study Group. 1998. Randomised double-blind placebo-controlled study of interferon beta-1a in relapsing/remitting multiple sclerosis. PRISMS (Prevention of Relapses and Disability by Interferon beta-1a Subcutaneously in Multiple Sclerosis) Study Group. *Lancet.*;352:1498-504.
134. Provinciali L, Ceravolo MG, Bartolini M, Logullo F, Danni M. 1999. A multidimensional assessment of multiple sclerosis: relationships between disability domains. *Acta Neurol Scand.*;100:156-62.
135. Purvin V. 1998. Optic neuritis. *Curr Opin Ophthalmol.*;9:3-9.
136. Rabins PV, Brooks BR, O'Donnell P, et al. 1986. Structural brain correlates of emotional disorder in multiple sclerosis. *Brain.*;109 :585-97.
137. Rae-Grant aD, Eckert NJ, Bartz S, Reed JF. 1999. Sensory symptoms of multiple sclerosis: a hidden reservoir of morbidity. *Mult Scler.*;5:179-83.
138. Ramirez-Lassepas M, Tulloch JW, Quinones MR, Snyder BD. 1992. Acute radicular pain as a presenting symptom in multiple sclerosis. *Arch Neurol.*;49:255-8.
139. Rao SM, Leo GJ, Bernardin L, Unverzagt F. 1991. Cognitive dysfunction in multiple sclerosis. I. Frequency, patterns, and prediction. *Neurology.*;41:685-91.
140. Rao SM, Leo GJ, Ellington L, Nauertz T, Bernardin L, Unverzagt F. 1991. Cognitive dysfunction in multiple sclerosis. II. Impact on employment and social functioning. *Neurology.*;41:692-6.
141. Remick RA, Sadovnick AD. Depression and suicide in multiple sclerosis. Thompson AJ, Polman C, Hohlfeld R, eds. 1997. *Multiple Sclerosis: Clinical Challenges and Controversies.* London: Martin Dunitz Ltd;:243-251.
142. Repka MX, Savino PJ, Reinecke RD. 1994. Treatment of acquired nystagmus with botulinum neurotoxin A. *Arch Ophthalmol.*;112:1320-4.
143. Richardson JT, Robinson A, Robinson I. 1997. Cognition and multiple sclerosis: a historical analysis of medical perceptions. *J Hist Neurosci.*;6:302-319.
144. Roelcke U, Kappos L, Lechner-Scott J, et al. 1997. Reduced glucose metabolism in the frontal cortex and basal ganglia of multiple sclerosis patients with fatigue: a 18F-fluorodeoxyglucose positron emission tomography study. *Neurology.*;48:1566-71.
145. Rolak LA, Brown S. 1990. Headaches and multiple sclerosis: a clinical study and review of the literature. *J Neurol.*;237:300-2.
146. Rothwell PM, McDowell Z, Wong CK, Dorman PJ. 1997. Doctors and patients don't agree: cross sectional study of patients' and doctors' perceptions and assessments of disability in multiple sclerosis. *BMJ.*;314:1580-3.
147. Rovaris M, Filippi M. 2000. MRI correlates of cognitive dysfunction in multiple sclerosis patients. *J Neurovirol.*;Suppl 2:S172-5.
148. Rushton DN. Sexual and sphincter dysfunction. Bradley WG, Daroff RB, Fenichel GM, Marsden CD, eds. 1991. *Neurology in Clinical Practice.* Boston: Butterworth-Heinemann;381-91.
149. Rymer WZ, Houk JC, Crago PE. 1979. Mechanisms of the clasp-knife reflex studied in an animal model. *Exp Brain Res.*;37:93-113.
150. Sailer M, Heinze HJ, Schoenfeld MA, Hauser U, Smid HG. 2000. Amantadine influences cognitive processing in patients with multiple sclerosis. *Pharmacopsychiatry.*;33:28-37.
151. Saint S, Lipsky BA. 1999. Preventing catheter-related bacteriuria: should we? Can we? How? *Arch Intern Med.*;159:800-8.

152. Samkoff LM, Daras M, Tuchman AJ, Koppel BS. 1997. Amelioration of refractory dysesthetic limb pain in multiple sclerosis by gabapentin. *Neurology.*;49:304-5.
153. Schapiro RT. 1999. Medications used in the treatment of multiple sclerosis. *Phys Med Rehabil Clin N Am.*;10:437-46, ix.
154. Schiffer RB, Caine ED. 1991. The interaction between depressive affective disorder and neuropsychological test performance in multiple sclerosis patients. *J Neuropsychiatry Clin Neurosci.*;3:28-32.
155. Schiffer RB, Wineman NM. 1990. Antidepressant pharmacotherapy of depression associated with multiple sclerosis. *Am J Psychiatry.*;147:1493-7.
156. Scott TF, Allen D, Price TR, McConnell H, Lang D. 1996. Characterization of major depression symptoms in multiple sclerosis patients. *J Neuropsychiatry Clin Neurosci.*;8:318-23.
157. Scott TF, Nussbaum P, McConnell H, Brill P. 1995. Measurement of treatment response to sertraline in depressed multiple sclerosis patients using the Carroll scale. *Neurol Res.*;17:421-2.
158. Sipski ML. 2000. The neurologic basis for sexual arousal and orgasm: effects of spinal cord injury. *Ann Neurol.*
159. Sipski ML, Alexander CJ. 1993. Sexual activities, response and satisfaction in women pre- and post-spinal cord injury. *Arch Phys Med Rehabil.*;74:1025-9.
160. Sipski ML, Alexander CJ, Rosen RC. 1999. Sexual response in women with spinal cord injuries: implications for our understanding of the able bodied. *J Sex Marital Ther.*;25:11-22.
161. Sipski ML, Rosen RC, Alexander CJ, Hamer RM. 2000. Sildenafil effects on sexual and cardiovascular responses in women with spinal cord injury. *Urology.*;55:812-5.
162. Smith SJ, Young CA. 2000. The role of affect on the perception of disability in multiple sclerosis. *Clin Rehabil.*;14:50-4.
163. Snow BJ, Tsui JK, Bhatt MH, Varelas M, Hashimoto SA, Calne DB. 1990. Treatment of spasticity with botulinum toxin: a double-blind study. *Ann Neurol.*;28:512-5.
164. Solaro C, Lunardi GL, Capello E, et al. 1998. An open-label trial of gabapentin treatment of paroxysmal symptoms in multiple sclerosis patients. *Neurology.*;51:609-11.
165. Spissu A, Cannas A, Ferrigno P, Pelaghi AE, Spissu M. 1999. Anatomic correlates of painful tonic spasms in multiple sclerosis. *Movement Disord.*;14:331-5.
166. Staerman F, Guiraud P, Coeurdacier P, Menard D, Edan G, Lobel B. 1996. Value of nocturnal penile tumescence and rigidity (NPTR) recording in impotent patients with multiple sclerosis. *Int J Impot Res.*;8:241-5.
167. Starck M, Albrecht H, Pollmann W, Straube A, Dieterich M. 1997. Drug therapy for acquired pendular nystagmus in multiple sclerosis. *J Neurol.*;244:9-16.
168. Stenager EN, Koch-Henriksen N, Stenager E. 1996. Risk factors for suicide in multiple sclerosis. *Psychother Psychosom.*;65:86-90.
169. Stenager EN, Stenager E. 1992. Suicide and patients with neurologic diseases. Methodologic problems. *Arch Neurol.*;49:1296-303.
170. Stenager E, Knudsen L, Jensen K. 1991. Acute and chronic pain syndromes in multiple sclerosis. *Acta Neurol Scand.*;84:197-200.
171. Stolp-Smith KA, Carter JL, Rohe DE, Knowland DP 3rd. 1997. Management of impairment, disability, and handicap due to multiple sclerosis. *Mayo Clin Proc.*;72:1184-96.
172. Tanaka M, Cummins TR, Ishikawa K, Dib-Hajj SD, Black JA, Waxman SG. 1998. SNS Na+ channel expression increases in dorsal root ganglion neurons in the carrageenan inflammatory pain model. *Neuroreport.*;9:967-72.
173. Taylor A, Taylor RS. 1998. Neuropsychologic aspects of multiple sclerosis. *Phys Med Rehabil Clin N Am.*;9:643-57, vii-viii.
174. The IFNB Multiple Sclerosis Study Group and the University of British Columbia MS/MRI Analysis Group. 1995. Interferon beta-1b in the treatment of multiple sclerosis: final outcome of the randomized controlled trial. *Neurology.*;45:1277-85.

175. The Optic Neuritis Study Group. 1997. Visual function 5 years after optic neuritis: experience of the Optic Neuritis Treatment Trial. *Arch Ophthalmol.*;115:1545-52.

176. Thompson AJ, Polman C, Hohlfeld R, eds. 1997. *Multiple Sclerosis: Clinical Challenges and Controversies.* London: Martin Dunitz.

177. Tilbery CP, Atra M, Oliveira AS, Calia LA, Schmidt B. 1989. [Histochemical study of the skeletal muscle in multiple sclerosis]. *Arq Neuropsiquiatr.*;47:337-45.

178. Trask PC, Esper P, Riba M, Redman B. 2000. Psychiatric side effects of interferon therapy: Prevalence, proposed mechanisms, and future directions. *J. Clin Oncology.*;18:2316-2326.

179. Valiquette G, Herbert J, Maede-D'Alisera P. 1996. Desmopressin in the management of nocturia in patients with multiple sclerosis. A double-blind, crossover trial. *Arch Neurol.*;53:1270-5.

180. Van den Burg W, van Zomeren AH, Minderhoud JM, Prange AJ, Meijer NS. 1987. Cognitive impairment in patients with multiple sclerosis and mild physical disability. *Arch Neurol.*;44:494-501.

181. Vas CJ. 1969. Sexual impotence and some autonomic disturbances in men with multiple sclerosis. *Acta Neurol Scand.*;45:166-82.

182. Vercoulen JH, Hommes OR, Swanink CM, et al. 1996. The measurement of fatigue in patients with multiple sclerosis. A multidimensional comparison with patients with chronic fatigue syndrome and healthy subjects. *Arch Neurol.*;53(7):642-649.

183. Vermote R, Ketelaer P, Carton H. 1986. Pain in multiple sclerosis patients. A prospective study using the Mc Gill Pain Questionnaire. *Clin Neurol Neurosurg.*;88:87-93.

184. Vidal J, Curcoll L, Roig T, Bagunya J. 1995. Intracavernous pharmacotherapy for management of erectile dysfunction in multiple sclerosis patients. *Rev Neurol.*;23:269-71.

185. Walther EU, Hohlfeld R. 1999. Multiple sclerosis: side effects of interferon beta therapy and their management. *Neurology.*;53:1622-7.

186. Waxman SG, Kocsis JD, Black JA. 1994. Type III sodium channel mRNA is expressed in embryonic but not adult spinal sensory neurons, and is reexpressed following axotomy. *J Neurophysiol.*;72:466-70.

187. Weiller C, May A, Limmroth V, et al. 1995. Brain stem activation in spontaneous human migraine attacks. *Nat Med.*;1:658-60.

188. Weinshenker BG, Penman M, Bass B, Ebers GC, Rice GP. 1992. A double-blind, randomized, crossover trial of pemoline in fatigue associated with multiple sclerosis. *Neurology.*;42:1468-71.

189. Wells KBSA, Hays RD, Burnam MA, et al. 1989. The functioning and well-being of depressed patients. Results from the medical outcomes study. *JAMA.*;262:914-919.

190. Werring DJ, Bullmore ET, Toosy AT, et al. 2000. Recovery from optic neuritis is associated with a change in the distribution of cerebral response to visual stimulation: a functional magnetic resonance imaging study. *J Neurol Neurosurg Psychiatry.*;68:441-9.

191. Whittle IR, Hooper J, Pentland B. 1998. Thalamic deep-brain stimulation for movement disorders due to multiple sclerosis. *Lancet.*;351:109-10.

192. Wikstrom J, Poser S, Ritter G. 1980. Optic neuritis as an initial symptom in multiple sclerosis. *Acta Neurol Scand.*;61:178-85.

# 4

# Disease Management and Measurement

The impact, management, and research needed on specific symptoms of multiple sclerosis (MS) are discussed in the previous chapter. This chapter discusses the conditions of life with MS from a more general perspective and emphasizes research that can improve the lives of people with MS. It covers psychosocial and physical adaptations, as well as a variety of health care issues. At the moment of being diagnosed, the patient is forever transformed into a "person living with MS." Even in the absence of signs or symptoms this person will forever after live with the knowledge that he or she can be unpredictably impaired. Sometimes the person will recover, sometimes not. For most, living with MS will become one of the major challenges of life. People with MS need to solve problems ranging from finding the right button hook, to getting dressed each morning with limited use of their hands, to specifying "reasonable accommodations" for continuing to work.

Improving the lives of people with MS rests on better understanding of their needs and their successes, specifically research into the conditions of life with MS, which requires objective, reliable research tools. The most essential tools for measuring the conditions of life with MS are the various survey instruments that measure abilities to function and quality of life, which are discussed in the latter half of this chapter. These tools not only provide for objective assessment of the needs of people with MS, they are also an essential element of measuring the effectiveness of any sort of therapeutic intervention—be it a rehabilitation process, a self-help program, or a disease-modifying therapy. Quality-of-life measures can also reveal aspects of the disease process that are not readily captured in standard clinical measures and might reveal insights into the underlying disease mechanisms. For example, pain, fatigue, and memory impairment are often among the earliest manifestations of the disease, yet they were virtually unrecognized as symptoms for many years. These symptoms are prevalent, troubling, and yet correlate only weakly, if at all, with neuropathology as revealed by current neuroimaging techniques. Quality-of-life measures might also provide more sensitive outcome measures of clinical efficacy of new therapies, and importantly, they measure the outcomes that concern patients the most.

Given the millions of people who will be living with MS now and in the future, it is important that the focus on curing MS not come at the expense of efforts to address the disruptions that pervade routine daily activities, personal relationships, family life, work responsibilities, and social involvement.[214]

## LIVING WITH MS

If a cure were found, would I take it? In a minute. I may be a cripple, but I'm only occasionally a loony and never a saint. Anyway, in my brand of theology, God doesn't give bonus points for a limp. I'd take a cure; I just don't need one. A friend who also has MS startled me once by asking, "Do you ever say to yourself, 'Why me, Lord?' " "No, Michael, I don't," I told him, because whenever I try, the only response I can think of is, "Why not?"

Nancy Mairs[124]

Many people with MS cope remarkably well, others less so. Understanding the traits and conditions that enable people to cope so well can provide insights necessary to help others, but obtaining these insights is complex. Conducting an investigation about people with MS similar in depth and scope to the multisite Medical Outcomes Study, a series of multisite studies funded by the Robert Wood Johnson Foundation in the early 1990s,[175] would be invaluable, but also methodologically and logistically challenging and enormously expensive.

A growing body of research describes the lives of average people living in the community with MS. Many of these studies involve surveys, the application of various psychometric instruments (functional status measures, quality-of-life indices, and other instruments targeting specific topics), and qualitative methods (reviews of in-depth interviews or focus groups). With the exception of the Expanded Disability Status Scale (EDSS; see Appendix D), there is little consistency in the survey forms or instruments used across studies. In addition, despite the experiential insight gained from well-conducted qualitative studies,[41] they rely on very small samples from specific subpopulations, and the results cannot be assumed to apply to the full range of people with MS. Some studies have involved large numbers, but they tend to focus on single, well-defined issues (for example, employment). Perhaps most importantly, most studies treat people with MS as a homogenous group, as opposed to groups of people with markedly different disease states.[51]

### "You Have MS"

Numerous studies have conclusively documented that communication between health professionals and patients is often problematic.[106,107] For people with lifelong conditions such as MS, initial contacts with health care professionals are especially important and can shape patients' attitudes about their disease and expectations about the role of clinicians. Sometimes problems result from general insensitivity, probably not specific to MS per se.

People with MS who write about their experiences invariably highlight the moment when they were first given their diagnosis. It is a pivotal, life-altering moment that remains vividly etched in their memories. Very often, these memories are filled with anger at the way the diagnosis was delivered. Sally Ann Jones, in her mid-fifties with MS, described how her doctor told her the diagnosis many years previously: [84]

> The doctor spent about a minute and a half with me and then he said, "The bad news is, Mrs. Jones, you have MS. The good news is, when I saw you before, I wrote down three potential diagnoses in my notes. If you'd had either of the other two diagnoses, you would be dead by now." Back then, he never mentioned that to me. I said, "Why didn't you tell me?" He said, "The symptoms of the other diagnoses would have been so bad, you would've had to return, and I didn't want to upset you unnecessarily." And with that, he left. He didn't tell me what to do. He didn't say, "Do X." He didn't say, "Come back in six weeks." He just left. Period. He spent about 10 minutes, beginning to end. I was absolutely in shock.

Because the symptoms are so often insidious, vague, and nonspecific, there can be a long period during which the patient knows something is seriously wrong but is unable to receive definitive answers. The uncertainty is highly stressful, and patients later often resent the long period of concerned waiting or the attitude of a physician who felt it was kinder to offer vague explanations when she or he was strongly suspicious the problem was MS.[130] In 1995, Murray wrote, "I have never heard a patient express gratitude for being kept ignorant of his or her diagnosis, but I have heard many express anger and disappointment for being kept in the dark. . . . While patients are in the dark about their diagnosis, they are unwell without legitimacy, expected to function normally without the physician-sanctioned 'sick role,' and often under the suspicion of family, friends, employers, and even themselves, of being hypochondriac or malingerers."[139]

One study identified four major themes of the experience of being diagnosed with MS: whispered beginnings (earliest signs and symptoms, understood only in retrospect); echoes of silence (worrying, wondering, and waiting, reinforced by relapsing and remitting patterns); hearing the words spoken and beginning to tell others; and refocusing their lives.[100] During the period of whispered beginnings, people often tried to minimize what they were experiencing, attributing it to stress. During the echoes-of-silence period, patients frequently felt anxious, lonely, and worried, sometimes trying various remedies (for example, multivitamins, stopping smoking, drinking lots of water, exercising). Finally, the actual moment of being told, "You have MS," was readily recalled by the participants. They described trauma-filled reactions such as "being in shock, feeling numb, and really stunned" when they heard the news. For some, the crisis of this response lasted for moments; for others, it lasted days to weeks. The experience of being told the diagnosis of MS brought the study participants to a time of being "emotionally wounded."[100]

These experiences emphasize not only the value of better diagnostic tools discussed in Chapter 2, but also the need for a better understanding of communicating with patients in the face of uncertainty at the initial stages of diagnosis and—once the diagnosis is confirmed—in the face of delivering devastating information.

Yet the issues surrounding diagnosis are changing. Patients today spend less time waiting for a diagnosis than they used to, largely due to improved magnetic resonance imaging (MRI) technology and its earlier, more frequent use. Once they receive their MRI results, however, they are faced with uncertainties and decisions that previous patients were not. One is the problem of interpreting abnormal MRI scans. Although the scans might confirm a diagnosis of MS, they still provide little information about the prognosis for impairment or disability. Another is the decision whether to start any of the disease-modifying therapies. Patients must weigh the immediate disadvantages of being yoked to a regular medication schedule with possible side effects that diminish their quality-of-life against the potentially great, but nonetheless uncertain, future benefit. In essence, it is impossible for a patient to make a fully informed decision. Patients can only guess, but the burden of decision rests with them. Therapies appear to be most effective if they are begun early in the disease—at a time when many patients might be most reluctant to assume the burden of treatment.

Disease-modifying therapies for MS were first approved in 1993 but have been widely used only in the last few years. In sum, much of the literature on the psychological aspects of living with MS, almost all of which predates the wide use of disease-modifying therapies, must be reconsidered in light of current options, which are themselves in flux. This does not, however, alter the fact that people with MS must adapt and readapt throughout their lives to MS.

## Psychosocial Adaptation

MS generally starts just as people are beginning their independent lives, families, and careers. Many will live with the disease across the full spectrum of their adult lives. Repeatedly over time, they adjust, with varying success, to its myriad disabling consequences. MS is a disease that teases with its unpredictably waxing and waning course—debilitating people one month, restoring function the next. Sometimes losses are insidious, gradually mounting and only dimly perceived until people finally recognize their presence and permanence. For some, living with MS can be like balancing, precariously, on a razor's edge. Others do well, experiencing only fleeting symptoms over many years. S. Kay Toombs, a philosophy professor who has had MS with progressive impairment over 25 years, observed:[214]

> When the body refuses my commands, it suddenly appears to have a will of its own. Rather than being that which enables me to carry out my projects in the world, my body is an obstacle that I must overcome. I may, for example, have to manually pick up my leg if I am to negotiate a small step, or pay exquisite attention to the way my body feels in terms of pain, fatigue, stiffness, if I am to engage in ordinary activities.

> Bodily attentiveness becomes an integral aspect of the illness experience. With permanent physical impairment, one must daily compensate for the body's disabilities and explicitly allow for its limitations. Even when there are lengthy periods of remission, the chronically ill remain uneasily attuned to the way the body feels and moves—always "on guard" for signs of an impending recurrence.

Research suggests that the experiences and feelings of people with MS are often more positive than clinicians or others expect. One study administered six instruments (Areas of Daily Functioning Questionnaire; Ways of Coping Checklist; Global Coping Scale; Thoughts About Suicide Probe; Anger-Fear-Depression Questionnaire; and Global Self-Esteem Scale) to 125 people with MS.[48] Although almost 60 percent reported having felt they needed professional psychological help at some point since their MS diagnosis and about 30 percent reported that they were not coping well and currently needed professional help, the most striking finding was that, despite the obvious challenges faced by people with MS, most successfully adapt to the disease. This finding was replicated across all the measures included in the study, including self-rated quality of marital, family, and friend relationships; objective measures of emotional functioning, thoughts of suicide, and self-esteem; and direct self-assessments of current coping with the disease.[48] Another study involving 629 women with MS found that compared to normative controls, they displayed significantly better interpersonal relationships and stress management, although they had significantly lower physical activity and spiritual growth compared to normative controls.[199] A study of 64 MS patients in Finland found that although they reported feeling physically limited and insecure, many also noted that having the disease helped clarify personal values and enhanced personal growth.[115]

People vary widely in their coping styles and in their perceptions of how much control they have over what happens to them.[160] Coping is defined by Lazarus and Folkman as "constantly changing cognitive and behavioral efforts to manage specific external and/or internal demands that are appraised as taxing or exceeding the resources of the person."[114] Styles of coping with stress are often dichotomized as "problem focused" or "emotion focused." Problem-focused behaviors entail confronting the problem, seeking information about how to manage it, and devising strategies to deal with it. Emotion-focused strategies generally involve denial and escape or avoidance, or reconfiguring the problem to make it more positive. While most people use both strategies, one style usually predominates. Studies in other diseases suggest that patients who use problem-focused techniques make better adjustments and have better outcomes than those who use avoidance and denial.[11,37,99,172,173,203,204]

Remarkably few investigators have inquired into the mechanisms that underlie success and failure in adapting to MS.[2] One prospective study that followed the adaptations and coping strategies of 27 patients found that escape avoidance coping strategies predicted future depression, but this was not a robust finding because the investigators reported that the correlation was not apparent in a follow-up study of the same patients.[2] Another study of 433 people with MS did not find a significant association between coping strategies and emotional well-being.[231] The same study noted that study subjects' coping styles depended on their level of uncertainty about their symptoms, treatment, relationships with caregivers, or future plans. Subjects used more emotion-focused coping when they were more uncertain and problem-focused coping when they were less so.

Psychological adjustment to MS is complex and multiply determined. Eklund and MacDonald[48] found that people with MS reporting better long-term adjustment tended to use "adaptive denial" as their coping mechanism at the time of diagnosis. By comparison, those reporting "confrontational coping" (obsession) and escape or avoidance (complete denial) adjusted relatively poorly. In addition, those who had thought through answers to the question, Why me?, were less likely to be depressed in the future. A study of 43 people who had MS for four years or longer (15 years on average) found no relationship between the extent of physical impairment and coping style.[12] Murray[139] suggests that MS patients use both problem- and emotion-focused coping styles, but the three most common strategies are problem focused: trying to maintain some sense of control; trying different problem-solving approaches; and looking objectively at problems from different angles. Coping strategies can change over time, with emotion-focused methods predominating when patients sense things are beyond their control.[139] One limitation of most studies on coping is that most study participants are identified well after the onset of MS so any consequences of adaptational style would have been in operation for a number of years.[42]

The chronic and uncertain nature of MS makes tremendous demands on the coping skills of people with MS and those who care for them. People adjust with varying degrees of success, relying on different coping strategies, often switching from one to another as their circumstances change. A better understanding of which of those strategies (and under which circumstances) foster more successful adaptations to life with MS would enable nurses, social workers, psychologists, physical therapists—indeed, anyone who counsels people affected by MS—to provide greater assistance in helping people manage their disease. Likewise, people with MS would directly benefit from information about what coping strategies will most enhance their personal sense of well-being.

### Change in Attitudes over Time

Finally, given the chronic nature of MS, patients' attitudes toward the disease—and even themselves—can vary widely and change over time. Toombs wrote:

> Bodily change may have different meanings for the same individual at different points in time. The inability to walk has a different significance for me now than it did when I first contemplated this loss of possibility as a thirty-year-old woman who was used to "standing on my own two feet." And the meaning of this change is different for me than it is for my friend who was a marathon runner before being diagnosed with MS.[214]

People of all ages with MS experience emotional distress and diminished sense of well-being when illness disrupts their life-styles, activities, and interests. However, older people with MS appear to be less adversely affected than their younger counterparts.[43] It is not known why this is so, but it could result from age differences in psychological disengagement, expectations about the age appropriateness of chronic disabling illness, or some other psychological processes. Little research has examined changes in people's attitudes over time or the factors associated with such shifts. These changes could alter perceptions of the value of medical therapy, the role of health care professionals, and interventions to address functional impairments.

Duration of disease does not appear to be associated with psychosocial adjustment: "longer duration is not manifested in greater psychological distress, worry, body image, depression, or guilt."[51,110] One interpretation is that the longer people have MS, the better they are at accepting the physical consequences and the less likely it becomes that MS will affect their emotional well-being.

### Impact of Self-Perceptions and Attitudes

Patients, regardless of their illness, also vary in their perceptions of how much control they have over their lives. People with a strong internal "locus of control" strive to exert influence over what happens to them. They believe they are responsible for what happens to them by their own efforts to control the situation. In contrast, those with an external "locus of control" tend to hold outside institutions, other people, or "fate" responsible for what happens to them. A study of 94 people with MS found that increasing sense of personal control was associated with better psychosocial well-being, and two-thirds of participants reported positive psychosocial adjustment.[42] An investigation involving 100 people with MS found that those with an internal locus of control were still largely ambulatory and self-sufficient after 25 years compared to externally focused patients.[226] These studies could not directly investigate the reason for those differences.

Self-perceptions and attitudes about their lives have important consequences. Toombs notes, "Negative societal attitudes towards illness and disability not only diminish self-esteem, making it hard to accommodate loss of bodily function, but such attitudes cause concrete hardships in terms of the disruption of personal relationships, loss of employment opportunities, inability to obtain health insurance, and so forth." [214] These self-perceptions might vary according to the cause of disability. In a study of 25 wheelchair users, Avillion[8] found much lower self-esteem among people disabled by MS than by spinal cord injury. Eklund and MacDonald,[48] however, found that self-esteem reported by their 125 respondents with MS did not differ significantly from that observed in samples of physically healthy people. Other studies also offer contradictory findings about self-esteem of people with MS.[139]

### Stress

Living with MS is indisputably stressful, but it does not follow from this that stress triggers exacerbations or hastens disease progression. This issue has been debated for more than a century with strong held views on both sides.[139,202] For many people, the link seems obvious. Psychological stress is known to alter immune response, but it should also be kept in mind that these changes are generally small and within normal ranges.[77] In June 1999, the American Academy of Neurology (AAN), through its Therapeutics and Technology Assessment Subcommittee, conducted a comprehensive review of studies on the impact of psychological stress on MS done up to that date.[66] The AAN committee concluded that research done up to the time of its review had not clearly established that psychological stress can trigger MS onset or exacerbation, but that this is possible. Most published studies attempting to demonstrate a causal link were methodologically flawed (reviewed in 1999 by Schwartz et al.[176]). Since the AAN review, a well-designed prospective study has been published indicating that patients who experience one or more stressful events have a small-to-moderate increased risk of disease progression.[176] However, the risk of stress following physical deterioration is even greater. In other words, patients with a faster rate of deterioration will also have a higher risk of stressful life events and, consequently, will be more likely to experience stress before an exacerbation. The link between stress and disease progression remains frustratingly unclear.

Many patients believe that stress will worsen their disease and blame themselves for exacerbations (or feel that others blame them) when they have not managed to eradicate stress from their lives. People with MS are frequently cautioned to "take it easy" and not "overdo it," sometimes leading to decreases in recreational and physical activity that are out of proportion to this level of impairment.[200] This inactivity can contribute to worsening functional capabilities, reducing endurance, and disturbing sleep patterns, perhaps also heightening stress. Indeed, Schwartz and her colleagues have suggested that limiting one's activities might actually leave people more vulnerable to stress.[176] The effect of this "vicious circle" on quality-of-life and disease progression has received little study. Even independently of a causal link between stress and disease progression, stress management would seem to be an obvious area in which interventions could improve quality-of-life for people with MS, as well as their caregivers.

### Family and Social Relationships

As for most people, relationships with family and friends are central to the lives of people with MS. Despite common assumptions, neurological impairment and physical handicap are not the major determining factors of quality of life for MS patients. Patients are affected primarily by their relationships to other people and secondarily by symptoms of fatigue, pain, and cognitive dysfunction.[139] Quality-of-life studies in MS patients suggest that there are seven primary factors affecting mental health and quality of life: loneliness-companionship, fatigue, degree of chronic pain, duration of symptoms, stressful life events, self-perceived cognitive deficits, and clinically assessed cognitive deficits.

Evidence about the effect of MS on relationships is somewhat contradictory. Conventional wisdom holds that the stresses of MS end marriages, especially those that are already tenuous, and that divorce rates are double those in the general population.[139] For marital relationships, three factors are particularly important: (1) both partners cannot equally "share" the illness experience, despite good intentions; (2) traditional gender roles may be compromised; and (3) having one's partner serve as caretaker raises a complex set of emotions on both sides.[115] In one study of 125 people with MS, slightly more than half reported that relationships with their spouses and other family members had changed as a result of the diagnosis (55 and 53 percent, respectively), and somewhat less so with close friends (39 percent).[48] However, respondents said that these changes were positive about half of the time. A study involving 629 women with MS found significantly better interpersonal relationships than for normative controls.[199] A study by Wassem[226] of 100 people with MS found that their divorce rate was less than one-third that of the general population. Several explanations are possible. Patients reported that the problems caused by having MS had brought them closer to their spouses and that they had more time to spend together than when both worked. Women reported less strain in their roles as mother and spouse when MS forced them to stay home rather than work full-time.[226] A study of 101 people with MS found they generally had small social networks of about four family members and two friends. Despite this, they perceived "moderate" to "quite a bit" of love, respect, or admiration from these people. Isolation grew with duration of disease.[145]

**Effect of Spousal Attitudes.** At the time of writing this report, only one recent publication has reported on the role of spousal attitudes in the psychosocial and physical functioning of the person with MS. Schwartz and Kraft[178] examined 44 people with MS and found, not surprisingly, that patients who saw their spouses as responding negatively to their impairment had poorer general mental health functioning and more symptoms of depression. In contrast, patients who viewed their spouses as encouraging of well behaviors were significantly less depressed. The authors of this study suggested that their findings be used to develop family-based treatment strategies but did not test any interventions. It should also be noted that cross-sectional studies such as this cannot establish causality, for instance, whether the spousal attitudes were a cause or a consequence of the mental health of their partners with MS.

**Caregiving.** When a partner, family member, or friend becomes the primary caregiver, complex issues arise.[139] While the person with MS is the one who needs the most help, the caregiver is inevitably affected, but the needs of the caregiver are often neglected by the health care system. Little information is available about the needs and preferences of caregivers who often must adapt to more restricted roles and heightened limitations on time, privacy, social activities, employment, and finances.[139]

One study that examined the experiences of nine caregiver wives of husbands with MS described how love and commitment for their husbands often coexist with anger toward the disease.[40] As one woman said, "I still love [husband's name] in spite of everything. And it's really hard to love someone so much and watch him deteriorate. I love him anyway. . . . I don't hate him, I hate the disease." Yet the demands of caregiving easily become overwhelming.[40] The wives sometimes admitted they had reached a breaking point. One observed, "There were times when I felt like throwing in the towel." The women sometimes felt the inequity of their marital relationships and the pressing need for "space." One woman said, "I just felt like . . . if I couldn't get away from the situation for just a little bit. . . . I felt like I was about to go stand on a corner and scream. It's not because I don't love him, or not because I resent what I am doing, it's just that I need some space." Another study of 146 people with MS and their caregiving spouses or partners revealed significant differences in coping styles, depending on the caregiver's gender and health, and the level of dependency of their partner with MS.[72]

More knowledge about the coping strategies and needs of caregivers can be used to provide information and counseling to help families cope more effectively with the demands of MS. There has been little research in this area or on ways to relieve caregiver burden. Yet relieving caregiver burden might, in fact, offer a strategy to reduce overall health care costs by supporting various interventions that might delay the time when an MS patient needs full-time institutional care or even forgo this need altogether. This might be achievable by relieving the burden of caregivers in a variety of ways such as by providing respite care as temporary relief for caregivers, household help, by providing counseling and social support to the caregivers, or by providing in-home health care visits. Identifying cost-effective measures to relieve caregiver burden would be of mutual benefit to caregivers, MS patients, and health care providers.

**Relationships with Children.** Parents with MS are especially concerned about the effect of their illness on their young children. Some research has described children of parents with chronic illnesses as constrained, repressed, and antisocial, whereas other studies have noted they are more empathetic and mature in their friendships. More research is needed about the children of parents with MS.[115]

Crist[35] videotaped interactions between 31 mothers with MS and their 8- to 12-year old daughters and compared them to those of 34 mothers without disabilities and their daughters. She found similar rates of receptive, directive, and dissuasive behaviors for mothers with MS and their daughters compared to the control group pairs. Another study examined 35 mothers with MS and their young children, paying particular attention to the effects of exacerbations of the disease.[38] When the mothers' symptoms were stable, both mothers and children described similar levels of physical affection. During exacerbations, however, their perceptions diverged. Mothers underestimated the impact of the exacerbations compared to the child's perception. One mother noted:

> Well, there's a lot of times, because my patience [is] short and . . . I'm more concentrating on myself, I'm self-centered at that time and they come in . . . my youngest daughter is very affectionate . . . when I am having an exacerbation and she wants to hug and she wants to kiss, I try to respond to her because I know she needs this. This is important to her and it's part of her make-up. There's times when I have to say to her, "Mommy's really not feeling well."[38]

Sometimes fathers or other family members take over family responsibilities from the mother, leaving mothers saddened and feeling less involved with their children than they would like.[38] Older children often overcome fears with knowledge of their own competence and increasing independence. As one older child said, "She deals with it pretty well and knows her limits. It doesn't really bother me because I don't rely on her for every need. She just needs to take care of herself and I will be fine."[38] Another child described her mother's frustration during exacerbations: "She complains all of the time and we have to get this and get that for her. Then she cries and gets mad because she can't do it. It's really hard to take when you just want a normal life like everybody else." Little research has examined strategies for working with parents who have MS and their children to handle fears and expectations.

## Navigating Community and Societal Attitudes

> One of the hardest things in living with MS is dealing with how other people
> react to your condition—this includes family, friends, caregivers and people in
> general.
>
>                          Anonymous survey respondent quoted by Clayton et al.[28]

The social stigma associated with disabling conditions is well recognized.[27,65,148,180,236] Charlton[27] argues that there is more discrimination worldwide toward people with mental health and hearing disabilities than those with physical impairments. In the United States, laws passed since the 1970s have attempted to redress systemic inequities against people with disabilities. The 1990 Americans with Disabilities Act followed such federal laws as Section 504 of the Rehabilitation Act of 1973, which made it illegal for organizations that received federal funding to discriminate against anyone "solely by reason of . . . handicap" and the Technology-Related Assistance for Individuals with Disabilities Act of 1988 (P.L. 100-407, the "Tech Act"), reauthorized in 1998, which aims to heighten access to products for improving function and independence.

The extent to which people with MS have litigated under these various provisions or faced overt discrimination is unclear. Despite federal and state laws, environmental and architectural barriers remain widespread.[157] Some communities are undoubtedly more accessible than others. Murray[139] believes that people with MS are more likely to have fulfilling lives when they reside in urban areas or near friends, theaters, museums, shopping areas, and community agencies, than when they live in isolated regions. The experience of rural residents with MS has been little studied.

People with MS, like others with disabilities, face negative societal attitudes that legislation cannot eradicate. Murray[139] observed, "The stigma of a disabling disease becomes a disturbing negative influence on MS patients as they become recognizable in the community. They are very conscious of their ataxia, aware that many will think them intoxicated; ashamed of their canes and wheelchairs, when a short time before they felt themselves healthy members of society." People with MS themselves have articulated these sentiments:

> When you kind of walk unbalanced and people think you're drunk and you start
> to stagger or you start to slur your words because the nerve ending in your
> mouth can't pronounce the right words, people look at you and cannot under-
> stand why you are acting that way. Some people also say that you are using the
> MS as an excuse for being tired, for getting out of things.[147]

> When strangers observe that I am in a wheelchair, they make immediate judg-
> ments about me as a person. Most assume that I am dependent on others and
> unable to engage in professional activities. In perceiving that my legs no longer
> work, strangers also conclude that my intellect has been likewise affected.[214]

How people with MS respond to these societal attitudes and whether their responses reflect life-style choices and participation in the community is unclear. Mairs is a writer who leads an active life and travels widely, including overseas. Toombs is a university professor who also travels and publishes scholarly works. Both women are "privileged," accomplished women with recognized achievements and reasonable financial resources. How others with MS, especially those with less education and lower incomes, face societal perceptions and potential discrimination is unknown.

## Critique of Research on Living with MS

An overarching view of the state of research in this area suggests the following:

- Studies are generally small and do not distinguish among different MS disease states, with authors noting that their results cannot be applied to the full spectrum of people with MS.

- Investigators come from various clinical and social science disciplines and tend to publish in journals specific to their disciplines, which are likely to be read primarily by people in those specific disciplines (such as neurology, physical medicine and rehabilitation, nursing, nursing rehabilitation, psychology, occupational therapy, sociology).

- Frequently, however, more than one study has targeted a particular topic, so results can be compared and preliminary opinions formed about the generalizability of conclusions. Yet it is unclear whether investigators are aware of or draw from studies performed by those in other fields because they often fail to cite each others' work.

- Most studies on coping and adaptation among people with MS rely on instruments developed and validated only among nondisabled populations.

In summary, although many studies address pertinent topics, the research community tends to operate within narrow disciplinary "silos," and relatively little cross-fertilization seems to have occurred. Given the breadth of the issues involved and the diversity of research techniques appropriate to exploring them, this situation is understandable. Nevertheless, these disciplinary boundaries obscure just how much is, in fact, known about the lives of people with MS. Multidisciplinary work is relatively rare.

Although many issues about living with MS have been addressed, important gaps remain. As noted below, some topics have received little attention. Obviously, the major area that has yet to be studied involves strategies for improving the lives of people with MS: although articles identify problems, they only speculate about how to address them. Trials of proposed interventions to ameliorate psychosocial and quality-of-life problems for people with MS and their families are rare.

Research strategies aimed at improving the ability of people with MS to adapt and function should be developed in partnership with research practitioners, managers, and beneficiaries; toward this end, the National Multiple Sclerosis Society (the MS Society) should convene a series of forums to identify the most pressing needs experienced by people with MS. The goal of such a series would be to define research needed to identify ways to help people with MS adapt to their illness and enhance their ability to function. The committee did not include the expertise to develop a research agenda to meet the needs experienced by patients. The committee recommends that the MS Society work in partnership with people with MS to better define their information needs and to guide the development of specific research strategies that will identify the most effective approaches to communicating this information. A series of forums could provide the needed perspective to defining these strategies and should include the following constituencies:

- patients and their families;
- health care providers;
- allied heath professionals, such as physical therapists, occupational therapists, and social workers;
- health services researchers, including survey scientists and clinical epidemiologists;
- social scientists, including sociologists, anthropologists, and psychologists; and
- representatives of organizations of patients with other disorders that present some of the same challenges faced by people with MS

## Employment

As a disabling disease of young adulthood, MS inevitably disrupts careers.[159,195] A 1992 survey of people with MS in the United States found that roughly 40 percent were employed.[24] Although the unemployment rate for people with MS is clearly high (even at the time of diagnosis), it is important to consider unemployment rates relative to the base rate for the general population. These rates vary over time, place, and general characteristics of the population, such as educational level, as well as disease-related characteristics such as level of impairment and form of MS. For instance, a community-based study conducted in 1991 that included almost all of the people with MS in Olmsted County, Minnesota, found that more than twice as many people with MS were employed (53 percent)[164] as reported in other U.S.[170] and Canadian surveys.[54,91] Two points are important to note. First, Olmsted County is an affluent community, with a low overall unemployment rate that was less than half of the national average at the time of the study. Second, it included all people in the region with MS, not just patients attending a specialized MS clinic. Many people with MS—most likely those who are coping most effectively and most likely to be employed—will not see neurologists regularly. Although it has often been reported that within five years of diagnosis, 70 to 80 percent of people with MS are unemployed,[147,170] it is important to know that this figure is based largely on data collected in 1975[101] and might be biased by the fact that fewer women were employed than during their childbearing years than is the case today. A 1998 study found 72 percent unemployment among people with MS in the United States, compared to 36 percent unemployment among the general adult population.[165] Forty-nine percent of unemployed people with MS in that survey indicated they were unemployed because of their disease rather than choice.

A number of factors are correlated with unemployment in MS. Women; people with severe physical impairment, visual impairments, ambulatory problems, or cognitive dysfunction; and people in lower socioeconomic strata are less likely to be employed than other people with MS.[159,170] In general, employment rates are lower for people in wheelchairs or for those with steadily progressive disease, both of which apply to people with MS.[48]

Recent research has focused on barriers to employment and factors that might allow people to continue working. Barriers to employment for people with MS can be divided into three categories: *personal* (disease characteristics and an individual's educational and employment background); *societal* (physical inaccessibility of job sites, public attitudes, and inadequate job accommodations); and *programmatic* (vocational rehabilitation and policies promulgated by programs such as Social Security or Medicaid in the United States).[147] Spastic paresis, which is slight or incomplete paralysis due to spasticity, is a major cause of the loss of ability to work.[57] Managing fatigue and workplace demands is also difficult, particularly when the job requires working on a deadline, excessive walking, handling and grasping objects, working a full eight-hour day, or standing. Strategies have been suggested for patients to help them manage fatigue at the workplace (see Box 4.1). Incoordination and sphincter disturbances are significant factors, with many patients having more than one impairment.[57] Other challenges include environmental factors such as excessive temperature; physical barriers such as entrances, stairs, and steps; and personal difficulties with remembering, writing, thought processing, vision, speaking, and communicating.[170] It has been suggested that more people with MS could work if there were better access to the workplace or if they could work from home.[57]

Work not only provides income, it often defines the adult identity.[212] A study of 604 people with MS described the emotional toll of having to leave work because of their illness.[115] Those who had left jobs commented they had "lost a part of me" or that they no longer felt "a sense of being needed and of purpose."[24] Often they felt "out of sync" with their employed peers or were forced to give up traditional roles that were important to them, such as when husbands with MS left

---

**BOX 4.1**
**Energy Conservation in the Workplace for Patients with MS**

- Work at a moderate pace.
- Schedule short rest periods.
- Organize tasks to avoid unnecessary steps.
- Work in a comfortable position.
- Maintain good posture during any activity.
- Organize your work areas.
- Avoid lifting or carrying heavy objects.
- Delegate work that is too stressful or fatiguing.
- Ensure appropriate temperature of the workplace.

SOURCE: Stolp-Smith et al.[195]

---

work and wives had to take a job. Some people reported positive aspects to retirement. For example, some respondents noted that retirement had decreased their stress and permitted more time with family and friends,[24] and women reported less strain in their roles as mother and spouse when MS forced them to stay home rather than work full-time.[226] The experience of being diagnosed with MS can cause a person to redefine attitudes and self-perceptions, and to some degree, the high unemployment rate among people with MS might reflect changes in their own attitudes more than barriers presented by others.

> For those with progressively degenerative disease the future becomes not only problematic but intensely threatening. . . . I have known many MS patients who have abandoned life goals and projects simply because they received the diagnosis of MS and without regard to actual physical incapacity.
>
> S. Kay Toombs[214]

One study of 72 people with MS reported a positive association between "learned helplessness" and unemployment, but no significant association with marital status or education.[129] As with other cross-sectional studies, the causes underlying this association cannot be inferred from these data.

Many people with MS who lose or change their jobs to accommodate their condition suffer associated financial losses:[24] 70 percent of the low-income families, 43 percent of the medium-income families, and 24 percent of the high-income families in one survey reported having trouble meeting health care needs, basic living needs, or both. Rodriguez and colleagues reported that 77 percent of the patients responding to their survey maintained their usual financial standard without external support.[164] Again, these data are from an affluent community, which might account for the relatively large percentage of people who were able to accommodate the financial burden of the disease.

Financial setbacks diminish not only the ability to live comfortably, but also the ability to afford medical care, services, home adaptations, or the equipment required to manage progressive impairment. Thus, the determination of when people qualify for disability compensation is paramount in MS, where disability can come and go and the decision process can take up to 18 months.[111,195] The U.S. Social Security Administration (SSA) is currently rethinking how it determines qualification for its much-criticized disability insurance (SSDI) and supplemental security income (SSI) programs (see appendix F). The 1990 Americans with Disabilities Act (P.L. 101-336) makes discrimination on the basis of disability illegal and guarantees equal employment opportunities and access to public accommodations for persons with disabilities. The U.S. Supreme Court has heard several cases from people claiming disabilities under the Americans with Disabilities Act (ADA), and has publicly struggled with how to define disabilities in these cases.[70] What these cases might portend for people with MS, especially those who primarily experience fatigue or sensory impairments, is unclear. It is also unclear whether this situation is worse for people with MS than for those with other disabilities. Physicians who provide services to people with MS often serve as sources of information and should be able to help patients deal with issues surrounding disability, employment, and the ADA.[195]

With the exception of developments that address the specific workplace needs of people with MS (see discussion of assistive technology), the most important advancements in employment issues will likely come through changes in national policies. While employment is an important contributor to individual well-being, it seems likely that the most effective way to improve employment opportunities for people with MS is within the broader context of the disability rights movement.

## MEASURING FUNCTIONAL STATUS AND QUALITY OF LIFE

Quantifying functional status and quality of life for persons with MS is essential for several reasons. Given the chronicity and uncertain course of MS, tracking its impact over time can assist with care of individual patients, suggesting short-term prognoses and the need for various interventions. Tabulating these findings across individuals offers insight into the burden of MS-related disability within populations—information that is increasingly used to set research, health, and social policy priorities. Examining the trajectory of functioning and quality of life over time defines the patterns of progression and expands understanding of the clinical epidemiology of MS. Finally, functional status and quality of life are critical end points in measuring the effectiveness of therapy, for both clinical trials and routine patient care. Although disease activity can be measured by biological markers (such as lesions identified by MRI), these are only surrogate measures for the ultimate goal of improving patients' lives.

Over the last several decades, researchers have developed hundreds of measures of functional status and quality of life. Although the boundaries between the two sets of measures blur, *functional status* measures typically focus on observable behaviors and might or might not incorporate the patient's viewpoint, whereas *quality-of-life* measures are designed to assess the perceptions and feelings of individuals in relation to their disease and, necessarily, rely on patient self-report.[64] Virtually all instruments used to measure health-related quality of life include a measure of physical function.[150] Indeed, some observers find such distinctions spurious, preferring global measures of patient well-being that cut across various dimensions, and categorize quality-of-life measures as any measure that defines health beyond traditional biological function indicators.[79,223]

Both functional status and quality of life can be measured using generic or disease-specific survey instruments.[152] Generic measures allow for broad comparison across studies, interventions, and types and stages of disease, while disease-specific measures focus on issues that are most relevant to individuals with the disease.[79] Disease-specific measures are likely, but not guaranteed, to be more responsive to changes in a patient's condition.[78]

The wide variety of approaches to outcome measurement used in MS leads to problems when comparing studies. For example, in clinical trials of disease-modifying drugs for MS, different investigators have used different outcome measures in different populations. Direct comparisons of the trials are thus intrinsically imprecise, with the result that comparisons of the drugs are based more on expert opinions than on evidence.[169] Functional status and quality of life are concepts that can be viewed in many different ways, and no single universally valid measure is likely to emerge.[13,151] Nevertheless, standardized assessment methods that are multidimensional, quantitative, and include cognition evaluation are needed, particularly for the evaluation of patients receiving therapy.[169] With these goals in mind, the National Multiple Sclerosis Society's Clinical Outcomes Assessment Task Force generated a list of the ideal characteristics of a clinical outcomes measure (Box 4.2).[56]

## Quality-of-Life Measurement

The modern outcomes movement, which developed in the 1980s, established the principle that the consequences of a medical intervention for its recipient should be a major criterion in determining its value.[162] This reflects the awareness that biological standards of evidence alone do not completely depict the effects of a medical procedure. The recent interest in assessing outcomes of care has increasingly sought the patient's own voice, coalescing into the burgeoning field of health status and quality-of-life assessment.

Eliciting patients' own values about their health states is central to quality-of-life measurement—the values that two people place on a given health state can differ widely. For example, older people tend to be health optimists, having more

---

**BOX 4.2**
**Characteristics of an Optimal MS Clinical Outcomes Measure**

| | |
|---|---|
| Valid | Validity refers to the extent to which an instrument measures what it was intended to measure. Different aspects of validity include *construct validity* (measures impairment directly attributable to MS), *concurrent validity* (correlates in predictable ways with established criteria at a single point in time), and *predictive validity* (subsequently correlates with established criteria). |
| Reliable | Reliability concerns the extent to which scores are free from measurement error. Instruments can be administered and scored in a standardized manner; scores should be reproducible over brief intervals both by the same examiner (intrarater reliability) and by different examiners (interrater reliability). |
| Responsive | Responsiveness means sensitivity to changes over relatively brief intervals, regardless of whether these are attributable to the patient's underlying disease or to an intervention. |
| Widely applicable | This refers to applicability across the full range of disease severity, without significant floor or ceiling effects. |
| Multidimensional, but nonredundant | Multidimensionality reflects the main independent clinical dimensions of MS. |
| Interval scale of measurement | Unit changes are of comparable magnitude across the entire range of the scale. |
| Practical | The measure should be brief and easy to administer, preferably by non-doctoral personnel, and acceptable to both patients and health care professionals. |

Adapted from Fischer et al.[56]

---

favorable health perceptions than their levels of physical functioning objectively allow.[105] One study of gravely ill patients found that their health values varied widely and could not be clearly predicted based on their current state of health.[215] Being heard is especially important for persons with disabilities. Those in what others may perceive to be "poor" health place a relatively high value on their own health since they have adjusted their life-styles and expectations to take account of their condition. This may be particularly true of young disabled men and women, since one-quarter of this group of respondents describe their health as "poor" yet value it as "good." Conversely. young people who describe themselves as "healthy" can be reluctant to value their health near the top because they have high expectations about what being in the "best imaginable health state" involves.[45] Health care professionals often see patients only in the setting of an office or hospital unit and might conclude that the effects of MS on the person's personal life will be measured by the elements in the neurological examination.[139] However, most aspects of health-related quality of life are only weakly related to measures of neurological impairment.[55] Interestingly, several studies have found that the duration of MS is not consistently related to quality of life—either positively or negatively.[6]

Health status measures generally rely on extensive data obtained directly from patients, encompassing numerous attributes such as severity of illness, physical capabilities, psychosocial and emotional functioning, sense of well-being, and health-related quality-of-life.[73,118,119,193,196,223] Numerous quality-of-life measures exist. A review of 75 articles involving quality-of-life measurement found that 159 different instruments were cited. Each article used anywhere from 1 to 19 instruments, with a mean of 3 per article.[64] Some are generic to the extent that they assess health concepts that represent basic human values (Box 4.3);[223] others are designed to capture the impact of specific diseases (Box 4.4).

The SF-36, a 36-item measure developed in the Medical Outcomes Study and comprised of eight dimensions, is the most widely used quality-of-life scale (Box 4.3).[192,193] However, four of its eight dimensions cover functional limitations, so it can also be considered a generic measure of functional status.

### Concerns About Quality-of-Life Measurement

Despite the obvious appeal of quantifying patients' experiences and perspectives, several caveats arise. First, the explicit effort to be inclusive frequently yields megavariable composite indices.[53] The importance of specific variables, such as particular symptoms that are especially troubling or of prognostic importance, can be overwhelmed by numerous other factors incorporated in the composite index. Further, many functional status measures contain subscales (for example, the SF-36 measures eight dimensions), and single numbers do not adequately capture the full range of functional problems. For instance, how should an overall health score be assigned to a person with a serious chronic disease such as diabetes who feels well and functions as a productive person with no role or social limitations?[193] As an example, three categories such as self-care, mobility, and physical activity could be satisfactorily combined into one functional status index, whereas personal and role functioning measures are not so satisfactorily collapsed into a single index.[194]

Certain quality-of-life measures have been developed specifically for patients with particular conditions, whereas others are generic. No single method suits all research needs,[152] and choosing an approach depends on the specific research question. Mosteller and colleagues recommend routinely using both condition-specific and generic methods,[137] while Patrick and Deyo recommend using standardized, generic instruments with disease-specific supplements.[152] The SF-36, a generic instrument, reportedly yields reliable and valid results when

---

**BOX 4.3**
**Examples of Generic Quality of Life (QoL)**
**Questionnaires Used in MS**

**MEDICAL OUTCOME STUDY SHORT FORM 36 (SF-36)[132,224]**

- Widely used generic measure of health status
- Contains 36 items in eight health dimensions: physical functioning, role limitations due to physical problems, bodily pain, general health perceptions, vitality, social functioning, role limitations due to emotional problems, and mental health.
- Categories were chosen from more than 40 that were studied in the Medical Outcome Study.
- Weak correlation between subscales and impairment measures, with one exception: SF-36 Physical Function subscale is well correlated with EDSS.
- MS patients score poorly in several domains, including physical functioning, energy/vitality, and role functioning, in comparison with both the general population and patients with other chronic diseases.
- Limited value for patients with advanced MS.

**SICKNESS IMPACT PROFILE (SIP)[14]**

- A behavior-based measure
- Contains 136 items in 12 categories: ambulation, mobility, body care and movement, social interaction, alertness behavior, emotional behavior, communication, sleep and rest, eating, work, and home management.
- The Sickness Impact Profile is either self-administered or administered through interview.

**NOTTINGHAM HEALTH PROFILE[82]**

- Based on patient-generated statements.
- Part I contains 38 items in six areas: sleep, physical mobility, energy, pain, emotional reactions, and social isolation.
- Part II relates to areas of life affected by health: paid employment, home management, social life, home life, sex life, hobbies and interests, and holidays.

---

tested in people with MS, although it fails to capture important information about their quality of life that can be captured in MS-specific measurements.[219] The authors of that study recommend supplementing generic measures of health-related quality of life with MS-specific scales.

Health status measures do not perform equally well across the entire spectrum of impairments or within selected patient populations. The Medical Outcomes Study general health survey (MOS-20) was largely designed and tested among ambulatory patients and is biased against documenting a decline in the

## BOX 4.4
## MS-Specific QoL Questionnaires

### DISABILITY AND IMPACT PROFILE (DIP)[108]

- Measures disability and its impact on human activities that might be affected by disease.
- Based on the International Classification of Impairments, Disabilities and Handicaps.
- Contains three symptom questions plus 36 questions in five domains: mobility, self-care, social activities, communication, and psychological status.
- Rates the importance of specific disabilities based on weighted scores.
- Evidence of validity was provided by a close correlation between open-ended questions concerning the most negative consequences of the disease and low-weighted scores.

### FUNCTIONAL ASSESSMENT OF MULTIPLE SCLEROSIS (FAMS)[26]

- The core of the FAMS is the Functional Assessment of Cancer Therapy QoL Instrument.
- Consists of 44 items in six subscales: mobility, symptoms, emotional well-being, general contentment, thinking/fatigue, and family/social well-being.
- Both samples provided evidence of validity; internal consistency and test-retest reliability were determined to be good.[209]
- Heavily weighted toward assessment of psychosocial aspects of MS and virtually omits assessment of visual, bladder and bowel, and sexual function.

### MULTIPLE SCLEROSIS IMPACT SCALE (MSIS-29)[80]

- Generated from patient interviews, focus groups, expert opinion, and literature review.
- 29-item instrument with physical and psychological scales.
- Variability, reliability, and validity have been assessed. Preliminary data on 55 people thus far indicate the scale is also responsive (Jeremy Hobart, personal communication).
- Correlates with SF-36, FAMS, Barthel Index.

### MULTIPLE SCLEROSIS QUALITY-OF-LIFE INVENTORY (MSQLI)[55]

- 137-item scale (requires 45 minutes to complete); 80 items in short version.
- Similar to QoL-54 (see below) and FAMS in that it uses generic health-related quality-of-life measures; QoL and MSQLI are based on SF-36. (The SF-36 was selected over the Sickness Impact Profile as the core instrument after testing for correlation between subscales and quantitative measures of function.)
- Unlike the QoL-54 and FAMS, in that it was formed by adding established scales rather than individual items, thereby permitting cross-disease comparisons on generic measures, but also on symptoms common to the conditions being compared.

*continues*

- Content validity, scale reliability, and construct validity were each formally tested.
- Most comprehensive coverage of common MS symptoms.

**MS QUALITY-OF-LIFE-54 (MSQOL-54)[220]**

- The SF-36 serves as the core of the 54-item MSQOL-54.
- Contains an 18-item supplement to the SF-36 in the areas of health distress, sexual function, overall quality-of-life, cognitive function, energy, pain, and social function.
- Validity and reliability were established by self-administration to three groups totaling 179 patients. The groups were defined by ability to walk, ability to walk with aid, or need to use a wheelchair.
- Limited coverage of visual, bladder, and bowel function.

health of severely ill patients, which would include many patients with advanced MS.[15,59] When baseline scores are already near the bottom (or floor) of the scale, indicating poor health, further declines are less likely to be captured by the scale. The SF-36, which is similar to the MOS-20 in that it was derived from the same Medical Outcomes Study survey, also has problems with elderly people, poorly educated or impoverished persons, disabled people, and patients with both medical and psychiatric comorbidity.[98,131] The SF-36 can produce ceiling effects for healthy, community-dwelling persons, even those who are elderly.[3] In general, such floor or ceiling effects are more likely to be found on instruments with small numbers of items.[15]

Another important issue involves what to do when patients cannot respond themselves for any number of reasons, such as poor health, cognitive impairment, or physical limitations. One common solution is to ask a family member or close friend to serve as a proxy.[17,190] The accuracy of a proxy's response in representing a patient's perceptions is, however, potentially suspect. Some studies find that although patients and proxies provide generally comparable assessments of overall health and physical functional status, proxies report significantly lower emotional health, social activity, and satisfaction than do patients.[188] Others find that proxies rate both physical and psychosocial dimensions of functional status as more impaired than do patients themselves.[21,122] Physicians also frequently underestimated patients' functioning.[167]

## Functional Status

Functional status is a component health status and refers to the ability to perform activities of daily living.[168,222] Researchers have developed measures of functional status that address either specific areas of functioning or a range of dimensions related to functioning (see Boxes 4.5 and 4.6). Core components of

---

**BOX 4.5**
**Generic Measures of Physical and**
**Social Functioning Used in MS**

**BARTHEL INDEX (BI)[123]**

- Developed in 1955 as an index of personal activities of daily living.
- Criticized for its lack of responsiveness, but studies do not confirm this.
- Only relevant to people with moderate to severe disability.
- Validity and reliability have been measured in severely disabled persons[67] and stroke patients.[69,74,117,184,221]

**FUNCTIONAL INDEPENDENCE MEASURE (FIM)[68]**

- Developed as an outcome measure for medical rehabilitation.
- The most widely used of all measures of disability.
- Measures disability and need for assistance on an 18-item observer-rated scale
- Highly correlated with BI, Incapacity Status Scale (ISS), Environmental Status Scale (ESS), and the Brief Symptom Inventory in assessing assistance needs and patient satisfaction in people with MS.
- Does not assess visual problems.
- Granger et al.[68] concluded that the FIM is more useful for predicting physical care needs of people with MS than the BI, ISS, or ESS.

**MEDICAL OUTCOMES STUDY SHORT FORM 36 (SF-36)[132,224]**

- Widely used generic measure of health status
- Contains 36 items in eight health dimensions: physical functioning, role limitations due to physical problems, bodily pain, general health perceptions, vitality, social functioning, role limitations due to emotional problems, and mental health.
- Categories were chosen from more than 40 that were studied in the Medical Outcomes Study.
- Weak correlation between subscales and impairment measures, with one exception: SF-36 Physical Function subscale is well correlated with EDSS.
- MS patients score poorly in several domains, including physical functioning, energy/vitality, and role functioning, in comparison with both the general population and patients with other chronic diseases.
- Limited value for patients with advanced MS.

---

functional status measures typically include basic activities of daily living (feeding, bathing, dressing, toileting, walking) and instrumental activities of daily living (shopping, cooking, cleaning house, telephoning, managing money, using transportation). Most comprehensive functional status measures also encompass cognitive abilities (level of alertness, orientation, long- and short-term memory, capacity for learning and computation), affective health (happiness, anxiety, de-

## BOX 4.6
## MS-Specific Measures of Physical and Social Functioning

### EXPANDED DISABILITY STATUS SCALE (EDSS)[104]

- The most commonly used MS clinical rating scale.
- Developed based on the clinical experience of a neurologist specializing in MS.
- Measures impairment and disability based on the ratings of an observer or neurologist through structured interview.
- Ordinal scale from 0 to 10 in 20 steps.
- Heavily weighted toward physical dysfunction.
- Ratings are not based on similar functions across the scale. For example, it measures symptoms and signs such as visual disturbance and ataxia at the lower end of the scale; at mid-range, it measures walking; at the higher range, it measures arm movements; and at the highest end, it measures the ability to talk or communicate.
- Criticized for poor interrater reliability and insensitivity to clinical change.

### FUNCTIONAL SYSTEMS SCALES (FSS)[104]

- Components of the EDSS.
- Individual scales to measure handicap in pyramidal function, cerebellar function, brainstem function, sensory function, bowel and bladder function, visual function, cerebral or mental function, and other functions.

### MULTIPLE SCLEROSIS FUNCTIONAL COMPOSITE (MSFC)[36,56]

- Developed by the National MS Society's Clinical Outcomes Assessment Task Force.
- Comprises quantitative functional measures of three clinical dimensions of MS: leg function/ambulation, arm/hand function, and cognitive function.
- The clinical dimensions have been shown to be relatively independent; it is sensitive to clinical changes over one- and two-year intervals, and predicts subsequent and concurrent EDSS change.

### MINIMAL RECORD OF DISABILITY (MRD)[90]

- Developed based on functional disabilities as well as other activities of daily living assessments.
- An effort to obtain a broad assessment of the impact of MS, covering impairment, disability, and handicap.
- Provides two rating scales for clinicians to supplement the EDSS and its component FSS, the Incapacity Status Scale (ISS) and the Environmental Status Scale (ESS).

### INCAPACITY STATUS SCALE (ISS)[55,90]

- 16-item scale.
- Component of the MRD.
- Measures disability.

*continues*

- Modification of the Barthel Index that assesses both specific MS symptoms (for example, vision, fatigue) and independence in performing activities of daily living such as bathing and grooming.
- Scores can be derived either through direct assessment and observation of the patient's performance or through a structured interview.

## ENVIRONMENTAL STATUS SCALE (ESS)[55,90]

- 7-item scale.
- Component of the MRD.
- Measures handicap.
- Includes items on employment, housing, and need for personal assistance.
- Derived through a structured interview.

## CAMBRIDGE MULTIPLE SCLEROSIS BASIC SCORE (CAMBS)[138]

- Contains four sections: disability and impairment, relapse, progression, and handicap.
- Each section has one item rated on a five-point scale.
- Ratings derived through a structured interview.
- CAMBS was not developed as a clinical outcome measure, but as a clinical profile record for routine practice.
- The CAMBS was a reliable (all four domains) and responsive (relapse and progression domains) outcome measure but had a limited validity (handicap domain).[183]

## GUY'S NEUROLOGICAL DISABILITY SCALE[181,182]

- Devised as a simple clinical disability scale that encompasses the whole range of disabilities associated with MS.
- 12 separate categories: cognition, mood, vision, speech, swallowing, upper limb function, lower limb function, bladder function, bowel function, sexual function, fatigue, and others.
- Valid when applied by neurologists or nonneurologists, over the phone, or by mail questionnaire.

## IMPAIRMENT SCALE FOR THE EUROPEAN DATABASE FOR MULTIPLE SCLEROSIS (EDMUS)[31]

- Simplified version of the EDSS developed for use with the EDMUS.
- Measures disability due to MS on a 10-item scale based on the ratings of an observer or neurologist.
- Reliability is adequate, but clinical data do not yet exist.

pression), and social activities (for example, visiting friends, sexual relationships). The context of measurement affects assessments of functional ability. "Capability" indicates what persons "can do" in controlled settings, whereas "performance" assesses what a person "does do" in everyday life. Capability typically exceeds performance.[235]

In response to the concern among MS researchers that no currently available outcome measure adequately measured changes in patients' conditions over time, the MS Society's Clinical Outcomes Assessment Task Force developed the Multiple Sclerosis Functional Composite (MSFC) (Box 4.6). The MSFC was designed to fulfill the optimal characteristics of clinical outcome measures previously developed by the task force (Box 4.2). Three measures (leg function and ability to walk, arm and hand function, and cognition) were derived from a statistical analysis of variables measured in six different natural history studies and in placebo groups from nine clinical trials. Preliminary results indicate that the MSFC is responsive to change over one- to two-year intervals, that it is reliable, and that the three dimensions are nonredundant.[56] Independent validation studies suggest that the MSFC is reliable,[29,30] has good construct and criterion validity,[92] and is moderately to strongly associated with quality-of-life as perceived by patients (see Box 4.2 for explanation of terms).[135] Wider use of the MSFC should facilitate collaborative data collections and comparison among clinical trials.

Measuring functional status raises several issues. First, as with other measures of health status, many functional status measures are generic in that they are independent of diagnoses or the cause of impairment. Although they do not permit comparisons among different treatments or conditions, condition-specific approaches are best for certain purposes. For instance, the Visual Analogue Pain Scale[128] pertains to pain syndromes; the Tinetti Balance and Gait Evaluation[211] assesses gait abnormalities; and the Activities of Daily Vision Scale (ADVS) focuses on visual function.[126] These condition-specific scales are generally more sensitive to change in specified functions than generic measures. As described above, most investigators believe that generic instruments do not capture the full range of functional status concerns for MS patients.[208]

The mode of administration (face-to-face interview, mail with self-administration, or telephone interview) can affect responses. In face-to-face interviews, respondents may be reluctant to reveal the extent of their dysfunction. One study using the SF-36 found significant differences in patients' reports over the course of a week, depending on the mode of administration. For four of the eight SF-36 dimensions, face-to-face administration elicited a more optimistic view of functioning than did self-administration.[227]

Finally, as described above, perceptions about functioning frequently vary depending on who is asked—patients, proxies, or physicians.

## Disability

The term disability is used in many conceptually different ways throughout the literature. The definition of disability has become so controversial that the World Health Organization published a draft report in 1997 proposing that the term disability be abandoned in favor of the more neutral term activity, to more comprehensively assess the following three different dimensions: body structures or function, personal activities, and participation in society.[233] At the time of this writing, the proposal had not been formally adopted, although the expanded concept of disability reflects current thinking.

Disability can generally be defined as inability or limitation in performing certain roles and tasks that society expects of an individual.[87,88,233] Thus, disability reflects the gap between a person's capabilities and the barriers posed by the environment and society, and his or her ability to carry out tasks in the face of these societal and environmental barriers.[88] Disability refers to much more than motor control, with which it is often equated. *Impairment*, which is defined as any abnormality of structure or function affecting the whole body, and *handicap*, which is any alteration in a patient's status in society, contribute to but are not synonymous with disability.

Not only is disability defined in different ways, it is measured and interpreted in ways that do not allow easy comparison. One problem is that the specific tasks or activities used to identify disability are not defined. As a result, scales that have been developed to measure disability contain different tasks, depending on the interpretation of the developers, and often intrude into the concepts of impairment, handicap, and quality-of-life.[208] Although reliability and validity have been established for many of these scales, these tests are performed in different ways on different populations. Comparison of studies that used different measures is therefore problematic.

Finally, functional status measures and disability measures have been criticized as too narrow to be used as outcomes measures by themselves because they do not address the impact of the disease on the patient. The effects of MS on relationships, family, employment, and other aspects of life are not covered by functional status measures but fall under the concept of health-related quality of life.[208] With respect to MS, no measure of disability has been shown to be superior to all others.

### Expanded Disability Status Scale

The EDSS is the most widely used measure of disability in MS to the extent that it has been used in almost every MS clinical trial for several decades. Yet it is widely disparaged as a flawed tool. The EDSS is not a linear scale; it is bimodal. Patient scores are generally at the low or higher ranges of the scale, with relatively few in the mid-ranges, and patients spend more time at some levels than at others.[208] It is not even strictly a measure of disability, because at different points on the scale, it mixes impairment (where it scores limb movement) with disability (where it scores ability to perform daily activities).

Several aspects of the EDSS make it insensitive to change. Once a patient has limited ambulation, other aspects of the neurological exam are not taken into account. Also the EDSS does not measure cognitive impairment, although this deficiency is common to all scales based on the standard neurological exam. As noted earlier, a patient with MS can be unable to sustain a full day's work due to fatigue or other factors and yet have an EDSS score of zero. The EDSS is also heavily criticized for poor reliability.[208] Consequently, even though its wide use should allow the advantage of comparing between studies, such comparisons should be made with caution.

Even though the EDSS is much criticized, there is no consensus on the usefulness of other disability measures for MS. Granger and colleagues[68] concluded that the most useful disability scale for MS is the Functional Independence Measure (FIM), but van der Putten and colleagues[217] concluded that the FIM and the Barthel Index (BI) were similar in their appropriateness and responsiveness in MS patients.[68] Marolf and colleagues reported that both are more responsive to changes in a patient's condition than the EDSS.[127] They measured the results of rehabilitation in 100 patients and found that about 30 percent of them showed improvements at the end of a four-week inpatient program, as measured by either the Extended Barthel Index or the FIM. However, only 5 percent of them showed any change in EDSS scores. The EDSS generally correlates with the physical function domains of the SF-36, but not with other aspects such as role functioning or mental health.[18,144]

The measurement of functional status and impairment is central to all aspects of clinical research on MS, and the development and validation of acceptable measures must remain a priority for MS research (see Recommendation 12).[217]

# ASSISTANCE

## Assistive Technology

Assistive technology refers to any technology that helps support the individual's independence by enhancing or assisting performance of the activities of daily living.[187] Assistive technology can be as simple as a bathtub shower grab bar or as complex as a motorized, voice-activated wheelchair. MS patients' needs for assistive technology are as variable and difficult to predict as the disease itself. Their needs can wax and wane with relapses, and the need for specific types of assistive technology will be determined by each patient's unique presentation and sequence of symptoms. The assessment of patients' needs and communication of the options available are thus especially important in MS.

### Access to Assistive Technology

Patient reluctance and high costs are factors that hinder individuals from making full use of existing assistive technologies. People can be reluctant to use assistive technology because of the social stigma associated with disability, the fear that reliance on assistive technology will promote further loss of function, and discomfort about assuming a new identity as a "handicapped person."[83,142]

The high cost of assistive technology limits its availability to persons who need it. Since reimbursement is limited even for durable medical equipment such as beds and wheelchairs, the patient may be forced to pay the cost of devices such as scooters or of home modifications such as installing ramps and widening doors.[24,83,142] Reimbursement for skilled occupational therapy services to match the needs of individuals with assistive technology is also limited, particularly for MS since the patient's needs vary over time[142] (Michael Weinrich, personal communication). Most neurologists do not routinely recommend the purchase of a scooter or wheelchair until lower extremity and balance problems affect mobility, whereas physical therapists generally recommend the use of large equipment much earlier.[33] It is not known which criteria will best match the level of individual capacity to the type of mobility aids for support of quality of life, safety, and long-range health needs.

It is important to note that assistive technology might pay for itself by affecting moneys in other areas, for example, when the individual is able to continue working as a result of technology.

Several technology databases are available on the internet to help clinicians and patients identify and locate appropriate technologies. ABLEDATA, sponsored by the National Institute on Disability and Rehabilitation Research, describes more than 25,000 assistive technology products, including the price and company information for each. REHABDATA, an online bibliography of publications, journals, and government reports on rehabilitation, provides information on assistive technology and is run by the National Rehabilitation Information Center and funded by the National Institute on Disability and Rehabilitation Research.[187] Several web sites provide recent information on research and events relevant to MS. In addition, telemedicine can help patients with wound management, self-injection support and training, education and support during the initial self-catheterization period, emotional and physical adaptation to increasing disability, and family education.

Technology can enhance independence through assistance with mobility control, environmental control, communication, and employment.[96]

### Mobility Control

Novelist Nancy Mairs, who cannot walk because of MS, travels the world in a motorized wheelchair:

> Relaxed and focused, I feel emotionally far more "up" than I generally did when I stood on two sound legs. . . . Certainly I am not mobility impaired; in fact, in my Quickie P100 with two twelve-volt batteries, I can shop till you drop at any mall you designate, I promise.[125]

Fatigue and impaired mobility are frequent problems in MS, and the use of technologies that enhance mobility can provide empowerment and relief to patients.[83,142] Mobility aids also reduce the risk of life-threatening and costly injuries, and can be an economical alternative to costly personal assistance and institutionalization.[96]

A variety of assistive technologies aid mobility for both ambulation and patient transfer.[187] For ambulation assistance, canes, walkers, power and manual wheelchairs, scooters, and a spectrum of wheelchair accessories that allow for voice control, a joystick, or head movement are available. Bathtub benches, shower chairs, grab bars on walls, and lift systems assist with transfers to and from the bed or in the bathroom. Aids for access to community include adapted vehicles, portable and permanent driving hand controls, portable and permanent ramps, and wheel chair lifts. Aids for accessing the upstairs of a home include stair lifts, small residential elevators, and wheelchairs that climb stairs. Functional electrical stimulation is a technology that stimulates muscles that are no longer motivated by nerve impulses.[153] This technology, originally conceived in the early 1980s, is relatively new, and research is needed to improve its functionality and reliability. Finally, portable and fixed cooling devices help with fatigue management and exercise participation, especially for pool therapy use.[103,142]

## Environmental Control

Technology can assist with environmental control in a variety of ways, including controlling the power and output from devices such as electric doors, fans, telephones, TVs, radios, stereos, lights, heating and air conditioning units, and drapes. Low-technology devices such as reachers, alternative types of door and drawer handles, buttonhooks, and kitchen items can be adapted or configured for more functionality. Mouthsticks and head pointers can assist individuals who cannot use their hands. High-technology devices such as electrically powered feeders, electrically powered page-turners, or environmental control units are also available. Permanent or temporary home environment modifications, such as lowering kitchen counters and cabinets to wheelchair height, can be helpful. Finally, voice-activated computers can be linked to robotic environmental controls and remote controls.

## Workplace

Since the onset of MS occurs in the years when most people are deeply involved with their careers, technologies that allow people with MS to keep their jobs are especially important. The most frequently cited reason that people with MS left their jobs was physical inability to perform job tasks; the use of a wheelchair by MS patients was also associated with unemployment.[170] Adaptive equipment has been related to continued employment among persons with increasing physical disabilities, as adaptive keyboards, voice control systems, and adaptations of the workstation expand the range of tasks that people can perform.[48] Aids for effective seating and positioning such as adapted desk chairs and chair cushions reduce pressure and fatigue, support posture, provide comfort, and enable function.[71]

## Communication Aids

Communication becomes increasingly difficult as MS progresses, particularly when vision, speech, and memory are affected. Visual problems are aided by magnifiers and eyeglasses as well as nonoptical aids such as enlarged print, high-intensity lamps, high-contrast objects, and enlarged and tactually labeled aspects of self-care and leisure items. Electronic aids, such as computer software that enlarges text and images, and closed-circuit television devices (CCTV), can increase image size, color contrast, and overall brightness.

In the later stages of MS, the patient's speech can be difficult for others to understand, and the ability to talk can be lost. Technologies that increase the ability of the patient to communicate include speech volume amplifiers, speech enhancers to clarify speech, and text-to-speech voice synthesizers. These devices can increase social interaction and, along with portable home emergency call systems, serve as important safety devices that can be used to call for help when an accident has occurred in the home.

**Internet.** The computer has opened the doors to enhancing communication for people with MS like no other technology before it. The Internet is the ultimate community access tool and information resource, with no restrictions on mobility or speech faculty beyond access to the technology. There are limitations, but they are surmountable. These limitations include screen size, the standard keyboard and mouse that are difficult to operate when fine motor control is impaired, and the need for a workstation to accommodate wheelchair use or use while in bed. In addition, the Internet can be used to spread false or misleading information, and consumers have to be careful in their search for information from reputable sources. Another limitation of this powerful tool is the digital divide. Many people cannot afford a home computer or lack the skills and knowledge to make use of one.

The Internet can serve health needs in a variety of ways. It can be a source of medical advice and information on the latest research results. It can be used to contact health care organizations for information, scheduling of appointments, and communication with physicians. It allows communication among members of support groups. Also, it is a source of information on goods and services, such as assistive devices, that are on the market. Tasks, such as ordering personal and household items, banking, and paying bills, can be accomplished through computers. Certain services, such as grocery shopping, are often limited to urban areas and are unaffordable for many people. Nonetheless, such a service might be cheaper than the cost of personal assistants.

## Research Needs in Assistive Technology

The greatest needs for the field of assistive technology in MS include strengthening the research on assessing and evaluating patient needs and improving the dissemination of information and equipment to patients to fully address their needs. Persons with MS frequently have little awareness of assistive technology options and professional support available in assistive technology (Peggy Neufeld, personal communication, Box 4.7).

Many specific research questions remain unanswered in the area of assistive technology and MS, and research should focus on ways to maximize the positive effects of available and emerging technologies on quality-of-life. Research on the satisfaction of consumers, therapists, and third-party payers with various products would provide direction for manufacturers of assistive technology to improve available technologies and new designs. Input from MS patients in the design of new technologies is crucial.

Development of effective educational methods for demonstrating the application and operation of assistive technology to health care professionals and people with MS would increase the use of available technologies and increase

---

**BOX 4.7**
**Assistive Technology That Would Be Particularly Useful to People with MS**

- Wheelchair and scooter designs that are effective in an environment built for people that stand; designs that can handle uneven floor surfaces or stairs.

- Effective transfer aids such as lifts to reduce stress on caregivers.

- Handicapped bathroom facilities in public buildings.

- Aids for ataxia or tremors, such as head control and hand control during functional activities.

- Options for MS patients with cognitive impairments. Currently available technologies include computer software for cognition rehabilitation, memory and problem-solving skills training, and perception skills rehabilitation.

- Assistive technology designs with fashionable and acceptable appearances.

- Assistive technology for recreation and leisure. Leisure activities and social participation are important aspects of a positive quality of life.

Source: Peggy Neufeld, personal communication.

patient safety (David Krebs, Peggy Neufeld, personal communication). Strategies to disseminate information, appropriate training methods, and self-help strategies to enhance the ability of persons with MS to select assistive technology will help educate both patients and care providers.

The optimal time for the introduction of assistive technology during the rehabilitation or therapy process should be studied. Strategies to reduce the social stigma associated with disability should be examined. Cost factors should be analyzed to determine when the use of assistive technology by people with MS results in economic benefit or loss. Finally, research should take place in natural environments using people with MS as subjects, and the MS consumer voice should be included in every aspect of assistive technology design, research, and policy development.

## Support Groups and Activities

There are several centers that provide life-enhancing experience for people with MS. For example, the committee met with Brian Hutchinson of the Jimmie Heuga center in Edwards, Colorado, in the Rocky Mountains. This center offers a variety of programs to promote general health for people with MS through exercise and psychological well-being. Charlotte Robinson, founder of Adventures Within, who also spoke to the committee, leads outdoor adventure tours where people with MS can go rock climbing, rappelling, horseback riding, and whitewater rafting. While participants in these programs enthusiastically extol their benefits, the impact of this type of program has not been measured. One can, of course, imagine innumerable benefits ranging from the rejuvenation offered by any pleasant vacation, to the companionship of other people with MS, to the discovery of unrealized capacities and learning new coping strategies.

Other types of group programs include "wellness" programs in which people with MS work on developing individual coping strategies and share their own knowledge with other participants.

## Patient Care Services

One of the greatest fears of the elderly and persons with disabilities is that they will eventually be "warehoused" in an institution where a life with dignity is impossible. As a person living with progressive neurological disease, my greatest fear is not unbearable pain, nor even death. Rather, I am most afraid that my illness will progress to a point where neither I nor my family will be able to cope.[214]

The options for care of someone disabled by MS range from in-home care provided and financed by the family to publicly funded care in an institutional setting. Most people prefer care that maximizes their independence and comfort, but the cost can be prohibitive for individuals. There are only a few published reports that analyze the cost-effectiveness of different modes of care. A British study reported that in-home care is more cost-effective than hospital care, even when home care includes a paid nurse.[229] However, any analysis of cost-effectiveness must take into account the health care financing system of a particular country. Observations for people with MS who live in countries where comprehensive health care is publicly funded will not necessarily apply to those living in countries where health care is privately funded or where there is a combination of public and private funding. These are national public health policy issues germane to all chronic, disabling conditions and must be addressed at that level and studied in the context of other chronic and disabling conditions.

This is an important and relevant issue in the management of MS because it incorporates acute hospital and neurorehabilitation services together with community-based activities and, in essence, has to bring together medical and social services in a way that meets the complex and ever-changing needs of the person with MS. The key components of such a service have been listed as including the following:

- it should offer support at the diagnostic phase;
- there should be a high level of expertise;
- it should be comprehensive and flexible;
- it should be accessible and coordinated; and
- it should be linked to a neuroscience center.

Ideally, most services should be community based, with supporting expertise from the acute hospital or rehabilitation center at times of particular need (for example, at diagnosis or at the time of a severe relapse) or complexity (when multiple symptoms interact and intensive inpatient rehabilitation is required). The optimum method of service delivery has not yet been defined, and little work has been done to compare existing services. A recently completed, though not yet published, study carried out in Rome compared two forms of service delivery in a randomized controlled trial of 201 patients with MS. One group (133 patients) received what was described as "hospital" home care, in which patients remained in the community but had immediate access to the hospital-based multidisciplinary team as and when required, while the other (68 patients) received routine care. The range of outcomes, which included EDSS, FIM, SF-36, and measures of anxiety and mood, were carried out at baseline and at 12 months. No difference was seen in the level of disability between the two groups, but the more intensively treated patients had significantly less depression and improved quality-of-life. Another study, comparing the benefits of multidisciplinary MS clinics, general neurology outpatient settings, and community-based general practice in 150 patients (50 in each group) has just commenced in the United Kingdom. Patients will be evaluated at baseline and at three-month intervals for one year, with a range of outcome measures from impairment to self-efficacy.

## Rehabilitation

Rehabilitation is often defined as the process of restoring or developing physical, sensory, and mental capacities in people with disabling conditions—in other words, reversing the disabling process.[88] However, this definition is too restrictive for MS or for any other degenerative condition. The World Health Organization has adopted a broader perspective that applies better to people with MS. It defines rehabilitation as an active process by which those impaired by injury or disease achieve a full recovery or, if a full recovery is not possible, realize their optimal physical, mental, and social potential and are integrated into their most appropriate environment. This definition expresses a philosophy that also emphasizes patient education and self-management and is ideally suited to meet the needs of such a complex and progressive disorder. An essential element of this definition is that an overarching goal of the rehabilitation process is to improve a patient's sense of well-being.[61]

The essential components of successful rehabilitation include expert multidisciplinary assessment (including an assessment of patients' perspectives and circumstances), goal-oriented programs, evaluation of impact on the patient, and evaluation of goal achievement. The wide range of coexisting symptoms in MS produces a complex pattern of disability, including the possibility that treating one symptom might worsen another. Any management strategy has to take this complexity into account. It is also apparent that comprehensive management will invariably require input from different treatment modalities, including the provision of information, patient education, therapy from a range of disciplines, and drug treatment. Finally, the variable and fluctuating nature of MS means that the needs of individual patients will change over time, often quite abruptly, and that these needs will tend to increase over time.

### *Evaluating Outcomes in Neurorehabilitation*

If there is to be ongoing improvement in the process and impact of rehabilitation, there must be an evaluation process. This essential component is probably also the most challenging. It requires the use of outcome measures that are scientifically sound (reliable, valid, and responsive to changes in a patient's condition), clinically useful (short and simple), and appropriate to the sample under study and the intervention being evaluated. In neurorehabilitation, improvements are not sought at the levels of pathology and impairment but rather in disability and handicap (or activity and participation, as proposed by the World Health Organization[233]) and in the broader, more patient-orientated areas of quality-of-life, coping skills, and self-efficacy. The standard outcome measure in MS therapeutic trials is the EDSS, but it is inappropriate for evaluating rehabilitation, not only because of its scientific limitations, but also because it does not measure many of the dimensions relevant to health-related quality-of-life such as mental and social function.[81] Indeed, the EDSS score can be zero even though a person is unable to sustain a full day of work. Consequently, a number of generic measures of disability and quality-of-life have been utilized in MS rehabilitation.

Integrated care pathways, which detail the expected interventions occurring within a given episode of clinical care, are used to monitor and audit both the process and the outcome of rehabilitation. They can be used to evaluate the rehabilitation process, including goal achievement, and serve as an excellent audit tool[206] that can document when goals are not achieved on time; more usefully, however, they can indicate why this has occurred (for example, because of underestimation of cognitive dysfunction or the impact of fatigue).

Evaluating any intervention within the context of a randomized double-blind placebo-controlled trial in a condition as variable and unpredictable as MS is inherently difficult. Yet evaluating interventions aimed at neurorehabilitation— an approach that encompasses such a broad range of approaches and that must, at the same time, be tailored to meet the specific needs of an individual patient— poses still another dimension of challenges for clinical trial design. Chief among these are a lack of detailed description of programs (for example, the number of disciplines involved or techniques employed) and inadequate standardization of an intervention including its duration and location (inpatient, outpatient, or community based). Therapists are reluctant to use control groups, and limited resources often prohibit the use of independent assessors, which is particularly important when masking a patient's identity is difficult. Finally, there is no consensus as to what the most appropriate outcome measures are, and until recently, limited and often-inappropriate tools have been used inconsistently.

Despite these obstacles, a number of recent studies have demonstrated that it is indeed possible to achieve some degree of evaluation for rehabilitation interventions, although many more studies are required. In order to assess the data that these studies have produced, it is useful to consider four distinct levels, moving from the broadest concept of (1) service delivery, to (2) packages of comprehensive rehabilitation, (3) individual components of that package, and finally the most specific, (4) the intrinsic components of the rehabilitation process such as assessment and goal setting. Most studies have focused on comprehensive packages of rehabilitation (predominantly inpatient), but some have addressed individual components including physical therapy and aerobic exercise, and recent studies have compared different forms of delivery of care. There are no published studies of the intrinsic components of rehabilitation as they apply to MS.

The following are two key questions that have to be answered:

1. Is comprehensive rehabilitation effective in reducing disability and handicap and improving quality of life?

2. If so, how long do these benefits last?

The majority of studies have evaluated inpatient rehabilitation programs, which are generally more accessible than outpatient programs to controlled studies. Two studies, both retrospective and relatively small, have compared inpatient rehabilitation with other forms of intervention. One study compared outcomes of 20 pairs of patients who were treated either in an inpatient rehabilitation hospital or in an acute care hospital.[161] Outcomes for the two groups were comparable at 16 months, although it should be noted that the acute care hospital was an MS center and thus provided more sophisticated care for MS patients than an average hospital. The other study compared the outcomes of 67 patients who received either inpatient services (in the same rehabilitation hospital as in the previous study) or outpatient treatment provided by visiting nurse services.[58] Three months after discharge, the inpatient group showed less disability, as measured by the Incapacity Status Scale (ISS), although both showed gradual worsening, and by 12 months there was no difference between the two groups.

Freeman and colleagues designed a randomized controlled trial that overcame some of the methodological issues discussed earlier.[60] Sixty-six patients with progressive MS were stratified at the beginning of the study according to their EDSS, and the treatment group received a short period of inpatient rehabilitation (mean of 20 days). A group of patients who were wait-listed for rehabilitation treatment served as a control. The two groups were matched in relation to age, sex, disease pattern, and duration. Disability (Functional Independence Measure) and handicap (London Handicap Scale, LHS) were measured at the beginning of the study and six weeks later. The treated group showed a significant benefit in both disability and handicap compared to the control group. No change in the EDSS was seen in either group.

A more recent randomized single-blind trial evaluated the benefit of a three-week inpatient rehabilitation program with a home exercise program in 50 moderately impaired ambulatory patients (EDSS 3.0-6.5).[189] The control group did only the home exercise program. Patients were evaluated with the EDSS, FIM, and a health-related quality-of-life measure, the SF-36, at the beginning of the study and at 3, 9, and 15 weeks. As in previous studies, neither group showed a significant change in impairment (as measured by the EDSS). Disability, as measured by all of the FIM motor domain scales, was significantly reduced in the rehabilitation group, and this benefit was sustained for six weeks after the three-week program ended (nine-week time point). However, only two subscales, self-care and locomotion, continued to be significantly different between the groups 12 weeks after the program ended. At the end of the three-week period, the rehabilitation group had received significantly greater benefit in the mental health components of the health-related quality-of-life measure. This beneficial difference between groups was still apparent 6 weeks after the end of the rehabilitation program but had disappeared by 12 weeks (15-week time point).

One study, in which 50 patients were studied at three-month intervals for one year after their discharge from an inpatient rehabilitation unit, illustrates the dependence of the observed outcome of rehabilitation on the measure used. In that study, improvements in disability and handicap were maintained for approximately 6 months, emotional well-being for 7 months, and the physical component of health-related quality-of-life for 10 months.[60]

Although few researchers have attempted to evaluate outpatient-based rehabilitation in MS, a 1998 study reported that fatigue and the frequency of other MS symptoms in progressive MS patients were significantly reduced after outpatient treatment.[44] A group of progressive MS patients was randomly assigned either to an active treatment group of 20 patients who received five hours outpatient therapy a week for one year or to a control group of 26 patients that was waitlisted for, but had not yet received, therapy. The range of outcome measures included an MS-related symptoms checklist composite score, a measure of fatigue frequency, and items from the Rehabilitation Institute of Chicago Functional Assessment Scale. The services provided in the study included therapy aimed at physical function but also involved support for the family as well as the patients, social support, assistance locating community resources, organized recreation, and counseling to improve coping skills. Indeed, the authors suggested that the observed therapeutic benefits might be attributable to the emphasis on social and emotional support.

All 11 studies summarized in a recent review of the outcome of comprehensive inpatient rehabilitation in people with MS indicate a potential benefit in the area of disability.[207] It is difficult, however, to combine the results of all these studies. There are major methodological differences among them, and few reach an adequate scientific level. Nevertheless, they all suggest that organized patient-centered multidisciplinary rehabilitation benefits MS patients. The degree of benefit and the extent of carryover have yet to be determined.

### Components of the Rehabilitation Package

Few studies have looked at therapy intervention in the management of MS, and the only specific modality examined has been physical therapy. A randomized control trial of inpatient physical therapy (6.5 hours over two weeks) was carried out on 45 patients.[62] Outcome measures used in the study included the Rivermead Mobility Index, the Barthel ADL Index, and a visual analogue scale of "mobility-related distress." The treatment did not show significant benefit on either mobility or ability to perform activities of daily living but did significantly reduce mobility-related distress. However, the same authors have recently demonstrated a significant benefit from outpatient or home-based physical therapy.[228] A second study went a step further and attempted to compare two forms of physical therapy.[120] This pilot study involved 23 patients, 20 of whom completed the study. They received what was described as an impairment-based "facilitation approach," while the other group received a more disability-based task-oriented approach. Patients received a minimum of 15 sessions over five to seven weeks.

The outcome measures were mobility based and included the 10-meter timed walk and the Rivermead Mobility Index. Not surprisingly, no difference was seen between the two small groups, but both improved from baseline ($p < 0.05$).

The impact of aerobic exercise was evaluated in a population of 46 patients with relatively mild MS (EDSS of 6 or less): 21 of the patients were randomly assigned to a 15-week exercise program, while 25 had no exercise over that period.[154] The wide range of outcome measures included aerobic capacity, isometric strength, the Fatigue Severity Scales (FSS), the EDSS, and the Sickness Impact Profile (SIP), which measures quality of life. Significant changes from baseline were seen in the exercise group over the 15 weeks in the physiological measures and the physical component of the SIP. There was little sustained change in the psychosocial domain of the SIP and none in the EDSS or FSS.

### Conclusion

Although there is good empirical evidence to support coordinated expert service delivery in other diseases, there is little evidence currently available to support this concept in the management of MS, and further studies are required. There are few adequately designed studies to support the role of rehabilitation therapy in MS, but recent studies have confirmed that such assessments are now feasible and urgently need to be carried out.

## INFORMATION AND COMMUNICATION

### What People Say

Problems of delivering the diagnosis MS were touched upon in the earlier section "You Have MS." Patients generally say they want concrete information about their diagnosis, even when it is uncertain. Although it has been common for physicians to euphemistically tell a patient he or she has an "inflammation of the nervous system" or something equally vague, this is not what patients say they want (reviewed in 1999 by McGuinness and Peters[130]). A retrospective study in Britain found that approximately 60 percent of the people with MS in Southampton felt they were not given enough information at the time of diagnosis.[133] They also reported being angry over the delay in the prompt provision of a diagnosis. At least part of that delay was due to the inherent difficulties in diagnosing MS, including the diagnostic requirement for more than one episode, and there are no published data to determine whether MS patients' anger at the delay is reduced when the difficulties are explained to them. It should also be kept in mind that most reports on patients' reactions to diagnosis do not reflect current approaches to diagnosing MS. Most of the studies were conducted in the mid-1990s or earlier and were done before MRI scans were as common as they are today and time to diagnosis was longer. Without more information, it is not possible to know whether patients' frustration arises from a failure to communicate on the part of their physicians or from the reality that MS is difficult to diagnose.

## Information for Newly-Diagnosed Patients

Effective communication about MS to the patient and family is especially crucial around the time of diagnosis. Not only is the patient wholly unprepared for such life-altering information, but after this point, many patients will see an MS specialist only rarely. Their experience with health care providers at this point will profoundly influence their future health care choices.

Withholding the diagnosis raises suspicions of physician dishonesty. These experiences may compromise patients' trust of their doctors, heightening fears that physicians will abandon them. Studies of other diseases have shown that such trust is essential to developing strong therapeutic relationships.[205,210] Koopman and Scheitzer[100] suggested that a supportive care model would help patients with MS and their families during the stresses surrounding the diagnosis, noting: "It is important for patients and their families to experience the first years of MS coupled with caring and consistent support from their MS team. . . . A case management or primary nursing delivery system may be the best option."[100] They did not test the role of a case manager-directed care model in delivering care to people with MS. Interestingly, another study found that patients who had not gone to an MS clinic in the prior two years were more likely than others to "have come to terms with" their disease.[6]

Although almost every study reports that patients say they would have preferred full disclosure during the diagnostic phase, these are retrospective views of people with MS.[57] However, one cannot assume that MS patients would have felt the same at the moment of diagnosis as they do many years later. To avoid the bias introduced by changes in people's perspectives over the passage of many years after their disease has progressed, studies on the outcome or effectiveness of different communications should be done prospectively. The committee found only one prospective study that measured the effect of diagnosis on patients suspected of MS.[146] They were divided into three groups, those with MS, without MS, and those whose diagnoses remained uncertain. Diagnostic testing benefited all three groups. It reduced patients' distress over their physical symptoms and their general anxiety, even in those with MS. However, while the study measured the impact of diagnostic testing, it did not provide specific information about how the diagnosis can be imparted most beneficially to patients and their families.

In 1993, the British Society of Rehabilitation Medicine with the support of the MS Society of Great Britain and Northern Ireland published guidelines for imparting the diagnosis (Box 4.8).[57] These guidelines represent the consensus of a committee of people with MS, their families, health care professionals, and service providers. Also, while an association with specific health or psychologi-

**BOX 4.8**
**Guidelines for Delivering the Diagnosis of Multiple Sclerosis**

- People with multiple sclerosis expect a clear explanation of their symptoms, which in the vast majority of cases involves communicating the specific diagnosis to the patient.
- Many people prefer a relative or friend to be with them.
- The doctor giving the diagnosis must have adequate knowledge of the disease and adequate time.
- It is thought to be helpful for the doctor to give a "working prognosis" for the next 12 months.
- A follow-up appointment to see the doctor who has discussed the diagnosis should be offered.
- Information should be given about the local MS society supplemented by appropriate written information about the disease.

Source: Ford and Johnson[57]

cal benefits has not been demonstrated, the guidelines are at least reasonable. It would be helpful to know what approach to communicating a diagnosis of MS is most conducive to successful adaptation to the illness and to establishing a productive relationship with one's physician. The MS Society developed a highly informative pamphlet, book, and Web page on information for the newly diagnosed. This information has been widely distributed and is generally believed to be very helpful, but its effectiveness has not been evaluated.

Given that the cause of MS remains unknown and the course of the illness is maddeningly unpredictable, one should consider the possibility that no amount of available information will satisfy. Patients will be frustrated by the lack of information, almost by definition. At the least, the background of unpredictability of the disease course should be considered as a potential factor in determining optimal forms of communication about health-related information.

Patients do not generally want to learn about demyelination when they are diagnosed.[10,140] They want to learn how to live. From the patient's point of view, while information about disease mechanisms might satisfy intellectual curiosity, it provides only marginally useful information for living with MS. At the time of diagnosis, it seems only reasonable to deal first with such practical concerns. Patients need to know the extent to which they can continue to fulfill their responsibilities at work and home; how and whether they should alter their family and career plans; reassess their needs, obligations, and desires; choose therapies; and—especially in the United States where health care coverage is fraught with uncertainty—how they are going to meet their future health care needs. Furthermore, with every change in their condition, they will have to solve each of these puzzles anew. Frequently, neither patients nor their doctors know where to go or whom to ask for advice. Only by understanding the specific hurdles that people face can initiatives be designed for improving the lives of people living today with MS.

## Parameters of Effective Communication Strategies

The desire of people with MS for more information is clearly a recurring theme, but there are many questions to answer before this general need is translated into effective communication strategies. What sort of information do people need most, and how is the available information most effectively shared? The first step in addressing these questions is to identify the communication goals— goals that might be defined somewhat differently by patients than by their physicians.

Many of the published reports implicitly assume the goal of short-term patient satisfaction in their consultation with their health care providers, but there are other goals. For example, a more ambitious goal of communicating information about MS is to foster long-term improvements in their health, ability to function, and psychological well-being for people with MS—in short, to facilitate patient adaptations to living with MS. Although this goal is not inconsistent with immediate patient satisfaction, it is also not necessarily a consequence of patient satisfaction with the physicians. This highlights the need to consider the temporal aspects of communication. Long-term goals are often best served by different approaches to communication than those that work best for short-term goals.

Important considerations in effective health communication include who defines the problem (or information need) and who defines the solution (what is to be communicated and how). Identification of both problem and solutions requires broad input—from patients and their families, as well as health care providers (physicians, nurses, physical therapists, and psychologists). While the perspectives of patients, physicians and other providers are likely to overlap in many respects, each will have a greater understanding of different elements of disease management. Ultimately, the most important outcome is improvement in the patient's quality of life.

An important principle that has emerged from recent advances in communication theory and practice is that communication is most effective when it is targeted to specific populations.[230] Different strategies work better for groups of different educational, ethnic, and economic backgrounds. This is even more important for people with MS, where the sheer variety and magnitude of the manifestations of the illness add to the already considerable differences among healthy populations. Another key principle of health communication is that no single communication or form of communication will be adequate. A pamphlet mailed to the patient or a scheduled visit with a physician will always be insufficient if it is the only information provided to someone with MS. Individual differences might also be important in determining optimal communication strategies. Some might absorb information best in group settings, whereas others might absorb information better in a private consultation or via written, videotaped, or computer material.

Other principles of effective communication stem from the specific features of MS, particularly the unpredictability of the disease course and changing levels of impairment. The information needs of people with MS change throughout their illness. As these needs change, optimal communication strategies will also likely change. For example, approaches to communication will be very different during periods of stability when information can be considered carefully, free of pressure to take immediate action, compared to periods of crisis when psychological stress is high and quick action is required. Examples of such periods include exacerbations when a person's ability to function declines, when a caregiver is suddenly unable to meet the person's needs and new arrangements have to be made on short notice, or during a transition state, such as when a person suddenly needs to use a wheelchair or scooter for the first time. (As discussed in the section on assistive technology, information on wheelchair use is sorely needed, but rarely easy to obtain.) Each of these difficulties brings with it new needs for information, and there has been almost no research to identify optimal modes of fulfilling the diverse information needs of people with MS. Finally, for people with MS an important consideration is that their access to information will vary, depending on their mobility (whether they can easily get to a group meeting or clinic), as well as on economic factors (whether they can afford a computer, internet access, scooter, or other adaptive devices).

Although there is a large body of research on optimal communication strategies, empirical research on the information needs of people with MS and effective communication strategies to meet these needs are starkly lacking. Because this is such an overarching need of people with MS, it should be an area of emphasis in MS research. The Institute of Medicine committee did not include the expertise to identify specific research strategies but suggests that the MS Society consider developing a request for proposals (RFP) to assess and address communication needs of MS patients. Ideally, the RFP would target researchers outside the field of MS, but would request that the project be a collaborative effort between experts in health communications and those whose research expertise includes knowledge of MS symptoms and measurement of the quality of life of people with MS. Much of the literature on health communication focuses on healthy populations and is unlikely to be particularly relevant to people with MS. Although the relapsing-remitting form of MS presents the distinctive challenges posed by unpredictable impairment, many of the problems faced by people with MS are also faced by others with other serious and chronic diseases. For example, the research that has been done on improving approaches to imparting the diagnoses of cancer and AIDS would likely add some insight to the communication challenges posed by MS. The depth of knowledge and rate of progress will improve if the research on communication is not restricted to MS but includes other relevant conditions.

At a minimum, the MS Society should work in an ongoing way with patients to evaluate their information needs and how the information should be presented, including *who* delivers it (physician, nurse, other), *when* (at diagnosis, follow-up, once, several times), and *how* (private consultation, mailings, pamphlets in doctors office, Internet chat groups, participatory group meetings).

## The Information Highway

The power of computers to deliver health information continues to accelerate. There is, of course, a quality problem. A recent National Research Council report concluded that it is not adequate for health care delivery per se, but the delivery of information is a distinctive aspect of health care, and for this, there is a wealth of excellent and clearly presented information that should be understandable to any college graduate, much of it supplied by the MS Society (United States), as well as the pharmaceutical companies that market the currently approved disease-modifying therapies (Berlex, Biogen, Serono, and Teva Marion Partners) and a number of research organizations. This information does not, however, cover all aspects of MS equally well. While there is an abundance of high-quality information about the biological aspects of the disease, as well as descriptions of the symptoms of MS, there is comparatively little information about specific adaptations to assist people with MS in adapting to their illness.

Of course, it is important to emphasize that this invaluable resource is not equally available to all. Only about 40 percent of the population of the United States and Canada were regular Internet users as of March 2000, although this figure is steadily increasing.[216] In Europe, the figure varies from country to country, but even in Sweden and Norway where Internet access is greatest, it is still only about 50 percent. Low-income, rural populations, and people with no college education have disproportionately less access to information posted on the Internet, and different approaches to meeting their information needs should be considered. A 1998 survey reported that 42 percent of people with MS surveyed in the United States have Internet access, suggesting that their access is somewhat greater than that of the general population.[165]

# HEALTH CARE

## Access to Health Care

Costs and payment policies present major barriers to obtaining mobility-related services. Health insurers typically restrict the numbers of physical therapy sessions, paying exclusively to restore patients to baseline function. Insurers, with some legitimacy, argue that financing therapy to maintain function or prevent its decline could generate insatiable demand. Despite its older and disabled population, Medicare, for example, limits coverage of interventions targeting functional status, and payment for rehabilitation services depends on continued functional improvements.[23] Many of these services have not yet garnered a rigorous "evidence base," which has seemingly become essential for insurance coverage.

Insurers often deny coverage of mobility aids. A 1990 national survey, not specific to people with MS, found that about 2.5 million Americans needed assistive technologies, including mobility aids, but 61.1 percent could not afford them.[109] Almost half of those using assistive devices paid for them entirely out-of-pocket. Improving home accessibility (for example, grab bars, ramps, widened doorways) is also expensive; 78 percent of these improvements came out-of-pocket.[109] Insurers routinely require doctors to certify the "medical necessity" of equipment. Despite this assurance, initial requests can be denied,[85] requiring lengthy and frustrating appeals. The experience for people with MS is unknown.

Even if coverage is approved, insurance payments may be incomplete. Medicare's Supplemental Medical Insurance (Part B) covers such mobility aids, but beneficiaries must pay 20 percent coinsurance.[1] Insurers sometimes deny payment for "lower-tech" equipment, arguing that the patient's rate of functional decline means more sophisticated, costly equipment will soon be needed,[225] for example, they might pay for a powered wheelchair but not for a scooter. Other payment policies affect the use of mobility aids. Medicare, for example, limits home health services to people confined to their homes except for medical appointments.[76] Medicare beneficiaries who obtain wheelchairs to leave their homes for other purposes will lose home health services. Whether financial barriers are impeding people with MS from obtaining assistive technologies is unknown. Quality-of-life could be diminished by inadequate access to these devices.

Attitudes and environment present barriers, even for health care services access. Justice Department investigations discovered persistent problems even with physical access to health care sites.[158] Iezzoni and colleagues[86] found low rates of Pap smear and mammography use among women with major mobility impairments; the study controlled for demographic characteristics and differences in access to health care. This fits with qualitative and anecdotal reports about barriers to primary and preventive care for people with disabilities.[16,19,39,63,156,197,198]

Toombs wrote that her primary care doctor questioned her need for bone density screening for osteoporosis, rationalizing that wheelchair users never fall.[213] One internist described her private practice in an upper middle class community, observing that although wheelchair users "probably could get into the building they would not have been able to get into the office and, certainly, would not have been able to get into the examining room."[4] When she moved to a Medicaid health maintenance organization (HMO), she encountered more patients with disabilities. One of her patients, a 45-year-old woman with MS, had never had a Pap smear; nobody had ever offered her one. When the internist and her assistants tried to move the patient onto the high, unadjustable examining table, they failed. The patient's daughter, familiar with the maneuver, transferred her mother. The internist next ordered a mammogram, but the facility could not serve her because she could not stand up.[4] Given the long lives of most people diagnosed with MS, more research on access to preventive and screening services, including physical access to care sites (for example, adjustable examining tables, mammography machines) is needed.

A 1990 survey of 604 families found that almost everyone with MS had some form of health insurance paying an average of 75 percent of the medical bills, but 28 percent reported that the coverage was inadequate for their health care costs.[24] Failure of insurance to pay for expensive drugs was particularly problematic, as were insurance exclusions for "preexisting" conditions. Some respondents reported staying in unhappy marriages to retain their health insurance.

**Participatory Style with Physicians.** The literature outside MS suggests that patients who participate more actively in decision making about their care may do better.[93-95,166] In one study, patients who assumed control of conversations (for example, asking more questions, attempting to direct the flow of the discussion and their doctors' behavior) during a baseline office visit reported fewer days lost from work, fewer health problems, lower functional limitations due to health, and improved health status at a follow-up visit. Patients seeking more conversational control had, at follow-up, lower blood glucose and blood pressure readings. Diabetes and hypertension management are, however, fairly clear-cut. Exactly how patients' interaction styles might affect treatment choices and outcomes in MS needs more study.

**Physicians Dealing with Emotional Distress and Psychosocial Issues.** Physicians can be trained to communicate more effectively with patients and, in particular, to deal with areas of emotional distress.[166] Physicians who are interested in the psychosocial aspects of disease are much more likely than other physicians to raise these issues.[116] Murray[139] observed that MS physicians often feel uncomfortable addressing such issues as marital and personal problems; unfortunately, they also do not refer MS patients to other clinicians for these issues. Furthermore, communication must also address patients' interests outside the focus on treating the disease. Little attention has been paid to health promotion activities for persons with MS to enhance their overall well-being and quality of life, although a study of 629 women with MS found that health promotion activities significantly improved quality of life along the spectrum of disability.[199]

Paradoxically, many health care professionals are ill-equipped to instill hope because they have a depressing view of the disease, perhaps because they often work in hospitals where only the most ill and therapeutically resistant and complicated patients are met. Most MS units now manage a large number of patients in an ambulatory setting, where most of the patients are getting along and the hospital-based medical student, physician, nurse, physical therapist, or social worker sees only the most difficult and most advanced problems in the wards. The availability of the new disease-modifying drugs has certainly increased the optimism of many physicians, but these drugs are still new. With time and experience, patients' and physicians' optimism could become more reserved or even greater. It is too early to know. Further, the new disease-modifying drugs have not been demonstrated to be helpful to the most ill patients.

The role of hope in patients with MS and the role of the physician in providing and supporting reasonable and appropriate hope have often been ignored. Hope is something physicians do not often discuss. Patients often called "hopeless" can be helped in many ways to cope with the ravages of the disease and to see the opportunity despite the limitations they face. We cannot yet cure, but we can help, and we can understand, and we can care.[139]

## Exercise

Physical activity has long been discouraged for people with MS, in part because they often experience fatigue and thermosensitivity, which causes their neurological symptoms to worsen during exposure to heat.[155] Exercise can be particularly difficult for patients with limited mobility and poor balance. Yet many people with MS are probably less active than they could be if they were given proper guidance and access to appropriate facilities. One study compared the activity levels of a group of ambulatory MS patients with those of sedentary control subjects who did not have MS. [143] (The median EDSS score of the MS patients was 3.0 [no assistance needed to walk], with a range of 1.5 [no disability] to 6.0 [assistance needed to walk]). When questionnaires asked them to recall their physical activity levels, the two groups reported similar activity levels. However, when their physical activity was measured over seven days using a motion detection device attached to their waists, the ambulatory MS patients were found to be significantly less active than the sedentary controls.

The benefits of exercise for people with MS are many and, conversely, lack of activity can contribute to fatigue and weakness and is a risk factor for many chronic diseases. Numerous studies have shown that physical activity in cancer patients enhances well-being in terms of physical and functional status, as well as psychological and emotional status (reviewed in 1999 by Courneya and Friedenreich[34]). Aerobic exercise training improves fitness, increases feelings of well-being, and reduces depression and anxiety in people with MS.[155] Some aspects of impaired muscle function observed in MS are similar to those seen in healthy people after prolonged periods of inactivity, and deconditioning due to reduced physical activity likely contributes to the loss of muscle function in MS.[97,143]

Exercise training might thus reduce the loss of muscle function, as well as decreasing fatigue.[97,143]

Although exercise programs can benefit MS patients, they should be undertaken with care and attention from exercise physiologists, physical and occupational therapists, and physicians. Different types of exercises are best for people with different types of MS and different types of impairment (reviewed in 1999 by Petajan et al.[155]). For example, patients with motor deficits need an exercise program that takes their impairment into account. Pools are helpful because they are safe and allow for a wider variety of exercises. They also increase body cooling, thereby reducing the problem of thermosensitivity. In general, because increased body temperature can block conduction in damaged nerves, exercise programs should be designed to avoid overheating. An assessment of exercise history, including activities of daily living, and a fitness evaluation should be obtained prior to the initiation of an exercise program. Exercises that increase flexibility, strength, coordination, and balance are particularly helpful. Lack of motivation to exercise is likely, especially when a person does not feel well, and a supportive, proactive, and pleasant exercise environment is especially important. Although exercise training does not appear to influence relapse rates, exercise programs should sometimes be modified or temporarily discontinued during relapses.[154]

Weakness, fatigue, spasticity, and ataxia make exercise difficult for people with MS, and even brief exercise bouts can cause symptoms to appear or increase, but improvement in fitness not only can help offset these difficulties, it can reduce fatigue and depression and improve quality-of-life.[155]

## Diet

All sorts of diets have been proposed to be of benefit in MS: low-saturated-fat with high-polyunsaturated-fat diets, megavitamins, liquid diets, and sucrose-free and gluten-free diets have all been advocated (see Appendix G).[185] However, none of them have been rigorously tested under clinical conditions, and none have been supported by an underlying immunological basis.[57,209]

The rate of MS is generally higher in countries where diets are commonly high in animal fat, animal protein, and meat from nonmarine mammals and lower in countries where people eat more vegetables and fish (reviewed in 1997 by Lauer[113]).[50,112] Yet despite the correlations, there are many confounding variables, and none of these dietary factors have been determined to be either risk factors or prognosticators for the disease.

Vitamin D has also been hypothesized to be related to MS.[75] Since needs for vitamin D are met through exposure to sunlight in addition to dietary intake, it has been suggested that vitamin D levels might be a factor in the geographic distribution of MS.[49] The evidence is circumstantial, and further investigation is needed. At least in EAE (experimental allergic encephalomyelitis) mice, exogenous vitamin D can prevent disease, supporting the idea that there might be some effect in humans, but this remains to be demonstrated.[22]

There are some data suggesting that large amounts of polyunsaturated omega-3 fatty acids, which are prevalent in fish, reduce the severity of relapses and the progress of disability in early cases (but not long-term disability) and some indicating that reduced intake of animal fat and increased intake of vegetable fat and seafood are beneficial. However, most of these data come from uncontrolled, methodologically flawed studies.

There is, however, an emerging body of evidence to indicate that dietary antigens might trigger autoimmune responses in diseases other than MS.[25,149,179,186] While this suggests a biological basis to predict an effect of dietary antigens in MS, as yet there are no conclusive data. If dietary influences are modest—which is highly likely considering the lack of clear-cut results to date—or if different foods interact in their effects on MS, obtaining such data would require an extensive clinical trial. In addition, since many patients are taking disease-modifying drugs, it would be statistically more difficult to detect the increased benefit of a modest improvement. Each treatment independently introduces some random variation, meaning that a clinical trial including both dietary changes and medication would have to be larger than a clinical trial with only one of these variables. While a healthy balanced diet is recommended for people with MS,[171] the evidence supporting a specific benefit from such for MS remains inconclusive.[113] Even if there were no specific benefit from dietary changes, if they resulted in generally improved health or well-being of people with MS, this would be reason alone to recommend them.

## Use of Alternative Medicine

Alternative medicine refers to a mix of practices as disparate as herbal medicine, therapeutic touch, imagery, and homeopathy. What unites such treatments is that they are not widely taught in medical schools and are not generally available through physicians or hospitals. The term "complementary medicine" is preferred by some people, because it indicates that alternative therapies can be integrated with conventional therapies. For simplicity, the single term "alternative medicine" is used here to include all aspects of non-traditional medicine. Despite the preferred concept of complementary medicine, the use of alternative therapies is not fully integrated into medical treatment. Most patients who use alternative therapies do not inform their doctors. In 1997, only 38 percent of U.S. users of these therapies informed their physicians.[46]

The distinction between alternative and conventional medicine is fluid. Over time, an unconventional practice, such as self-hypnosis or yoga, might become conventional and many formerly conventional treatments such as blood-letting have fallen out of favor. One constant of alternative therapies, however, is that they are not subject to the same regulatory protections as conventional drugs.

They are not tested in clinical trials; manufacturer's claims of safety and efficacy are not reviewed by independent parties; and there is no product standardization. For example, in an analysis of ginseng products, even though different brands were labeled as containing equal amounts of the active ingredient, the actual amounts varied as much as tenfold; some brands contained no ginseng at all.[5]

## Prevalence of Use

Despite its medically uncertain status, alternative medicine is an integral part of Western health care systems, if only because it is so widely used. A study of the U.S. population estimated that the number of visits to alternative therapy practitioners was 243 million *more* than the number of visits to all primary care physicians.[46,52] Estimates vary among countries, but independent surveys of Australia and of North American and European countries generally report that more than 40 percent of the general population in the countries surveyed use alternative medicine.[46,121,174] Many patients use more than one therapy at a time.[136,218] Prevalence of use varies among the population. Twenty-five to 49 year-olds are more likely to use alternative medicine than people who are younger or older, and African-Americans are less likely than other ethnic groups to use alternative medicine.[47] Different surveys report different age groups as those who use alternative therapies most extensively.[46,134] This inconsistency might reflect international differences, population differences in health status, or differences in the way alternative therapies were described in survey questions.

Use of alternative therapies is not only widespread among healthy people; once people are diagnosed with a serious illness, their use is likely to increase.[136,163,174,218] For example, in a study of 480 women with newly diagnosed breast cancer, 28 percent of them began to use alternative therapies.[20] On the bright side, and unlike the general population, most of these women informed their doctors.

People with chronic illness consult alternative care providers about three times more often than people without chronic illness,[7,134,163] and those with disabilities are 50 percent more likely than the general population to use alternative therapies.[102] Compared to people without disabilities, those with disabilities seek alternative therapies significantly more often for treatment of pain, depression, and anxiety.[7,102]

Not surprisingly, the use of alternative therapies is more widespread among MS patients than among the general population. Although estimates vary, probably three-quarters use an alternative therapy, often more than one.[52,141,177,191,232] (Note that some studies report visits to alternative therapy providers, whereas others report the use of alternative therapies. In general, the number of people who visit alternative therapy providers is about half that of those who use alternative therapies, many of whom do so without consulting an alternative therapy provider.)

Because MS is a long-term disease for which conventional medicine has no cure or completely effective treatment, one might reasonably ask, "Why not try alternative therapies?" Even though most herbal remedies have not been proven effective, most are probably not dangerous (reviewed in Angell and Kassirer, 1998),[5] but there are other concerns. Because MS symptoms typically wax and wane, false positives are particularly likely. For instance, when a symptom is relieved after some therapeutic intervention, many patients are convinced that the intervention was responsible, even when they know that MS symptoms can wane with no treatment at all. In addition to the illusion of benefit when symptoms spontaneously subside, the placebo response can give patients the illusion that their sense of improvement is due to the specific treatment they tried, when in fact, the placebo effect could have arisen from any treatment. If placebo effects and illusions of benefit have no impact on the disease, they are harmless, but if they encourage the patient to forgo effective treatments, then these effects can be medically harmful. In addition to illusory effects, there are also medical concerns about using unregulated products whose contents are unverified. Finally, MS patients should be particularly cautious about substances that are relatively benign in people without immune disorders but might have negative impacts on the immune responses of MS patients.

The widespread use of alternative therapies has implications for both treatment and research in MS. There are endless varieties of alternative therapies, and it is important to know which of these are used most often and most heavily by MS patients. The use of alternative therapies should be taken into account in all aspects of treatment and assessment—from prescription of symptomatic treatments, to research on health status and quality of life, to identifying the most pressing health information needs of people with MS. Proven or not, alternative therapies are a pervasive dimension of health care among people with MS.

### Specific Alternative Therapies

Of all forms of alternative treatment, herbal medicine is the most common (reference 15 in Angell and Kassirer[5]). Appendix G offers a critique of more than 50 alternative therapies that have been claimed to be beneficial for treating MS. Approaches not included there are described below.

**Marijuana.** Many MS patients, as well as patients with spinal cord injury, smoke marijuana to relieve spasticity. Controlled studies of the effects of marijuana or THC (tetrahydrocannabinol), the primary active ingredient in marijuana, have generally been inconclusive in MS patients, but none of those studies have included more than 13 MS patients (reviewed in 1999 by the IOM).[89] These studies neither disprove nor support claims of the therapeutic value of marijuana's active ingredients. Many MS patients are convinced that marijuana relieves their spasticity and pain. One survey reported that 97 percent of MS patients reported using marijuana to relieve one or more of their MS symptoms, but it is important to note that the target population of this survey was marijuana users.[32] The degree to which these results apply to the general population of people with MS is impossible to know. Further, marijuana and THC can reduce both anxiety and pain, and this might reduce the discomfort associated with spasticity or tremor, although with no direct effect on spasticity. Experiments in EAE mice indicate that THC and related compounds can reduce spasticity and tremor.[9] As of this writing, clinical trials testing the effects of marijuana extracts on MS patients are being conducted in Britain. The results of these trials should help clarify the effects of marijuana and its constituent compounds on MS symptoms.

**Traditional Chinese Medicine.** A variety of approaches—primarily herbal treatments, but also acupuncture—are used in traditional Chinese medicine to treat symptoms of MS, but their effectiveness has not been tested in rigorous clinical trials, and their descriptions are limited to Chinese-language publications.[234] There are reports that Chinese herbal treatments can reduce the neuropathology associated with EAE in guinea pigs, but these reports have to be validated through experiments published in journals that are more widely accessible for critical review.

**Hypnosis.** Hypnosis has been proposed as an approach to improve muscular control in MS patients, but at present, the committee is aware of only scattered case reports of improvement after hypnosis.[201] As with every individual case of improvement after some experimental treatment, there is a strong possibility that improvement might be a placebo effect or might have occurred in the absence of any treatment.

## REFERENCES

1. Medicare and Medicaid Statistical Supplement, 1999. *Health Care Finan Rev.*;(No volume listed on publication):3-4.
2. Aikens JE, Fischer JS, Namey M, Rudick RA. 1997. A replicated prospective investigation of life stress, coping, and depressive symptoms in multiple sclerosis. *J Behav Med.*;20:433-45.
3. Anderson C, Laubscher S, Burns R. 1996. Validation of the Short Form 36 (SF-36) health survey questionnaire among stroke patients. *Stroke.*;27:1812-6.
4. Andriacchi R. 1997. Primary care for persons with disabilities. The internal medicine perspective. *Am J Phys Med Rehabil.*;76:S17-20.
5. Angell M, Kassirer JP. 1998. Alternative medicine—the risks of untested and unregulated remedies. *N Engl J Med.*;339:839-841.
6. Aronson KJ. 1997. Quality of life among persons with multiple sclerosis and their caregivers. *Neurology.*;48:74-80.
7. Astin JA. 1998. Why patients use alternative medicine: results of a national study. *JAMA.*;279:1548-1553.
8. Avillion AE. 1986. Barrier perception and its influence on self-esteem. *Rehabil Nurs.*;11:11-4.

9.  Baker D, Pryce G, Croxford JL, et al. 2000. Cannabinoids control spasticity and tremor in a multiple sclerosis model. *Nature.*;404:84-7.

10. Baker LM. 1998. Sense making in multiple sclerosis: the information needs of people during an acute exacerbation. *Qual Health Res.*;8:106-20.

11. Balbin EG, Ironson GH, Solomon GF. 1999. Stress and coping: the psychoneuroimmunology of HIV/AIDS. *Baillieres Best Pract Res Clin Endocrinol Metab.*;13:615-33.

12. Beatty WW, Hames KA, Blanco CR, Williamson SJ, Willbanks SL, Olson KA. 1998. Correlates of coping style in patients with multiple sclerosis. *Mult Scler.*;4:440-443.

13. Bergner M. 1989. Quality of life, health status, and clinical research. *Med Care.*;27:S148-56.

14. Bergner M, Bobbitt RA, Pollard WE, Martin DP, Gilson BS. 1976. The sickness impact profile: validation of a health status measure. *Med Care.*;14:57-67.

15. Bindman AB, Keane D, Lurie N. 1990. Measuring health changes among severely ill patients. The floor phenomenon. *Med Care.*;28:1142-52.

16. Bockenek WL, Mann N, Lanig IS, DeJong G, Beatty LA. Primary care for persons with disabilities. DeLisa JA, Gans GM, eds. *Rehabilitation Medicine: Principles and Practice.* Philadelphia: Lippincott-Raven Publishers; 1998:905-928.

17. Branch LG, Meyers AR. 1987. Assessing physical function in the elderly. *Clin Geriatr Med.*;3:29-51.

18. Brunet DG, Hopman WM, Singer MA, Edgar CM, MacKenzie TA. 1996. Measurement of health-related quality of life in multiple sclerosis patients. *Can J Neurol Sci.*;23:99-103.

19. Burns TJ, Batavia AI, Smith QW, DeJong G. 1990. Primary health care needs of persons with physical disabilities: what are the research and service priorities? *Arch Phys Med Rehabil.*;71:138-43.

20. Burstein HJ, Gelber S, Guadagnoli E, Weeks JC. 1999. Use of alternative medicine by women with early-stage breast cancer. *N Engl J Med.*;340:1733-9.

21. Calkins DR, Rubenstein LV, Cleary PD, et al. 1991. Failure of physicians to recognize functional disability in ambulatory patients. *Ann Intern Med.*;114:451-4.

22. Cantorna MT, Hayes CE, DeLuca HF. 1996. 1,25-Dihydroxyvitamin D3 reversibly blocks the progression of relapsing encephalomyelitis, a model of multiple sclerosis. *Proc Natl Acad Sci U S A.*;93:7861-4.

23. Cassel CK, Besdine RW, Siegel LC. 1999. Restructuring Medicare for the next century: what will beneficiaries really need? *Health Aff (Millwood).*;18:118-31.

24. Catanzaro M, Weinert C. 1992. Economic status of families living with multiple sclerosis. *Int J Rehabil Res.*;15:209-18.

25. Cavallo MG, Fava D, Monetini L, Barone F, Pozzilli P. 1996. Cell-mediated immune response to Beta casein in recent-onset insulin-dependent diabetes: implications for disease pathogeneris. *The Lancet.*;348:926-928.

26. Cella DF, Dineen K, Arnason B, et al. 1996. Validation of the functional assessment of multiple sclerosis quality of life instrument. *Neurology.*;47:129-39.

27. Charlton JI. *Nothing About Us Without Us : Disability Oppression and Empowerment.* Berkeley, CA: University of California Press; 1998.

28. Clayton DK, Rogers S, Stuifbergen A. 1999. Answers to unasked questions: writing in the margins. *Res Nurs Health.*;22:512-22.

29. Cohen JA, Cutter GR, Fischer JS, et al. In Press. *Arch Neurol.*

30. Cohen JA, Fischer JS, Bolibrush DM, et al. 2000. Intrarater and interrater reliability of the MS functional composite outcome measure. *Neurology.*;54:802-6.

31. Confavreux C, Compston DA, Hommes OR, McDonald WI, Thompson AJ. 1992. EDMUS, a European database for multiple sclerosis. *J Neurol Neurosurg Psychiatry.*;55:671-6.

32. Consroe P, Musty R, Rein J, Tillery W, Pertwee R. 1997. The perceived effects of smoked cannabis on patients with multiple sclerosis. *Eur Neurol.*;38:44-8.

33. Copperman L, Hartley C, Scharf P, Hicks RW. 1994. Fatigue and Mobility. *J Neuro Rehab.*;8:131-136.
34. Courneya KS, Friedenreich CM. 1999. Physical exercise and quality of life following cancer diagnosis: a literature review. *Ann Behav Med.*;21:171-9.
35. Crist P. 1993. Contingent interaction during work and play tasks for mothers with multiple sclerosis and their daughters. *Am J Occup Ther.*;47:121-31.
36. Cutter GR, Baier ML, Rudick RA, et al. 1999. Development of a multiple sclerosis functional composite as a clinical trial outcome measure. *Brain.*;122:871-82.
37. Dakof GA, Taylor SE. 1990. Victims' perceptions of social support: what is helpful from whom? *J Pers Soc Psychol.*;58:80-9.
38. Deatrick JA, Brennan D, Cameron ME. 1998. Mothers with multiple sclerosis and their children: effects of fatigue and exacerbations on maternal support. *Nurs Res.*;47(4):205-210.
39. DeJong G. 1997. Primary care for persons with disabilities. An overview of the problem. *Am J Phys Med Rehabil.*;76:S2-8.
40. DesRosier MB, Catanzaro M, Piller J. 1992. Living with chronic illness: social support and the well spouse perspective. *Rehabil Nurs.*;17:87-91.
41. Devers KJ, Sofaer S, Rundall TG, eds. 1999. Qualitative methods in health services research. SA special supplement to HSR. *Health Services Research.*;34:1083-1263.
42. Devins GM, Seland TP, Klein G, Edworthy SM, Saary MJ. 1993. Stability and determinants of psychosocial well-being in multiple sclerosis. *Rehabilitation Psychology.*;38.
43. Devins GM, Styra R, O'Connor P, et al. 1996. Psychosocial impact of illness intrusiveness moderated by age in multiple sclerosis. *Psychology, Health & Medicine.*;1:179-191.
44. Di Fabio RP, Soderberg J, Choi T, Hansen CR, Schapiro RT. 1998. Extended outpatient rehabilitation: its influence on symptom frequency, fatigue, and functional status for persons with progressive multiple sclerosis. *Arch Phys Med Rehabil.*;79(2):141-146.
45. Dolan P. 1996. The effect of experience of illness on health state valuations. *J Clin Epidemiol.*;49:551-64.
46. Eisenberg DM, Davis RB, Ettner SL, et al. 1998. Trends in alternative medicine use in the United States, 1990-1997: results of a follow-up national survey. *JAMA.*;280:1569-75.
47. Eisenberg DM, Kessler RC, Foster C, Norlock F.E., Calkins DR, Delbanco TL. 1993. Unconventional medicine in the United States: Prevalence, costs, and patterns of use. *New Engl J Med.*;328:246-252.
48. Eklund V-A, MacDonald ML. 1991. Description of persons with multiple sclerosis, with an emphasis on what is needed from psychologists. *Professional Psychology: Research and Practice*;22:277-284.
49. Embry AF, Snowdon LR, Vieth R. 2000. Vitamin D and seasonal fluctuations of gadolinium-enhancing magnetic resonance imaging lesions in multiple sclerosis. *Ann Neurol.*;48:271-2.
50. Esparza ML, Sasaki S, Kesteloot H. 1995. Nutrition, latitude, and multiple sclerosis mortality: an ecologic study. *Am J Epidemiol.*;142:733-7.
51. Evers KJ, Karnilowicz W. 1996. Patient attitude as a function of disease state in multiple sclerosis. *Soc Sci Med.*;42(8):1245-1251.
52. Fawcett J, Sidney JS, Riley-Lawless K, Hanson MJ. 1996. An exploratory study of the relationship between alternative therapies, functional status, and symptom severity among people with multiple sclerosis. *J Holist Nurs.*;14:115-129.
53. Feinstein AR. 1992. Benefits and obstacles for development of health status assessment measures in clinical settings. *Med Care.*;30:MS50-6.
54. Finlayson M, Impey MW, Nicolle C, Edwards J. 1998. Self-care, productivity and leisure limitations of people with multiple sclerosis in Manitoba. *Canadian Journal of Occupational Therapy.*;65:299-308.
55. Fischer JS, LaRocca NG, Miller DM, Ritvo PG, Andrews H, Paty D. 1999. Recent developments in the assessment of quality of life in multiple sclerosis (MS). *Multiple Sclerosis.*;5:251-9.

56. Fischer JS, Rudick RA, Cutter GR, Reingold SC. 1999. The Multiple Sclerosis Functional Composite Measure (MSFC): an integrated approach to MS clinical outcome assessment. National MS Society Clinical Outcomes Assessment Task Force. *Mult Scler.*;5:244-50.
57. Ford HL, Johnson MH. 1995. Telling your patient he/she has multiple sclerosis. *Postgrad Med J.*;71:449-52.
58. Francabandera FL, Holland NJ, Wiesel-Levison P, Scheinberg LC. 1988. Multiple sclerosis rehabilitation: inpatient vs. outpatient. *Rehabil Nurs.*;13:251-3.
59. Freeman JA, Hobart JC, Langdon DW, Thompson AJ. 2000. Clinical appropriateness: a key factor in outcome measure selection: the 36 item short form health survey in multiple sclerosis. *J Neurol Neurosurg Psychiatry.*;68:150-156.
60. Freeman JA, Langdon DW, Hobart JC, Thompson AJ. 1999. Inpatient rehabilitation in multiple sclerosis: do the benefits carry over into the community? *Neurology.*;52:50-6.
61. Fuhrer MJ. 1994. Subjective well-being: implications for medical rehabilitation outcomes and models of disablement. *Am J Phys Med Rehabil.*;73:358-64.
62. Fuller KJ, Dawson K, Wiles CM. 1996. Physiotherapy in chronic multiple sclerosis: a controlled trial. *Clin Rehabil.*;10:195-204.
63. Gans BM, Mann NR, Becker BE. 1993. Delivery of primary care to the physically challenged. *Arch Phys Med Rehabil.*;74:S15-9.
64. Gill TM, Feinstein AR. 1994. A critical appraisal of the quality of quality-of-life measurements. *JAMA.*;272:619-26.
65. Goffman E. *Stigma: Notes on the Management of Spoiled Identity.* New York: Simon & Schuster; 1963.
66. Goodin DS, Ebers GC, Johnson KP, Rodriguez M, Sibley WA, Wolinsky JS. 1999. The relationship of MS to physical trauma and psychological stress: report of the Therapeutics and Technology Assessment Subcommittee of the American Academy of Neurology. *Neurology.*;52:1737-45.
67. Granger CV, Albrecht GL, Hamilton BB. 1979. Outcome of comprehensive medical rehabilitation: measurement by PULSES profile and the Barthel Index. *Arch Phys Med Rehabil.*;60:145-54.
68. Granger CV, Cotter AC, Hamilton BB, Fiedler RC, Hens MM. 1990. Functional assessment scales: a study of persons with multiple sclerosis. *Arch Phys Med Rehabil.*;71:870-875.
69. Granger CV, Dewis LS, Peters NC, Sherwood CC, Barrett JE. 1979. Stroke rehabilitation: analysis of repeated Barthel index measures. *Arch Phys Med Rehabil.*;60:14-7.
70. Greenhouse L. Justices hear disability cases on vision. *New York Times.* April 29, 1999:(A20).
71. Gulick EE. 1991. Reliability and validity of the work assessment scale for persons with multiple sclerosis. *Nurs Res.*;40:107-12.
72. Gulick EE. 1995. Coping among spouses or significant others of persons with multiple sclerosis. *Nurs Res.*;44:220-5.
73. Guyatt GH, Feeny DH, Patrick DL. 1993. Measuring health-related quality of life. *Ann Intern Med.*;118:622-9.
74. Harwood RH, Gompertz P, Ebrahim S. 1994. Handicap one year after a stroke: validity of a new scale. *J Neurol Neurosurg Psychiatry.*;57:825-9.
75. Hayes CE, Cantorna MT, DeLuca HF. 1997. Vitamin D and multiple sclerosis. *Proc Soc Exp Biol Med.*;216:21-7.
76. Helbing C, Sangl JA, Silverman HA. 1992. Home health agency benefits. *Health Care Financ Rev Annu Suppl.*;125-48.
77. Herbert TB, Cohen S. 1993. Stress and immunity in humans: a meta-analytic review. *Psychosom Med.*;55:364-379.
78. Hobart J.C. 1997. Measuring health outcomes in multiple sclerosis: why, which, and how? Thompson A.J., Polman C., Hohlfeld R. *Multiple Scerosis: Clinical Challenges and Controversies.* London, England: Martin Dunitz Ltd;:211-225.

79. Hobart JC, Freeman JA, Lamping DL. 1996. Physician and patient-oriented outcomes in progressive neurological disease: which to measure? *Curr Opin Neurol.*;9:441-4.
80. Hobart JC, Lamping DL, Fitzpatrick R, Thompson AJ. 2000. The Multiple Sclerosis Impact Scale (MSIS-29): a New Patient Based Measure of the Physical and Psychological Impact of MS: *Quality of Life Research.*
81. Hobart J, Freeman J, Thompson AJ. 2000. Kurtzke scales revisited: the application of psychometric methods to clinical intuition. *Brain.*;123:1027-40.
82. Hunt SM, McEwen J, McKenna SP. 1985. Measuring health status: a new tool for clinicians and epidemiologists. *J R Coll Gen Pract.*;35:185-8.
83. Iezzoni LI. 1996. When walking fails. *JAMA.*;276:1609-13.
84. Iezzoni LI. 1998. What should I say? Communication around disability. *Ann Intern Med.*;129:661-5.
85. Iezzoni LI. 1999. Boundaries. What happens to the disabled poor when insurers draw a line between what's "medically necessary" and devices that can improve quality of life? *Health Aff (Millwood).*;18:171-6.
86. Iezzoni LI, McCarthy EP, Davis RB, Siebens H. 2000. Mobility impairments and use of screening and preventive services. *Am J Public Health.*;90:955-61.
87. Institute of Medicine. Pope AM, Tarlow AR, eds. *Disability in America.* Washington, D.C.: National Academy Press; 1991.
88. Institute of Medicine. Brandt EN, Pope AM, eds. *Enabling America.* Washington, D.C.: National Academy Press; 1997.
89. Institute of Medicine. Joy JE, Watson Jr. SJ, Benson Jr. JA, eds. *Marijuana and Medicine: Assessing the Science Base.* Washington, D.C.: National Academy Press; 1999.
90. International Federation of Multiple Sclerosis Societies. 1984. Minimal Record of Disability—1983. *Acta Neurol Scand Suppl.*;101:169-190.
91. Jackson MF, Quaal C, Reeves MA. 1991. Effects of multiple sclerosis on occupational and career patterns. *Axone.*;13:16-7, 20-2.
92. Kalkers NF, de Groot V, Lazeron RH, et al. 2000. MS functional composite: relation to disease phenotype and disability strata. *Neurology.*;54:1233-9.
93. Kaplan SH, Gandek B, Greenfield S, Rogers W, Ware JE. 1995. Patient and visit characteristics related to physicians' participatory decision-making style. Results from the Medical Outcomes Study. *Med Care.*;33:1176-87.
94. Kaplan SH, Greenfield S, Gandek B, Rogers WH, Ware JE Jr. 1996. Characteristics of physicians with participatory decision-making styles. *Ann Intern Med.*;124:497-504.
95. Kaplan SH, Greenfield S, Ware JE Jr. 1989. Assessing the effects of physician-patient interactions on the outcomes of chronic disease. *Med Care.*;27:S110-27.
96. Karp G. Life on wheels. For the active wheelchair user. Sebastopol, CA: O'Reilly and Associates; 1999.
97. Kent-Braun JA, Sharma KR, Miller RG, Weiner MW. 1994. Postexercise phosphocreatine resynthesis is slowed in multiple sclerosis. *Muscle Nerve.*;17:835-41.
98. Kersten P, Mullee MA, Smith JA, McLellan L, George S. 1999. Generic health status measures are unsuitable for measuring health status in severely disabled people. *Clin Rehabil.*;13:219-28.
99. Kneier AW, Temoshok L. 1984. Repressive coping reactions in patients with malignant melanoma as compared to cardiovascular disease patients. *J Psychosom Res.*;28:145-55.
100. Koopman W, Schweitzer A. 1999. The journey to multiple sclerosis: a qualitative study. *J Neurosci Nurs.*;31(1):17-26.
101. Kornblith AB, LaRocca NG, Baum HM. 1986. Employment in individuals with multiple sclerosis. *Int J Rehabil Res.*;9:155-65.
102. Krauss HH, Godfrey C, Kirk J, Eisenberg DM. 1998. Alternative health care: its use by individuals with physical disabilities. *Arch Phys Med Rehabil.*;79:1440-1447.

103. Ku YT, Montgomery LD, Wenzel KC, Webbon BW, Burks JS. 1999. Physiologic and thermal responses of male and female patients with multiple sclerosis to head and neck cooling. *Am J Phys Med Rehabil.*;78:447-56.

104. Kurtzke JF, Page WF. 1997. Epidemiology of multiple sclerosis in US veterans: VII. Risk factors for MS. *Neurology.*;48:204-13.

105. Kutner NG, Ory MG, Baker DI, Schechtman KB, Hornbrook MC, Mulrow CD. 1992. Measuring the quality of life of the elderly in health promotion intervention clinical trials. *Public Health Rep.*;107:530-9.

106. Laine C. 1997. Should physicians discourage patients from playing the sick role? *CMAJ.*;157:393-4.

107. Laine C, Davidoff F, Lewis CE, et al. 1996. Important elements of outpatient care: a comparison of patients' and physicians' opinions. *Ann Intern Med.*;125:640-5.

108. Lankhorst GJ, Jelles F, Smits RC, et al. 1996. Quality of life in multiple sclerosis: the disability and impact profile (DIP). *J Neurol.*;243:469-74.

109. LaPlante MP, Hendershot GE, Moss AJ. 1992. Assistive technology devices and home accessibility features: prevalence, payment, need, and trends. *Adv Data Vital Health Stat.*;217:1-11.

110. Larsen PD. 1990. Psychosocial adjustment in multiple sclerosis. *Rehabil Nurs.*;15:242-6; discussion 246-7.

111. Lassmann H, Raine CS, Antel J, Prineas JW. 1998. Immunopathology of multiple sclerosis: report on an international meeting held at the Institute of Neurology of the University of Vienna. *J Neuroimmunol.*;86:213-7.

112. Lauer K. 1995. Environmental associations with the risk of multiple sclerosis: the contribution of ecological studies. *Acta Neurol Scand Suppl.*;161:77-88.

113. Lauer K. 1997. Diet and multiple sclerosis. *Neurology.*;49:S55-61.

114. Lazarus RS, Folkman S. *Stress, Appraisal and Coping.* New York: Springer; 1984.

115. Leino-Kilpi H, Luoto E, Katajisto J. 1998. Elements of empowerment and MS patients. *J Neurosci Nurs.*;30(2):116-123.

116. Levinson W, Roter D. 1995. Physicians' psychosocial beliefs correlate with their patient communication skills. *J Gen Intern Med.*;10:375-9.

117. Loewen SC, Anderson BA. 1988. Reliability of the Modified Motor Assessment Scale and the Barthel Index. *Phys Ther.*;68:1077-81.

118. Lohr K, ed. 1989. Advances in health status assessment, conference proceedings. *Medical Care.*;27:S1-294.

119. Lohr K, ed. 1992. Advances in health status assessment: Fostering the application of health status measures in clinical settings: Proceedings of a conference. *Medical Care.*;30:MS1-293.

120. Lord SE, Wade DT, Halligan PW. 1998. A comparison of two physiotherapy treatment approaches to improve walking in multiple sclerosis: a pilot randomized controlled study. *Clin Rehabil.*;12:477-86.

121. MacLennan AH, Wilson DH, Taylor AW. 1996. Prevalence and cost of alternative medicine in Australia. *Lancet.*;347:569-573.

122. Magaziner J, Simonsick EM, Kashner TM, Hebel JR. 1988. Patient-proxy response comparability on measures of patient health and functional status. *J Clin Epidemiol.*;41:1065-74.

123. Mahoney FI, Barthel DW. 1965. Functional evaluation: the Barthel Index. *Maryland St Med J.*;14:61-65.

124. Mairs N. Saxton M, Howe F, eds. On being a cripple. *With Wings: An Anthology of Literature by and About Women With Disabilities.* New York: Feminist Press at the City University of New York; 1987:118-127.

125. Mairs N. Waist-high in the world. A life among the nondisabled. Boston, MA: Beacon Press; 1996.

126. Mangione CM, Phillips RS, Seddon JM, et al. 1992. Development of the 'Activities of Daily Vision Scale'. A measure of visual functional status. *Med Care.*;30:1111-26.

127. Marolf MV, Vaney C, Konig N, Schenk T, Prosiegel M. 1996. Evaluation of disability in multiple sclerosis patients: A comparative study of the functional independence measure, the extended barthel index and the expanded disability status scale. *Clinical Rehabilitation.*;10:309-313.

128. McDowell I, Newell C. *Measuring Health: A Guide to Rating Scales and Questionnaires.* New York: Oxford University Press; 1987.

129. McGuinness S. 1996. Learned helplessness in the multiple sclerosis population. *J Neurosc Nurs.*;28(3):163-170.

130. McGuinness SD, Peters S. 1999. The diagnosis of multiple sclerosis: Peplau's Interpersonal Relations Model in practice. *Rehabil Nurs.*;24:30-3.

131. McHorney CA, Ware JE, Jr, Lu JF, Sherbourne CD. 1994. The MOS 36-item Short-Form Health Survey (SF-36): III. Tests of data quality, scaling assumptions, and reliability across diverse patient groups. *Med Care.*;32:40-66.

132. McHorney CA, Ware JE Jr, Raczek AE. 1993. The MOS 36-Item Short-Form Health Survey (SF-36): II. Psychometric and clinical tests of validity in measuring physical and mental health constructs. *Med Care.*;31:247-63.

133. McLellan DL, Martin JR, Roberts MHW, Spackman A, McIntosh-Michaelis S., Nichols S. 1989. *Multiple Sclerosis in the Southampton District.* University of Southampton: Rehabilitation Research Unit and Department of Sociology and Social Policy.

134. Millar WJ. 1997. Use of alternative health care practitioners by Canadians. *Can J Public Health.*;88:154-158.

135. Miller DM, Rudick RA, Cutter G, Baier M, Fischer JS. 2000. Clinical significance of the multiple sclerosis functional composite: relationship to patient-reported quality of life. *Arch Neurol.*;57:1319-24.

136. Miller M, Boyer MJ, Butow PN, Gattellari M, Dunn SM, Childs A. 1998. The use of unproven methods of treatment by cancer patients. Frequency, expectations and cost. *Support Care Cancer.*;6:337-347.

137. Mosteller F, Ware JE, Jr., Levine S. 1989. Finale Panel: Comments on the conference on advances in health status assessment. *Medical Care.*;27:S282-294.

138. Mumford CJ, Compston A. 1993. Problems with rating scales for multiple sclerosis: a novel approach—the CAMBS score. *J Neurol.*;240:209-15.

139. Murray TJ. 1995. The psychosocial aspects of multiple sclerosis. *Neurol Clin.*;13:197-223.

140. Murray TJ. 2000. Personal time: the patient's experience. *Ann Intern Med.*;132:58-62.

141. Murray TJ. Alternative therapies used by MS patients. Polman CH, Thompson AJ, Murray TJ, McDonald WI, eds. In Press. *Multiple Sclerosis: The Guide to Treatment and Management.* 5th ed. New York: Demos Publications.

142. Neufeld P. Assistive Technology—Occupational Therapy. 2000.

143. Ng AV, Kent-Braun JA. 1997. Quantitation of lower physical activity in persons with multiple sclerosis. *Med Sci Sports Exerc.*;29:517-23.

144. Nortvedt MW, Riise T, Myhr KM, Nyland HI. 1999. Quality of life in multiple sclerosis: measuring the disease effects more broadly. *Neurology.*;53:1098-103.

145. O'Brien MT. 1993. Multiple sclerosis: the role of social support and disability. *Clin Nurs Res.*;2:67-85.

146. O'Connor P, Detsky AS, Tansey C, Kucharczyk W. 1994. Effect of diagnostic testing for multiple sclerosis on patient health perceptions. Rochester-Toronto MRI Study Group. *Arch Neurol.*;51:46-51.

147. O'Day B. 1998. Barriers for people with multiple sclerosis who want to work: A qualitative study. *J Neuro Rehab.*;12:139-146.

148. Oliver M. Understanding disability: From theory to practice. New York: St. Martin's Press; 1996:97.

149. Ostenstad B, Dybwad A, Lea T, Forre O, Vinje O, Sioud M. 1995. Evidence for monoclonal expansion of synovial T cells bearing VO2.1/VJ5.5 gene segments and recognizing a synthetic peptide that shares homology with a number of putative autoantigents. *Immunology.*;86:168-175.
150. Painter P, Stewart AL, Carey S. 1999. Physical functioning: Definitions, measurement, and expectations. *Advances in Renal Replacement Therapy.*;6:110-123.
151. Patrick DL, Chiang YP. 2000. Measurement of health outcomes in treatment effectiveness evaluations: conceptual and methodological challenges. *Med Care.*;38:II14-25.
152. Patrick DL, Deyo RA. 1989. Generic and disease-specific measures in assessing health status and quality of life. *Med Care.*;27:S217-32.
153. Peach L. 1998. Electronics get muscles moving. *Design News.*;96-100.
154. Petajan JH, Gappmaier E, White AT, Spencer MK, Mino L, Hicks RW. 1996. Impact of aerobic training on fitness and quality of life in multiple sclerosis. *Ann Neurol.*;39:432-41.
155. Petajan JH, White AT. 1999. Recommendations for physical activity in patients with multiple sclerosis. *Sports Med.*;27:179-91.
156. Peters L. 1982. Women's health care: approaches in delivery to physically disabled women. *Nurse Pract.*;7:34-7, 48.
157. Pierce LL. 1998. Barriers to access: Frustrations of people who use a wheelchair for full-time mobility. *Rehabil Nursing.*;23:120-125.
158. President's Advisory Commission on Consumer Protection and Quality in the Health Care Industry. Consumer bill of rights and responsibilities. Washington, DC: 1997:45-49.
159. Rao SM, Leo GJ, Ellington L, Nauertz T, Bernardin L, Unverzagt F. 1991. Cognitive dysfunction in multiple sclerosis. II. Impact on employment and social functioning. *Neurology.*;41:692-6.
160. Redelmeier DA, Rozin P, Kahneman D. 1993. Understanding patients' decisions. Cognitive and emotional perspectives. *JAMA.*;270:72-6.
161. Reding MJ, LaRocca NG. 1987. Acute-hospital care versus rehabilitation hospitalization for management of nonemergent complications in multiple sclerosis. *Journal of Neurologic Rehabilitation.*;1:13-17.
162. Reiser SJ. 1993. The era of the patient. Using the experience of illness in shaping the missions of health care. *JAMA.*;269:1012-7.
163. Risberg T, Wist E, Melsom H, Kaasa S. 1997. [Use of alternative medicine among Norwegian hospitalized cancer patients]. *Tidsskr Nor Laegeforen.*;117:2458-2463.
164. Rodriguez M, Siva A, Ward J, Stolp-Smith KA, O'Brien P, Kurland L. 1994. Impairment, disability, and handicap in multiple sclerosis: a population-based study in Olmsted County, Minnesota. *Neurology.*;44:28-33.
165. Roper Starch Worldwide I. *The National MS Society: An Analysis of Non-Members.* New York: Roper Starch Worldwide, Inc.; 1998.
166. Roter DL, Hall JA, Kern DE, Barker LR, Cole KA, Roca RP. 1995. Improving physicians' interviewing skills and reducing patients' emotional distress. A randomized clinical trial. *Arch Intern Med.*;155:1877-84.
167. Rothman ML, Hedrick SC, Bulcroft KA, Hickam DH, Rubenstein LZ. 1991. The validity of proxy-generated scores as measures of patient health status. *Med Care.*;29:115-24.
168. Rubenstein LV, Calkins DR, Greenfield S, et al. 1989. Health status assessment for elderly patients. Report of the Society of General Internal Medicine Task Force on Health Assessment. *J Am Geriatr Soc.*;37:562-9.
169. Rudick RA. 1999. Disease-modifying drugs for relapsing-remitting multiple sclerosis and future directions for multiple sclerosis therapeutics. *Arch Neurol.*;56:1079-84.
170. Rumrill PD, Roessler RT, Cook BG. 1998. Improving career re-entry outcomes for people with multiple sclerosis: A comparison of two approaches. *Journal of Vocational Rehabilitation.*; 10:241-252.

171. Schapiro RT. Models of care in progressive multiple sclerosis. Thompson AJ, Polman C, Hohlfeld R, eds. *Multiple Sclerosis: Clinical Challenges and Controversies.* London, UK: Martin Dunitz Ltd.; 1997:325-334.

172. Scheier MF, Carver CS. 1987. Dispositional optimism and physical well-being: the influence of generalized outcome expectancies on health. *J Pers.*;55:169-210.

173. Scheier MF, Weintraub JK, Carver CS. 1986. Coping with stress: divergent strategies of optimists and pessimists. *J Pers Soc Psychol.*;51:1257-64.

174. Schraub S. 2000. Unproven methods in cancer: a worldwide problem. *Support Care Cancer.*;8:10-15.

175. Schroeder SA. 1999. The legacy of SUPPORT. Study to Understand Prognoses and Preferences for Outcomes and Risks of Treatments. *Ann Intern Med.*;131:780-2.

176. Schwartz CE, Foley FW, Rao SM, Bernardin LJ, Lee H, Genderson MW. 1999. Stress and course of disease in multiple sclerosis. *Behav Med.*;25:110-6.

177. Schwartz CE, Laitin E, Brotman S, LaRocca N. 1999. Utilization of unconventional treatments by persons with MS: is it alternative or complementary? *Neurology.*;52:626-629.

178. Schwartz L, Kraft GH. 1999. The role of spouse responses to disability and family environment in multiple sclerosis. *Am J Phys Med Rehabil.*;78:525-32.

179. Scott FW. 1996. Food-induced type 1 diabetes in the BB rat. *Diabetes/Metabolism Reviews.*;12:341-359.

180. Shapiro JP. *No Pity: People With Disabilities Forging a New Civil Rights Movement.* New York: Times Books; 1994.

181. Sharrack B, Hughes RA. 1999. The Guy's Neurological Disability Scale (GNDS): a new disability measure for multiple sclerosis. *Mult Scler.*;5:223-33.

182. Sharrack B, Hughes RAC, Soudain S. 1996. Guy's Neurological Disability Scale. *J Neurol.*;243:S32.

183. Sharrack B, Hughes RA, Soudain S, Dunn G. 1999. The psychometric properties of clinical rating scales used in multiple sclerosis. *Brain.*;122:141-59.

184. Shinar D, Gross CR, Bronstein KS, et al. 1987. Reliability of the activities of daily living scale and its use in telephone interview. *Arch Phys Med Rehabil.*;68:723-8.

185. Sibley WA. Therapeutic claims in multiple sclerosis. New York, NY: Demos Publications; 1992:202.

186. Singh VK, Yamaki K, Donoso L, Shinohara T. 1989. Yeast histone H3-induced experimental autoimmune uveitis. *Journal of Immunology.*;142:1512-1517.

187. Smith RO. Technological Approaches to Performance Enhancement. Christiansen C, Baum C, eds. *Occupational Therapy: Overcoming Human Performance Deficits.* Throfare: Slack Incorporated; 1990.

188. Sneeuw KC, Aaronson NK, Osoba D, et al. 1997. The use of significant others as proxy raters of the quality of life of patients with brain cancer. *Med Care.*;35:490-506.

189. Solari A, Filippini G, Gasco P, et al. 1999. Physical rehabilitation has a positive effect on disability in multiple sclerosis patients. *Neurology.*;52:57-62.

190. Sprangers MA, Aaronson NK. 1992. The role of health care providers and significant others in evaluating the quality of life of patients with chronic disease: a review. *J Clin Epidemiol.*;45:743-60.

191. Stenager E, Stenager EN, Knudsen L, Jensen K. 1995. The use of non-medical/alternative treatment in multiple sclerosis. A 5 year follow-up study. *Acta Neurol Belg.*;95:18-22.

192. Stewart AL, Greenfield S, Hays RD, et al. 1989. Functional status and well-being of patients with chronic conditions. Results from the Medical Outcomes Study. *JAMA.*;262:907-13.

193. Stewart AL, Ware JE, eds. Measuring Functioning and Well-Being: The Medical Outcomes Approach. Durham, NC: Duke University Press; 1992.

194. Stewart AL, Ware JE Jr, Brook RH. 1981. Advances in the measurement of functional status: construction of aggregate indexes. *Med Care.*;19:473-88.

195. Stolp-Smith KA, Carter JL, Rohe DE, Knowland DP 3rd. 1997. Management of impairment, disability, and handicap due to multiple sclerosis. *Mayo Clin Proc.*;72:1184-96.
196. Streiner D.L., Norman GR. *Health Status Measurement Scales. A Practical Guide to Their Development and Use.* 2nd ed. Oxford, UK: Oxford University Press; 1995.
197. Stuifbergen AK, Becker HA, Ingalsbe K, Sands D. 1990. Perceptions of health among adults with disabilities. *Health Values.*;14:18-26.
198. Stuifbergen AK, Becker H, Sands D. 1990. Barriers to health promotion for individuals with disabilities. *Fam Community Health.*;13:11-22.
199. Stuifbergen AK, Roberts GJ. 1997. Health promotion practices of women with multiple sclerosis. *Arch Phys Med Rehabil.*;78(12 Suppl 5):S3-S9.
200. Stuifbergen AK, Rogers S. 1997. Health promotion: an essential component of rehabilitation for persons with chronic disabling conditions. *ANS Adv Nurs Sci.*;19:1-20.
201. Sutcher H. 1997. Hypnosis as adjunctive therapy for multiple sclerosis: a progress report. *Am J Clin Hypn.*;39(4):283-290.
202. Taylor A, Taylor RS. 1998. Neuropsychologic aspects of multiple sclerosis. *Phys Med Rehabil Clin N Am.*;9:643-57, vii-viii.
203. Temoshok L. 1985. Biopsychosocial studies on cutaneous malignant melanoma: psychosocial factors associated with prognostic indicators, progression, psychophysiology and tumor-host response. *Soc Sci Med.*;20:833-40.
204. Temoshok L, Heller BW, Sagebiel RW, et al. 1985. The relationship of psychosocial factors to prognostic indicators in cutaneous malignant melanoma. *J Psychosom Res.*;29:139-53.
205. Thom DH, Campbell B. 1997. Patient-physician trust: an exploratory study. *J Fam Pract.*;44:169-76.
206. Thompson AJ. 1998. Multiple Sclerosis: rehabilitation measures. *Semin Neurol.*;18(3):397-403.
207. Thompson AJ. 2000. The effectiveness of neurological rehabilitation in multiple sclerosis. *J Rehabil Res Dev.*;37:455-61.
208. Thompson AJ, Hobart JC. 1998. Multiple sclerosis: assessment of disability and disability scales. *J Neurol.*;245:189-96.
209. Thompson AJ, Polman C, Hohlfeld R, eds. Multiple Sclerosis: Clinical Challenges and Controversies. London: Martin Dunitz; 1997.
210. Thorne SE, Robinson CA. 1988. Reciprocal trust in health care relationships. *J Adv Nurs.*;13:782-9.
211. Tinetti ME, Williams TF, Mayewski R. 1986. Fall risk index for elderly patients based on number of chronic disabilities. *Am J Med.*;80:429-34.
212. Toombs SK. 1988. Illness and the paradigm of lived body. *Theor Med.*;9:201-26.
213. Toombs SK. Sufficient unto the day. A life with multiple sclerosis. Toombs SK, Barnard D, Carson RD, eds. *Chronic Illness. From Experience to Policy.* Bloomington and Indianapolis: Indiana University Press; 1995.
214. Toombs SK. 1998. "Where would she like to sit?" The personal and societal challenge of chronic illness and disability. Unpublished.
215. Tsevat J, Cook EF, Green ML, et al. 1995. Health values of the seriously ill. SUPPORT investigators. *Ann Intern Med.*;122:514-20.
216. 2000. State of the Internet 2000.
217. Van der Putten JJ, Hobart JC, Freeman JA, Thompson AJ. 1999. Measuring change in disability after inpatient rehabilitation: comparison of the responsiveness of the Barthel index and the Functional Independence Measure. *J Neurol Neurosurg Psychiatry.*;66:480-4.
218. Verhoef MJ, Hagen N, Pelletier G, Forsyth P. 1999. Alternative therapy use in neurologic diseases: use in brain tumor patients. *Neurology.*;52:617-622.
219. Vickrey BG, Hays RD, Genovese BJ, Myers LW, Ellison GW. 1997. Comparison of a generic to disease-targeted health-related quality of life measures for multiple sclerosis. *J Clin Epidemiol.*;50:557-69.

220. Vickrey BG, Hays RD, Harooni R, Myers LW, Ellison GW. 1995. A health-related quality of life measure for multiple sclerosis. *Qual Life Res.*;4:187-206.
221. Wade DT, Hewer RL. 1987. Functional abilities after stroke: measurement, natural history and prognosis. *J Neurol Neurosurg Psychiatry.*;50:177-82.
222. Ware JE Jr. 1991. Conceptualizing and measuring generic health outcomes. *Cancer.*;67:774-9.
223. Ware JE Jr. 1995. The status of health assessment 1994. *Annu Rev Public Health.*;16:327-354.
224. Ware JE Jr, Sherbourne CD. 1992. The MOS 36-item short-form health survey (SF-36). I. Conceptual framework and item selection. *Med Care.*;30:473-83.
225. Warren CG. 1990. Powered mobility and its implications. *J Rehabil Res Dev Clin Suppl.*;74-85.
226. Wassem R. 1991. A test of the relationship between health locus of control and the course of multiple sclerosis. *Rehabil Nurs.*;16:189-93.
227. Weinberger M, Oddone EZ, Samsa GP, Landsman PB. 1996. Are health-related quality-of-life measures affected by the mode of administration? *J Clin Epidemiol.*;49:135-40.
228. Wiles CM, Newcombe RG, Fuller K.J, Furnival-Doran, Pickersgill TP, Morgan A. In Press. A controlled randomised crossover trial of the effects of physiotherapy on mobility in chronic multiple sclerosis. *J. Neurol. Neurosurg. Psychiatry.*
229. Wilson A, Parker H, Wynn A, et al. 1999. Randomised controlled trial of effectiveness of Leicester hospital at home scheme compared with hospital care [see comments]. *BMJ.*;319:1542-6.
230. Windahl S, Signitzer BH, Olson JT. *Using Communication Theory: An Introduction to Planned Communication.* London, UK: Sage Publications, Ltd.; 1992.
231. Wineman NM, Durand EJ, Steiner RP. 1994. A comparative analysis of coping behaviors in persons with multiple sclerosis or a spinal cord injury. *Res Nurs Health.*;17:185-94.
232. Winterholler M, Erbguth F, Neundorfer B. 1997. [The use of alternative medicine by multiple sclerosis patients—patient characteristics and patterns of use]. *Fortschr Neurol Psychiatr.*;65:555-561.
233. World Health Organization. ICIDH-2: International Classification of Impairments, Activities and Participation: A manual of dimensions of disablement and functioning. Geneva: World Health Organization; 1997.
234. Yi S, Xiaoyan L. 1999. A review on traditional chinese medicine in prevention and treatment of multiple sclerosis. *Journal of Traditional Chinese Medicine.*;19:65-73.
235. Young NL, Williams JI, Yoshida KK, Bombardier C, Wright JG. 1996. The context of measuring disability: does it matter whether capability or performance is measured? *J Clin Epidemiol.*;49:1097-101.
236. Zola IK. 1982. Missing pieces: A chronicle of living with a disability. Philadelphia, PA: Temple University Press;228.

# 5

# Strategies for Future Research
# on Disease Mechanisms

## NEUROBIOLOGY

Even though the histology of multiple sclerosis (MS) was described in early texts of neurology more than a century ago, the full repertoire of cellular players, and their roles in the disease process (which cells are actors, and which are victims?) are incompletely understood.

Oligodendrocytes, astrocytes, and neurons can, in a sense, all be regarded as the "victims" in multiple sclerosis. It is clear that oligodendrocytes and the myelin sheaths they form are damaged, astrocytes respond by forming a glial scar, and in some cases, axons (which are outgrowths of neurons) degenerate in MS. Although this much is known, additional questions remain, and their answers have important implications for therapy.

### Understanding Injury of Neurons

Even the earliest descriptions of multiple sclerosis mentioned axonal degeneration. Recent studies, using contemporary methods such as magnetic resonance imaging (MRI) and confocal microscopy, have more definitively demonstrated the degeneration of axons, both within plaques in multiple sclerosis and in normal-appearing white matter in this disorder (Figure 5.1). It has been speculated that axonal injury contributes to the development of irreversible neurologic deficits as in multiple sclerosis.[23,60,66,93,99] If this turns out to be true, it will be important because the prevention of axonal loss might then prevent persistent

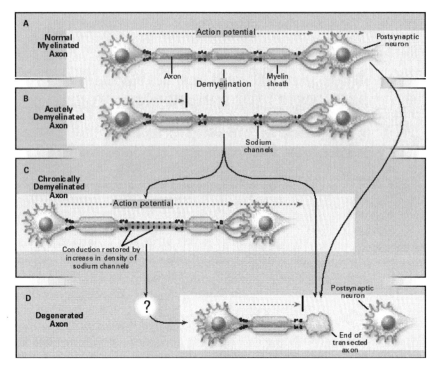

**FIGURE 5.1** Demyelination and axonal degeneration in multiple sclerosis.
(A) In a normal myelinated axon, the action potential (dashed arrow) travels, with high velocity and reliability, to the postsynaptic neuron. (B) In acutely demyelinated axons, conduction is blocked (black bar). (C) In some chronically demyelinated axons that acquire a higher-than-normal density of sodium channels, conduction is restored. (D) Axonal degeneration, by contrast, interrupts action potential propagation in a permanent manner. SOURCE: Waxman, SG, 1998.[99] Copyright 1998 Massachusetts Medical Society. All rights reserved. Reprinted with permission.

disability. Synapses are not formed onto axons, so that the excitotoxic theory of neuronal death, which almost certainly applies to diseases of gray matter such as stroke, may not play an important role in multiple sclerosis.[80]

It is not yet known whether axonal injury is a consequence of demyelination, or the immune processes underlying demyelination, or is an independent process. There are some results suggesting that inflammation results in axonal damage in MS.[60,93] This provides an important angle for further investigation. Cytokines are likely candidates as mediators of inflammatory-induced axonal damage, and their possible role in MS should be investigated. Another approach is suggested by demonstrations that ion channels and exchangers together form a "final common pathway" that can be modulated by neurotransmitters and that underlies axonal degeneration after various insults.[13,25,26,91,92] Neuroprotective interventions can preserve axonal function and integrity after acute insult in two ways. Axons can be protected either by agents that block or modulate the various injurious ion fluxes that occur during this molecular death cascade or by agents that interfere with "downstream" degenerative events, such as activation of calpains and other destructive enzymes.[24,32,92]

It is well established that axonal transection can trigger dramatic changes in the neuronal cell body, but with a few exceptions, the effects of demyelination on the neuronal cell body have not been examined. The available evidence suggests that demyelination may produce significant molecular changes in the neuronal cell body, including changes in gene activation.[9] Since these changes are likely to interfere with neuronal function, they should be studied.

Details of the molecular mechanisms underlying various pathological changes in neurons in MS remain to be elucidated. Rather than reflecting a pessimistic scenario, recognition of neuronal changes in the "demyelinating" diseases presents new therapeutic targets and opportunities. We know a lot about injured neurons, including injured axons, and about how to alter their behavior. Neuronal injury in demyelinating diseases is therefore not necessarily bad news. More information about neuronal dysfunction in MS and related disorders might provide inroads in the search for more effective therapies that will preserve function in people with MS.

## How Oligodendrocytes and Myelin Are Injured

Demyelination is the hallmark of multiple sclerosis, and it is also known that oligodendrocytes degenerate in this disorder. Yet we still do not understand the primary target of MS. Is it the oligodendrocyte or the myelin sheath it forms? Much is known about the "death cascade" in neurons, which leads from initial insults, via a series of molecular steps, to the ultimate death of the cell. Less is known about the degenerative cascade in oligodendrocytes. Recent evidence suggests that excitotoxic mechanisms, possibly involving glutamate acting via AMPA/kainate receptors, may injure oligodendrocytes (Figure 5.2).[47] (The AMPA/kainate receptor is one of several glutamate receptors in the brain; it also binds to kainic acid and AMPA.) If the details of mechanisms that injure oligo-dendrocytes and axons were better understood, it might be possible to protect oligodendrocytes, or their myelin sheaths, so that they are not injured in MS.

There is also the important question of whether oligodendrocyte progenitors (stemlike cells that can give rise to oligodendrocytes with the potential to form new myelin) are present within the adult brain. If they are, can these cells be awakened or activated, so that they will, in fact, form new myelin in multiple sclerosis? Evidence from animal models indicates that it is, in fact, possible to promote remyelination by endogenous cells by exposing oligodendrocytes to various factors. If this could be accomplished in humans, it might be possible to promote recovery of function in people with MS.

## Astrocytes: Glial Cells Are More than "Glue"

Astrocytes are star-shaped glial cells that do not form myelin. They have traditionally been viewed only as "scarring" elements in multiple sclerosis. Yet there is evidence that these cells are much more complex than this. Astrocytes are capable of presenting antigens and promoting T-cell proliferation, which indicates that they might play a role in reactivation and regulation of inflammatory process in the brain.[2,16,46] They may play an important role in the etiopathogen-

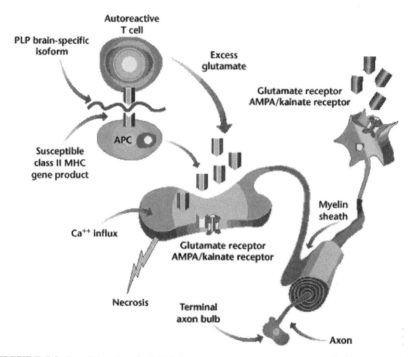

**FIGURE 5.2** Possible role of AMPA/kainate receptors on neurons and glia. Activation of T lymphocytes (in this case, a T lymphocyte reactive to the brain-specific loop of the myelin protein, PLP [proteolipid protein]), macrophages, and resident microglia at the site of inflammation in the white matter of the central nervous system causes release of glutamate. The increased extracellular glutamate binds to AMPA/kainate receptors on neurons and on oligodendrocytes. This leads to increased calcium fluxes and death of oligodendrocytes and neurons. NOTE: MHC = major histocompatibility complex. SOURCE: Steinman L, 2000.[89] Reprinted with permission.

esis of MS. More information is needed about the degree to which astrocytes can serve as antigen-presenting cells and, if so, about the role they play in triggering, driving, or amplifying the immune assault on myelin in MS.

The permeability of the blood-brain barrier reflects, to a major degree, the tightness of the junctions between endothelial cells. Astrocytes are the brain cells that are the nearest neighbors to these cells. Astrocytes send out "feet" that cover much of the surface of the endothelial barrier cells. While astrocytes play a role in brain permeability, this can be modified by many other factors, including a range of inflammatory mediators secreted by leukocytes.[1,83] It is important to determine whether it is possible to modulate the leakiness of the blood vessels that occurs in multiple sclerosis by modifying the behavior of astrocytes.

It has also been suggested that astrocytes may play a role in axonal plasticity. Although astrocytes do not generate action potentials and have classically been considered "nonexcitable" cells, they produce sodium channels and insert them in their membranes.[7,35] These astrocytic sodium channels have physiological and molecular properties very similar (if not identical) to those of neuronal sodium channels.[4,87]

The role of astrocytic sodium channels is not known. Interestingly, astrocytes extend finger-like processes that contact sodium channel-rich parts of the axon membrane, for example, at the node of Ranvier. It has been speculated that astrocytes might serve as subsidiary sites for the synthesis of sodium channels, which they donate to nearby axons, thereby helping to restore conduction.[7] The last step in this hypothetical sequence, transfer of sodium channels from astrocytes to axons, has not been demonstrated however. Given the critical role that sodium channels play in restoration of conduction in demyelinated axons and the intimate spatial relationship that develops between astrocytes and demyelinated axons, there is a need to understand the role of astrocytic sodium channels, and thus of astrocytes, in MS.

## Mechanisms of Recovery

The nervous system exhibits a remarkable degree of plasticity, and it seems likely that reorganization at several levels, ranging from the molecular to the circuit level, contributes to remissions.

### *Neuronal Plasticity at the Molecular Level*

MS is unique among diseases of the brain and spinal cord in that many patients display remissions, in which lost functions (such as vision, ability to walk, tactile sensory function) are regained. Gaining a fuller understanding of the mechanisms underlying remissions is important for several reasons:

First, even if a totally effective immunotherapy were to be developed tomorrow, so that the immune assault on the myelin could be halted, 250,000 patients in the United States alone would be left with multiple sclerosis, and the disease would have left its footprints on their nervous systems, along with resultant neurologic deficits; if remissions could be induced in these patients, this might restore function.

Second, very few neurological diseases exhibit the degree of functional recovery that is seen during remissions in patients with MS. Thus, remissions might provide a unique model that could teach us important lessons about principles underlying recovery of function after various types of assaults on the nervous system. Although it has been demonstrated that, in principle, remyelination of denuded axons within the brain and spinal cord can promote restoration of conduction, this does not seem to provide a basis for remission in MS. There is, in fact, very little remyelination within the core of the plaques that characterize this disorder.

## *Molecular Plasticity of Demyelinated Axons*

Neurons are remarkably dynamic cells, and it has recently become clear that even in the healthy nervous system, they are constantly rebuilding and retuning themselves, so as to meet functional needs. There is a constant background turnover, for example, of ion channels including sodium channels and potassium channels. Following injury to the nervous system, the magnitude and rate of changes in channel deployment appear to be even greater.

It is now well established that conduction block occurs in demyelinated axons, in part, because they do not possess an adequate number of sodium channels within the internodal (previously myelinated but denuded after demyelination) part of their membranes. Following loss of the overlying myelin insulation, electrical current is lost through this sodium channel-poor membrane, and the density of current through sodium channel-rich parts of the axon membrane falls. As a result, the conduction of action potentials is impaired and, in some cases, abolished.[98] It has been well demonstrated in a number of animal models that in some chronically demyelinated axons, the denuded axon membrane, however, can acquire a higher-than-normal number of sodium channels, which is sufficient to support conduction.[10,20,21,29,65] Experimental methods for demonstrating this sodium channel plasticity require access to demyelinated tissue, and to date, most demonstrations of this phenomenon have been confined to laboratory models of MS. It would be useful, in the future, to develop methods for "sodium channel scanning" that might permit the visualization of sodium channel plasticity in humans. Now that nearly a dozen different genes for sodium channels with distinct molecular structures have been cloned (eight of which are expressed in the nervous system), there is also the opportunity to study their promoter regions and to learn about the molecular control mechanisms that regulate their synthesis.

The edge of the demyelinated plaque is a critical zone in that events there can also contribute to remissions. Even if an adequate density of sodium channels is present in a demyelinated axon, conduction from the normally myelinated region to the demyelinated zone must traverse a critical transition region where the geometry of the nerve fiber changes as the myelin is lost. This produces a phenomenon called "impedance mismatch," which is well-known to electrical engineers who study wires that have different properties at different points along their course. To overcome impedance mismatch, there must be a mechanism for "impedance matching." This probably occurs, in some demyelinated fibers, as a result of the production of short myelin segments at the juncture between normally myelinated and demyelinated parts of the axon.[97] This is an elegant example of impedance matching in the biological domain, but if it does not occur, conduction will be blocked. Thus, it is important for us to learn how the myelin-forming cell "knows" to form a myelin sheath of the appropriate length and to be able to control this process.

## Neuroplasticity at the Cell and Systems Levels

The concept of neural plasticity is varied but usually means a change in the neural response. This change can include either increases or decreases in neural responsivity, due to some modification of the environment, or in the input or output of the neurons involved. After the occurrence of lesions in the central (CNS) or peripheral nervous system (PNS), neurons display plastic changes in response properties that can range from subtle to dramatic. Altered neural responses can occur quickly or progress over many years. For example, after a long-term deafferentation of the nerve supply to the upper limb (several years) or after amputation, neurons in the primary somatosensory cortex that normally responded to the missing arm discharge after stimulation to the face.[74,77-79] This phenomenon reflects a substantial reorganization in the response properties of neocortical neurons distributed over many millimeters (a long distance in cortex) and is not seen after shorter periods of deafferentation. A quicker alteration in neural organization can be seen in patients with syndactyly.[64] Before surgery to separate their fingers, maps of primary somatosensory cortex showed an abnormal organization, with the representation of all fingers focused in a restricted cortical site. After surgery, a rapid reorganization of the finger representation occurred so that the digits were more normally distributed across the somatosensory cortex. Whether the changes after a lesion occur rapidly or over long periods of time, neurons acquire the ability to respond to stimuli that were previously ineffective in producing a response.

Recent evidence suggests that neural reorganization might also contribute to recovery from MS relapses. An MRI study of a group of seven MS patients showed that their patterns of neural activation were altered after they had recovered from a single episode of optic neuritis.[102] Visual stimulation of the recovered eye activated various areas of the brain that do not normally respond to visual stimulation (lateral temporal and posterior parietal cortices, thalamus, and insula-claustrum), whereas stimulation of the unaffected eye showed normal activation patterns.

In relation to MS, the question is, How do neurons change their responses in the presence of lesions, and how can the potential for positive neuronal change be harnessed to promote restorative recovery of function? Although the lesions in MS are clearly related primarily to glial cells, it is now accepted that axonal damage accompanies the lesions, which will impact on neural function. Presented below is a synopsis of the more commonly accepted manifestations of neural plasticity and ideas about the mechanisms that may underlie their occurrence.

**Changes in the Balance of Excitation and Inhibition.** Neuroplastic changes can occur within minutes or can evolve over extended periods of time, from weeks to years. In many instances after an acute lesion, neurons at different levels of the CNS quickly alter their responses so that cells previously responding to a restricted region on one side of the body can expand their responsiveness dramatically to include input from widespread regions, including the contralateral side.[13] One idea underlying the rapid changes is that they occur so quickly that only an immediate alteration in the balance of excitation and inhibition can account for the new level of activity. These changes are often referred to as an "unmasking" of responses, due to removal of a suppression or excitation, allowing a new type of activity to emerge. A delicate balance exists between excitatory and inhibitory inputs so that if a component is removed from the equation, a new response capability emerges rapidly. Several dramatic examples of these types of changes appear in reports dating back decades. One classic example is a study in which reversible blockade of the dorsal columns at a level in the spinal cord receiving input from the leg revealed neuronal responses to stimuli of remote parts of the body including the abdomen, which would not normally activate these neurons. After the blockade was removed, the neural responses returned to normal.[63] The unmasking of latent responses suggests the existence of dormant or normally suppressed pathways that might be tapped for functional restoration. More recent studies report that subtle and experimental alterations in the balance of excitation and inhibition can produce changes in receptive field organization and in motor behavior. For example, small injections of $GABA_A$ (gamma-aminobutyric acid) agonists into motor cortex, which increase inhibition, result in severe incoordination and deficits in motor dexterity of primates, suggesting the necessity of proper inhibition for smooth and coordinated movements.[84]

Relatively longer-term changes after cortical lesions, which reflect continued alterations in the balance of excitation and inhibition, include hyperexcitability of neurons accompanied by enhancement of receptors known to mediate long term excitation of a subset of glutamate receptors (NMDA [*N*-methyl-D-aspartate] receptors), and downregulation of $GABA_A$ receptors.[68] Numerous triggers for functional reorganizations of maps, primarily in the cerebral cortex, have also been reported over the past several decades. Maps can be altered after minor (practice at a skill) to major (removal of an input, such as blindness) changes in system inputs. Over time, the altered properties of neurons continually refine to result in neuronal representations that reflect numerous factors, including the ensuing experiences of the patient or subject.

**Changes in Synaptic Strength.** At its most elemental, the concept underlying altered synaptic strength is that a stimulus that previously elicited a relatively small neuronal response, now elicits a larger response, or an even smaller response. Several mechanisms for such a change have been proposed. One is activity dependence, in which the output of a given cell depends on both the quantity and the quality of the input. Much of this notion stems from the pioneering work of Hebb,[37] who postulated in 1949 that synaptic strength can be increased when neurons receive inputs that are temporally or physically correlated (reviewed in 1998 by Buonomano and Merzenich[12]). Understanding the mechanisms underlying synaptic strength has been approached experimentally through the phenomena of long-term potentiation (LTP) and long-term depression (LTD). These processes were first identified in the hippocampus but have since been identified in many other loci of the CNS, including the cerebral cortex (reviewed in 1999 by Malenka and Nicoll[56]). Researchers initially observed that stimulation of afferent fibers in the hippocampus at a specific frequency resulted in a long-lasting enhancement of postsynaptic cell activity. Similarly, LTD can be elicited by a reversal of the neural mechanisms producing LTP. The mechanisms essential to LTP production are too numerous to consider in depth here. Several conditions are considered fundamental to the implementation of LTP; these include postsynaptic activation of NMDA receptors and subsequent inflow of calcium into the cell.

Although the experimental procedures that produce LTP may not be physiological, since the stimuli used are generally of a higher frequency than that normally active in the CNS, many researchers agree that a similar phenomenon may produce plastic changes in neural responses. For example, rats trained in a motor task subsequently display increased field potentials in the motor cortex, which are reminiscent of the electrophysiological enhancements occurring in LTP.[81] In a different paradigm, cellular conditioning can be produced in visual and auditory cortex, by pairing a given cell's preferred stimulus with a decrease in activity and a nonpreferred stimulus with an increase in activity by manipulating current injected into the cell. This procedure also results in a change in synaptic strength because the conditioned cell often responds to the nonpreferred stimulus.[12]

**Changes in Morphology of Neurons-Axonal Growth or Sprouting.** Many types of CNS lesions result in morphological changes, particularly axonal growth or sprouting. Such changes have been observed after lesions in multiple regions and levels of the CNS, without further special treatment. The possibility of axonal regrowth obviously represents a potentially important mechanism for repair in MS. Although it has long been known that substantial morphologic reorganizations of major fiber tracts occur in young animals in response to central or peripheral manipulations, such dramatic patterns of regrowth do not occur in adults. For nearly half a century, however, evidence has accumulated reporting that various levels of the adult CNS attempt self-repair, which is difficult to correlate with changes in function (see, for example, Chambers et al.[14]). More recently, studies find that at specific levels of the nervous system, structural changes in response to specific deprivations or lesions occur in adults, which correspond more clearly to alterations in functional responses (see, for example, Kossut and Juliano[44]). For example, the ability to display morphologic reorganization appears impossible for thalamic axons terminating within the neocortex after a certain critical period, whereas structural reorganizations at the level of the neocortex itself continue to occur into adulthood.[95] These observations encouraged researchers to search for properties present in young brains that allow axonal growth and for properties in adult brains that inhibit axonal reorganization. Several potential molecules and genes have been identified on both sides, and their capacity is beginning to be exploited. For example, growth factors are important molecules that appear to encourage axonal growth. The support of these molecules is withdrawn as the CNS develops. More detail about this family of neurotrophic and gliotrophic molecules is given in other sections. On the other side, proteoglycans such as chondroitin sulfate are molecules that appear to block axonal growth and may prevent successful attempts at reorganization.[8,18,27]

In summary, all the manifestations of neural plasticity described above hold the potential to be harnessed for recovery of function in diseases such as MS. More than likely, they are interdependent, so that the long-term changes, such as those occurring after amputation or deafferentation, may reflect sprouting or axonal growth, whereas the more quickly occurring reorganizations may reflect unmasking of responses due to a change in excitatory and inhibitory balance. Furthermore, structural alterations, such as local sprouting, may result from the changes in synaptic strength that occur during normal or repetitive stimulation. Another point to consider is that some manifestations of plasticity may be functionally maladaptive. For example, after long-term amputations the massive cortical reorganization that occurs may not be helpful to function. Other types of axonal sprouting have also been reported to result in impaired behavior.[88] In relation to MS, it is possible that attempts at sprouting or axonal growth may contribute to a pattern of paresthesias or other dysesthesias that occur. On the other hand, it is likely that the redistribution of the finger representation that occurs after surgery to release individual digits in patients with syndactyly, will present as a positive functional change. It is important to distinguish the mechanisms responsible for alterations in functional responses and to harness their most useful components, whether axonal growth or modification of excitation and/or inhibition.

# IMMUNOLOGY

MS appears to result from an autoimmune attack against myelin initiated by autoreactive T cells (see Chapter 2). However, there is no formal proof of an immunopathogenesis of MS. The classic experiment to reproduce the disease by transferring autoreactive T cells from affected to unaffected individuals is not ethically permissible in humans.

There are, however, reasons to suspect that MS is not a "pure" T-cell autoimmune disease. In animal models, T cells are able to cause autoimmune inflammation, but they are unable by themselves to create large-scale demyelination, the hallmark of the MS plaque.[48] Demyelination, however, is produced by the addition of B-lymphocyte-derived autoantibodies, which then bind to the surface of myelin sheaths or myelin-forming oligodendrocytes. Both T cells and B cells are needed to produce demyelination in these animal models.

To determine how MS lesions are generated, it is essential for future research to sort out the precise roles of T cells, B cells, their target antigens, and other immune mechanisms. Greater understanding of immunopathology is pivotal for identifying new molecular and cellular targets for treatment. One key question is, Which cells are the actual pathogenic effector cells in the disease? Newly identified effector cells become candidates for immunospecific therapy.

Finally, the destruction of axons in MS lesions has gained attention, but how this destruction occurs is unknown. It remains unclear whether axons and the neuron cell bodies from which they extend are damaged by direct attack by CD8+ cytotoxic T cells, by other activated immune cells (microglia or macrophages), by soluble mediators of cytotoxicity, such as those contained in cytotoxic granules (for example, perforin and granzymes), or by cytokines and neurotransmitters. Axons and neuronal cell bodies can be induced to express MHC class I and thus, in principle, could be recognized by cytotoxic T cells (CTLs). Neurons can also be damaged by perforin released from cytotoxic T cells,[57,61] but the potential target autoantigen and the mode of autoimmune attack remain completely unknown. Experimental systems for studying neuronal injury in MS will have to be developed further to answer these questions.

## Identification of Pathogenic T Cells

Studies in healthy humans and primates have shown that peripheral blood lymphocytes normally contain numerous T-cell clones that are autoreactive to myelin antigens.[58,70,72] More importantly, two studies showed that some, but not all, of these myelin autoreactive T cells isolated from healthy primates have the potential to induce experimental autoimmune encephalomyelitis (EAE) upon transfer.[31,62]

As a consequence, assays must be developed for the identification and enumeration of pathogenic—as distinguished from merely autoreactive—T cells in the blood of MS patients. One possible approach is the construction of "humanized" animal models to allow monitoring of the pathogenic potential of individual T-cell clones. These could be transgenic rodents with a suitable complement of human immune genes[55] or immunodeficient mice carrying human tissue grafts serving as targets for potentially autoaggressive T cells. (*Autoreactive T cells* recognize an autoantigen but do not necessarily attack the autoantigen-presenting cells; an *autoaggressive T cell* is autoreactive, and, at the same time, will attack the autoantigen-presenting cells.) Alternatively, tissue culture systems could be developed to assess autoaggressive T-cell potential. Any technique that allows the identification of pathogenic T cells would provide a surrogate marker for assessing therapeutic efficacy.

### Direct Visualization of Autoantigen-Specific T Cells

Myelin autoreactive T cells have been identified in the peripheral blood or the cerebrospinal fluid (CSF) of MS patients using microculture techniques.[70,72] These techniques allowed the isolation and characterization of T-cell clones reactive against a variety of brain autoantigens. However, comparable clonal yields were found in the blood of MS patients and healthy donors. Unfortunately, cloning assays do not provide a reliable estimate of the absolute number of autoreactive T cells present within a particular blood sample, and they are of limited use in estimating fluctuations of brain-specific T-cell clones in MS patients over time.

Additional methods are required to correlate disease activity with the number of recirculating autoimmune T cells. These may include the use of recombinant MHC class II proteins complexed with autoantigenic peptide epitopes. These complexes resemble the MHC-peptide complexes formed on the surface of an antigen-presenting cell and therefore are bound to a specific T-cell receptor. Myelin basic protein (MBP) specific, class II restricted CD4 T cells, for example, bind recombinant complexes of appropriate MHC class II and peptide to their membrane receptors, and this binding can be visualized by fluorescence staining. The number of antigen-specific T cells can thus be quantified by cytofluorometry.

Recombinant MHC class I-peptide complexes have been used successfully to monitor the dynamics of T cells in microbial infection.[3] Complexes of class II with suitable peptide are now available.[15] To be of use in MS, complexes have to be tailored to contain both individual class II proteins (for example, those of the DR, DQ, or DP subclasses) and autoantigenic peptides suspected to have a role in the development of disease in a particular patient. Similar approaches, along with intracellular cytokine determination, ELISPOT (Enzyme-Linked ImmunoSPOT, an assay used to enumerate individual cytokine-secreting T cells), and T-cell receptor spectratyping technologies, will be of use in determining the number of T cells responding to altered peptide ligands and predicting their therapeutic effect in an individual.

## Identification of Target Autoantigens

For many years, it was assumed that MBP was the dominant, if not the only, myelin autoantigen in EAE and perhaps in MS. Later it became clear that numerous other CNS proteins, myelin or nonmyelin, can serve as targets of T-cell-mediated EAE. The ever-growing list of candidate autoantigens includes proteolipid protein (PLP), heat shock proteins, myelin oligodendrocyte glycoprotein (MOG), myelin-associated oligodendrocyte basic protein (MOBP), and S100b—a calcium-binding protein produced by astrocytes.

However, recent evidence indicates that not all autoantigens are equal: the antigen specificity of T cells may mediate EAE syndromes of different lesion locations, and different degrees of inflammation and clinical severity.[6] For example, T cells specific for MBP often mediate highly aggressive EAE in rodents, with lesions dominated by activated macrophages. In contrast, MOG- and S100b-specific T cells often induce huge infiltrates composed mainly of T cells, but with only marginal neurological deficits.[6]

It will be critically important, therefore, to identify all CNS autoantigens that can act as targets in MS and then to determine if there is a dominant autoantigen in individual patients and whether there are differences in clinical presentation with different principal autoantigens. Different autoantigens might predominate in different people because of individual variation in T-cell repertoire or in genetic makeup, or they might vary with different stages of disease. The significance of different CNS autoantigens is not yet known.

At present, the repertoire of strategies and technologies to determine potential target autoantigens is limited. Phage display technology refers to the insertion of a mutation at an appropriate location within the gene of a virus, resulting in the display of a mutation-encoded peptide on the surface of the virus.[82] Large-scale growth of the viral particle results in a library of peptides that are physically linked to the encoded DNA, allowing for identification of a single peptide, whose presence has been increased with the help of viral replication. Phage display libraries have been used to directly test potentially binding target autoantigens of B-cell-derived autoantigens.[17] In the case of T cells, which recognize peptide segments embedded in suitable MHC class I or class II products rather than native proteins, modified approaches must be developed. One example is the screening of large-scale libraries of synthetic peptide variants, which implies laborious determination of T-cell responses in multiple microcultures.[38] In any event, identification of autoantigens is crucial for designing more powerful and specific immunomodulatory therapies.

## Triggers of Autoimmune Attack

Studies of T-cell-mediated models of EAE have shown that brain-specific T cells are able to mediate EAE only when transferred directly after activation. However, the mechanisms that lead to the activation of an autoreactive T-cell population can be diverse. They can include presentation and recognition of the nominal antigen, as well as erroneous recognition of structurally similar microbial protein components ("mimicry"), microbial "superantigens," or global T-cell mitogens (such as phytohemogglutinin [PHA] and concanavalin A [ConA]).[100] T-cell mitogens activate lymphocytes by binding to carbohydrate components of T-cell receptors, which they do independently of antigens. They are thus "polyclonal" activators, because they activate many, if not all, T-cell clones at the same time.

Microbial factors can be critical in triggering an autoimmune attack. Indeed, in one model of transgenic mice with MBP-specific T-cell receptors, EAE developed only in animals exposed to a heavy microbial load, while unexposed mice remained healthy.[34] However, the further course of the autoimmune disease involves regulatory controls inherent in the immune system. Evidence for self-regulatory T cells has been identified in several transgenic EAE models. An early study pointed to CD8+ T cells,[43] while more recent work showed that CD4+ T cells could prevent spontaneous exacerbations of EAE.[69] In future MS research it will be important to identify precisely the self-tolerogenic regulatory T cells (especially of human equivalents), and to determine their mode of action and the location of the regulatory interactions. Regulatory T cells, also known as "suppressor cells," downregulate ongoing immune responses against self- or foreign antigens. Although the nature of these cells is still incompletely understood, they are important in fine-tuning the immune response. Certain regulatory cells might recognize peptide antigens, whereas others act independently of antigens. The entire field of regulation and suppression is still subject to debate.

Although it is likely that downregulation of autoimmune responses takes place in the immune tissues, the location of T-cell activation, for example by exposure to autoantigen, is less established. The development of local lesions in the CNS means of course that the autoantigen must be presented locally in the CNS. However, additional events, such as export of autoantigen via macrophages or dendritic cells warrant consideration. This possibility has recently received further attention because of the demonstration that dendritic cells preferentially engulf apoptotic parenchymal cells (such as oligodendrocytes), and then "home" to immune organs where they present their antigenic load to specific T cells.[90] The expansion of target epitopes, or epitope spreading, observed in some (but not all) models of EAE might involve presentation of autoantigen by dendritic cells. Thus, one hypothesis is that dendritic cells engulf apoptotic brain cells, then migrate out of the CNS into the peripheral immune system (lymph nodes), where they present protein components of these engulfed cells as autoantigens to specific autoreactive T cells. Such spreading of an autoimmune response might cause a relapse or exacerbation of the clinical disease.

## Clarifying the Role of B Cells and Antibodies

New emphasis is being placed on the role of B cells in MS. Upon transfer of T cells, most animal models display the inflammatory changes seen in the active MS plaque, but importantly, they do not exhibit large-scale demyelination. In rodent EAE, fully demyelinating, plaque-like lesions have been created by co-transferring autoimmune T cells along with autoantibodies bound to the surface of myelin, or oligodendrocytes, or both. These studies heralded MOG as a prominent target autoantigen for demyelinating autoantibodies (and B lymphocytes, implicitly).[48] The pathogenic role of antibodies to MOG was spotlighted by a recent study that found MOG-specific antibodies bound to myelin debris in active lesions in people with MS.[30]

These findings, along with evidence of antigen-driven clonal expansion of B lymphocytes in the MS brain,[76] urge new investigations into the physiological and pathological roles of B cells in inflammatory demyelination. Such investigations could include suitable transgenic experimental models with demyelinating B cells,[50] the development of technologies allowing the establishment of antigen-specific B-cell lines, and B-cell receptor grafting techniques, which have been successfully used in studies of T lymphocytes.[19] Further, these new approaches would be of help in learning more about the role of autoantigen-presenting B cells in inducing T cells toward a pro-inflammatory (Th1) or anti-inflammatory (Th2) cytokine-secreting phenotype.

## Neurotoxic T Cells

As discussed earlier in this chapter, axonal damage is a common feature of the MS lesion and it appears to be responsible for brain atrophy and long-term, irreversible neurological deficits, although the mechanisms leading to neuronal damage are unknown. Two recent reports described a protective effect of glutamate receptor antagonists in preventing destruction of myelin and axons in mouse models of EAE.[36,73] These observations are possibly related to the earlier discovery that neuroreactive T cells profoundly interfere with the electrical conductance of axons in optic nerve explant cultures, a process requiring histocompatibility between lymphocytes and CNS tissue.[104] In addition, cytotoxic CD8+ T cells are able to kill neurons by release of perforin, possibly also a process involving glutamate cytotoxicity.[57]

Clearly, the new field of T-cell neurotoxicity will require much attention. The conditions of antigen presentation by neurons must be better understood, and there are important deficits in our knowledge of the mechanisms by which T cells mediate damage to neurons.

Importantly, it now appears that neurons are by no means just passive targets of immune destruction. It has become apparent that neurons have an essential role in regulating immune reactivity within the CNS. Intact neurons efficiently suppress the induction of immunologic molecules (MHC products, as well as humoral mediators), not only in surrounding glia cells but also in the neurons themselves. Nerve growth factor seems to be one mediator involved in this regulation.[67] Conversely, areas with failing neuronal function preferentially attract immune cells and favor local inflammatory responses, as in Alzheimer's disease and other cases of neurodegeneration.

Research into the interactions between neurons and immune cells thus may shed light on the generation of MS lesions and generate new therapeutic targets.

## Gene Expression in MS Lesions: Microarrays and Proteomics

Thus far, most explorations of autoimmune interactions have relied either on global, morphological descriptions of CNS lesions or on the study of isolated cell cultures. Both approaches have quite narrow technical limits. More recently, techniques are emerging that allow direct and detailed investigation of the cellular microenvironment in situ. They combine the advantages of in vitro and in vivo approaches.

One example is the isolation of single cells from tissue sections followed by exploration of the expressed genome using microarrays.[54] This new technology, also known as gene chip technology, can profile gene expression patterns for thousands of genes simultaneously. Microarrays, especially if combined with biological markers,[28] may lead to better understanding of cell-to-cell interactions in MS CNS lesions. Microarrays are useful to identify and quantify genes involved in a response—but the actual function of these activated genes must be verified via functional tests.

Another emerging technology to be used in determining disease-related changes in the CNS and immune organs comes from proteomics. In contrast to a global genetic approach, proteomics uses microtechniques to first separate protein units of a particular tissue (or cell populations) and then identify these molecules by microsequencing methods. Proteomics yields information about protein concentrations and posttranscriptional chemical modifications, neither of which can necessarily be predicted on the basis of mRNA expression via microarrays. Thus, proteomic approaches are the ultimate tool to characterize the *expressed* gene repertoire.

## Therapeutic Perspectives

Initial strategies to design immunotherapies were aimed at physically eliminating, or functionally blocking, pathogenic T cells. One such strategy, vaccination, was tested as a possible approach to activate immunoregulatory mechanisms that could suppress the autoimmune T-cell response. Vaccinations with inactivated, "mitigated" autoreactive T-cell lines[5] or peptide segments representing their antigen receptors were tested.[94] There have also been attempts to "blindfold" pathogenic T cells, for example, by injecting either peptide antagonists that bind to restricting MHC loci or soluble MHC class II proteins complexed with autoantigenic peptide.

More recently, researchers have attempted to modify the pathogenic potential of autoreactive T cells by exposing them to altered peptide ligands. Under optimal conditions, they may reeducate the T cells to produce anti-inflammatory cytokines instead of their natural pro-inflammatory products. However, it is not clear whether these T-cell modulatory therapies will work. Although such treatments may benefit some patients, they might aggravate the disease in others. As pointed out earlier, diagnostic tests allowing the exact monitoring of immune status will be indispensable to safe application of these approaches.

A more radical therapy uses brain-specific T cells merely as vehicles to transport therapeutically effective transgenes through the endothelial blood-tissue barrier into the brain. For example, recombinant plasmid DNA and retroviruses have been used to express genes for neurotrophins or anti-inflammatory cytokines.[45,59,85] This approach must be tailored for each individual patient because it requires the isolation and engineering of T-cell clones from that patient.

## Cytokines in MS

Cytokines are intercellular signaling proteins produced by cells of the immune system and CNS. They are involved in various aspects of disease processes, including altering the permeability of blood-brain barrier, recruitment of inflammatory cells, cytotoxicity, but also stimulating repair processes.

### *Blood-Brain Barrier Permeability*

MS is characterized by significant infiltration of leukocytes into the CNS. Normally, the CNS is protected from leukocyte infiltration by the blood-brain barrier. This barrier consists of a layer of specialized endothelial cells, that are interconnected by tight junctions and foot-like projections of astrocytes, and it is responsible for the brain's "immunoprivileged" status. Only some highly activated lymphocytes pass through the resting blood-brain barrier. Among these are the freshly activated MBP-specific T cells that initiate the pathological processes culminating in EAE.[101]

After T cells reach and recognize their CNS targets, they become activated, thereby triggering a complex series of inflammatory events that enhance the permeability of the blood-brain barrier. The mediators of this complex process are pro-inflammatory cytokines (for example, interleukin-1 [IL-1] and tumor necrosis factor-α [TNF-α]) and chemokines produced and released locally within the CNS by activated glia cells (also by endothelial cells).[39] As a consequence of their release, endothelial cells acquire a new set of cell adhesion molecules, to which recirculating lymphocytes and monocytes adhere in order to gain access to the CNS. One adhesion molecule is VCAM-1, which binds to the receptor, VLA-4, that is expressed on activated lymphocytes and serves as a signal to recruit activated lymphocytes into the brain. In EAE, the interaction between endothelial cells and lymphocytes leads to a massive invasion of inflammatory cells into the CNS, a process that results in a general permeabilization of the blood-brain barrier. Leukocyte enzymes, including matrix metalloproteinases and glycosidases, digest the extracellular blood-brain barrier matrix, including the basement membrane, thereby loosening the inter-endothelial junctions.[53] The critical importance of adhesion molecules and chemokines has been demonstrated in animal models in which immunization with antibodies against adhesion molecules and chemokines prevented the onset of EAE.[41] Other cytokines, such as transforming growth factor-β (TGF-β) and IL-10, might be involved in reversing the process of blood-brain barrier permeability.

It is well established that the blood-brain barrier becomes more permeable during inflammatory attacks in MS, yet the cytokines, chemokines, and other molecular mechanisms underlying enhanced permeability are just beginning to be defined.[33] Greater understanding of key events that initiate blood-brain barrier permeability and trafficking of immune cells into the CNS may lead to means for preventing the development of MS lesions or controlling the degree of inflammation once an MS attack is in progress. Fresh experimental and clinical studies are required to identify the best therapeutic targets.

## Cell-Cell Interactions in Inflammation

In the active MS lesion, cytokines appear to be responsible for recruitment of inflammatory cells, astrocytes, and microglia into the inflammatory process by causing their migration, proliferation, and activation. Production of TNF-α, IL-1, and interferon-γ (IFN-γ) for instance, has been implicated in the production of EAE in rodents and in the progression of MS. Other cytokines that have been demonstrated to be elevated in MS patients also possess anti-inflammatory properties. These include TGF-β, IL-6, IL-4 and IL-10. In EAE models, administration of IL-4, IL-10, TGF-β, or IL-13 can ameliorate clinical and histological disease by downregulating aspects of the inflammatory response.

## Cytotoxicity

Cytokine signaling contributes to cell dysfunction and death by inducing antibody and complement production, direct activation of cell death signaling pathways, and induction of antigen-presenting class II MHC molecules on both glial and inflammatory cells. Cytokine signaling also contributes to the generation of toxic intermediaries such as hydrogen peroxide and nitric oxide in macrophages, glia, and astrocytes. Direct toxicity of cytokines to oligodendroglial cells has not been convincingly demonstrated.

## Induction of Restorative Processes

Paradoxically, several cytokines can also induce what can be considered protective, restorative, or reparative processes in the brain. Several cytokines, including IL-6, TGF-β, and ciliary neurotrophic factor (CNTF), both protect and support the proliferation of oligodendroglia. Pro-inflammatory cytokines, such as IL-1, perpetuate lesion production, yet they also induce the production of counter-regulatory cytokines that dampen the immune response and stimulates the production of neurotrophic factors. For example, TGF-β is a potent chemotactic factor for inflammatory cells, yet it also inhibits aspects of immune function. It is also an important differentiation factor for oligodendrocytes. It is thus vital to understand the precise temporal patterning of cytokine release, interactions, and responses, as well as the nature and localization of cytokine receptors and the specificity of intracellular signaling pathways that they command. The precise roles of various cytokine and cytokine-related molecules in dampening the inflammatory process and initiating restorative mechanisms in the MS plaque is a fertile area for future research.

## Cytokine Production as a Systemic Marker of Disease Activity

Cytokine levels and the production of cytokines by circulating peripheral blood cells have reportedly been increased in MS patient sera and CSF. Increased TNF levels have been observed in the prodromal period before an attack, but they do not correlate with disease activity as shown by MRI. Careful, prospective longitudinal profiling of cytokine activity in the periphery may give clues to predict the pattern of disease activity in patients.

## Cytokines and Cytokine Antagonists as Therapeutic Agents

The demonstrated utility of beta-interferon in the clinical management of MS is presumably due to its ability to downregulate inflammatory cytokine activity and perhaps to enhance the activity of anti-inflammatory cytokines such as IL-

10. Other anticytokine approaches have not yet proven their utility. Agents with promising results in animal models (for example, IFN-γ and anti-TNF, which are effective in EAE models) have not been successful when tested in humans with MS. Many cytokine-based strategies are currently under development. There are currently no cytokine-based strategies other than the use of corticosteroids, which appear to alter the course of individual MS attacks. In the absence of completely effective disease course-modifying agents, the availability of anticytokine therapies with the ability to interrupt the acute disease process would be desirable.

## IDENTIFICATION OF INFECTIOUS AGENTS IN MS

Standard and conventional approaches to the isolation of pathogens in MS have failed to find any consistent and convincing result. For this reason, it seems appropriate to pursue new directions with respect to the identification of an etiologic agent. These approaches should pursue cultivation-independent methods primarily involving the identification of genomic information relevant to the pathogen. The methods include polymerase chain reaction (PCR), differential sequence analysis based on subtraction or display, and sequence screening using the host immune response. These new directions are especially attractive since the powerful methods that will be employed in these studies have not yet been applied to investigations of MS tissues in any concerted and organized way.

One method of differential sequence analysis, representational difference analysis, has recently been used successfully to identify a new pathogenic herpesvirus in Kaposi's sarcoma. Representational difference analysis employs PCR to amplify DNA fragments that are present in the diseased tissue, but not in healthy tissue from the same patient. The identification of even a small amount of sequence information may be sufficient to characterize the agent.

In addition, it might be valuable to probe tissues for transcription expression profiles that are associated with particular pathogens. This will involve microchip array approaches.

The use of phage display libraries as a screen for the antigenic target of oligoclonal immunoglobulin G (IgG) is a valuable method, however, there may be problems interpreting these studies. The antigenic targets of the oligoclonal IgG may be merely a result of immunodysregulation rather than relevant from an etiological point of view.

Methods similar to those used to probe the antigenic target of oligoclonal IgG can be used to identify the antigenic targets of T cells that are present in the MS brain. The results are more difficult to interpret in the case of T cells than B cells, since the antigenic targets that are identified in the case of the T-cell target epitopes might have little sequence identity with the actual sequence of the antigen within the MS brain.[103] Isolation of peptides from human leukocyte antigen (HLA) class I molecules followed by purification and Edman sequencing or mass spectrometry should also be valuable as a means of identifying cytolytic T-cell epitopes. In some situations, however, the application of these techniques can be time-consuming and problematic because of the complexity and low abundance of the epitopes presented.

## IDENTIFICATION OF DISEASE SUBTYPES

Identification of specific biologic or surrogate markers that characterize each of the different disease subtypes will help determine whether the different disease subtypes represent distinct entities or are, instead, a spectrum of single pathogenic disorders. If the latter is true, it will be important to determine what modifies disease expression. The identification of markers of disease phenotype would also permit one to identify these forms prior to full clinical expression and to determine the effectiveness of therapy.

Improved identification of different disease subtypes could be derived from clinical observations, neuroimaging, and genetic or acquired biological markers. The biological markers to be considered would include those related to products of the immune system (immunological) and products of the nervous system (neurobiological). The latter could reflect tissue injury or repair.

### Clinical Data Collections

Organized clinics focused on MS have been in existence for more than 25 years. Most have attempted to adopt standardized measures to document neurological status, clinical disease course, and occurrence of clinical relapses. National and international clinical databases have been and continue to be developed (EDMUS in Europe, Costar in Canada). No one uniform database has been adopted, although measures of neurological disability have become standardized. Emerging data from these databases are providing important information on the relation between early clinical patterns of disease and subsequent disease course. The overall scope of existing databases in different regions of the world remains to be documented. Comparative studies would help confirm observations already reported and identify regional differences (see also discussion of data registries in Chapter 6).

### Neuroimaging

In the context of disease heterogeneity, one would wish to know whether lesion frequency and topography as defined by current MRI techniques correlate with specific clinical or pathologically defined disease phenotypes. MRI studies indicate that single clinical episodes have markedly different prognoses with regard to recurrent disease, depending on the presence or absence of multifocal lesions. Further data are needed to define the imaging correlates of either human cases of MS or animal demyelinating models with distinct pathologies. Neuroimaging could facilitate the classification of patients with regard to their prognosis and the identification of subgroups of patients that would respond best to different treatment strategies. If patterns of neuropathology revealed by neuroimaging could be linked to biochemical, immunological, or genetic markers, it might become possible to understand the variation among patients in the clinical course of their disease. In general, neuroimaging should play a critical role in bridging the gap between understanding the underlying biological mechanisms of the disease and the resulting damage to the brain and spinal cord.

New methods in neuroimaging are described in a later section.

## Biological Markers

One would like to develop markers that reflect or serve as surrogates for the actual biology of the disease process. We do not yet know what the critical biological mediators of the disease process are. One would have to establish whether such markers also serve as surrogates for the clinical disease course.

The interpretation of measures of biological markers during clinical trials can be complex. One could theoretically derive the following during a clinical trial with a new agent (Table 5.1).

### Genetic Markers

Specific genetic markers are covered in greater depth in Chapter 2. Genes related to immune function are candidate markers of disease susceptibility or progression. Precedent exists in animals for the importance of genes regulating

**TABLE 5.1** Hypothetical Results of a Clinical Trial

| Clinical Response | Biological Marker | Implications |
|---|---|---|
| Positive | Correlates with clinical response | One would still have to determine whether there is a true cause-effect relation, but such a result would encourage seeking more selective agents that act on this marker |
| Positive | Does not correlate with clinical response | No conclusion is possible |
| Negative | Altered by therapy response | Biological marker is not central to the disease |
| Negative | No change | No conclusion |

blood-brain barrier permeability and antigen presentation within the CNS. In the EAE model, disease susceptibility and disease course are highly dependent on which mouse strain is studied.

## Acquired Markers

One has to consider both what to measure and from which body compartment one can obtain the necessary samples to perform the measure. The site of injury in MS, namely the CNS tissue, is not routinely available for clinical correlative-type studies. The CSF is considered to more closely reflect events that occur in the CNS than does the peripheral blood compartment, but it is also not readily available, especially for serial analyses.

## Immunologic Markers

The most accepted postulate regarding MS pathogenesis is that the disease process is initiated by autoreactive T cells that migrate from the systemic compartment into the CNS. The status of the overall immune environment may be a critical factor in determining the extent and persistence of the initial response. As the disease evolves, this initial immune response may expand to involve additional antigens (determinant spreading). The actual effectors of tissue injury could involve a wide array of immune mediators derived from the adaptive ($\alpha\beta$ T cells, antibody) and innate (macrophages, NK [natural killer] cells, $\gamma\delta$ T cells) immune systems.

Immunologic markers would be relevant in MS with regard to defining a disease-related antigen, that is, identifying the presence of a T-cell or B-cell population in MS patients that reacts with a candidate disease-relevant antigen, and demonstrating ongoing immune activation or altered immune regulation that contributes to autoimmunity.

## T-Cell-Related Markers

The molecular events associated with antigen presentation, cell activation, and migration have increasingly been defined. Studies of disease-specific immune responses—the measurement of antigen reactive T cells—are dependent on having a candidate disease-relevant antigen. Most studies continue to focus on myelin antigens, although the same assay techniques could be applied to any such candidate. These assays are considered in terms of whether they require in vitro manipulation of the cells or whether they are based on ex vivo analysis of harvested cells.

**In Vitro Manipulation Required.** Repeated cycles of stimulation with the selected antigen is the classic technique used to generate and determine the frequency of antigen-specific T cells. At issue is whether the properties of the derived cells, such as their T-cell receptor (TCR) phenotype and cytokine production profiles, are representative of the in vivo situation. Memory T-cell stimulation assays can be done in which memory cells are enriched either by addition of IL-7 or by preselecting cells that have undergone somatic mutation (HPRT mutant T cells).[51]

**Analysis of Harvested Ex Vivo Cells.** These techniques remain to be established and standardized. Single-cell PCR techniques are used to sequence the TCR of individual T cells and compare them to the sequence of myelin-reactive T-cell clones derived by in vitro cell culture (as above).

Tetramer technology allows one to assess the direct binding of labeled peptide-MHC constructs to T cells. The MHC tetramer technology is a general, robust and extremely powerful method for the precise and rapid measurement of T cell responses to a broad range of antigens. (MHC tetramers consist of four complexes of an antigenic peptide, beta-2 microglobulin and a biotinylated MHC class I molecule conjugated to streptavidin linked to a fluorescent marker, hence the name *tetramer.*) The ability to link multiple MHC class I/peptide complexes together allows for identification of specific receptor-bearing T cells by flow cytometry. In addition, investigators can use tetramers to quickly and efficiently purify a specific T-cell population using fluorescent activated cell sorting (FACS).

Other T-cell related markers include assays for antigen presentation, T-cell activation, and T-cell migration.

**Antigen Presentation.** T-cell activation by antigen is dependent on antigen presentation in context of MHC molecules in the presence of costimulatory molecules (CD40/CD40L; CD80:86/B27:CTLA-4) expressed on the antigen-presenting cell (monocytes, dendritic cells, B cells). Levels of expression of many of these molecules are themselves subject to regulation by cytokines. MHC and costimulatory molecules can be monitored by antibody fluorescence-activated cell sorter (FACS) analysis techniques.

**T-Cell Activation.** When activated, T cells upregulate an array of surface molecules that contribute to their capacity to proliferate (IL-2 receptor) and migrate (adhesion molecules, chemokine receptors). These cell surface molecules can be assayed by immunostaining and FACS analysis as described in the previous section.

Activated T cells increase the production of soluble molecules (cytokines) that promote communication between cells of the immune system, between immune cells and cells that form the vascular barriers, and between immune cells and cells within specific body compartments. Families of cytokines are identified that promote (pro-inflammatory or Th1—IFNγ and TNF) or inhibit (anti-inflammatory or Th2—IL-4, 5, and 13) the inflammatory response. Antigen-presenting cells also produce cytokines that can regulate immune function (TNF, IL-10, TGF, IL-12, IL-1).

Cytokines can be assayed in terms of either protein or mRNA by a number of methods. The former includes the techniques of intracellular cytokine staining (ICS) and ELISPOT. The latter involve PCR or RNA protection assays. DNA microarray techniques, focused on the immune system, are beginning to be used as a means to survey for a wide array of known and unknown genes. The ideal would be to analyze immune cells directly ex vivo, but the low level of cytokines has often required the use of in vitro activation techniques to amplify the signal. In vitro, one can apply enzyme-linked immunosorbent assay (ELISA) measures to the supernatant in which cells are cultured. Measures of serum cytokine levels do not permit one to determine what cell is the source of the molecule being measured.

Measures of cytokine levels in the CSF have been technically difficult to perform due to the paucity of cells present in MS cases and the low levels that can be detected in the fluid.

**T-Cell Migration.** This property can be assessed either in functional assays or in terms of participating molecules. In the context of migration of lymphocytes into the CNS, in vitro models of blood-brain barrier have been used. These include assessment of lymphocyte adherence to isolated microvessels or migration through barriers comprised of extracellular matrix proteins or endothelial cells. The molecular families involved in the migration process include chemokines and chemokine receptors, adhesion molecules (such as integrins and selectins), and proteases such as the matrix metalloproteinases that digest the extracellular matrix.

There is an extensive literature indicating that the release of immunoregulatory molecules described above correlates with clinically or MRI-defined disease activity in MS. There are significant differences related to disease phase (for example, IL-12 and IFN-γ levels are higher in mononuclear blood cells from primary progressive MS patients than in those from relapsing-remitting MS patients) and disease phenotype (for example, lymphocyte migration rate and IFN-γ production are increased in primary progressive patients with high lesion volume compared to primary progressive patients with low lesion volume).[75]

## B-Cell-Related Markers

In terms of disease-specific immune responses, the direct approach has been to look for the presence of antibodies in the serum or CSF that may directly participate in the MS disease process. The search has focused largely on myelin-directed antibodies. These can be assayed directly from serum or CSF. An alternative approach has been to determine whether stimulated blood or CSF-derived cells produce such antibodies in vitro.

There has long been recognition of the oligoclonality of the immunoglobulin fraction of the CSF in MS (oligoclonal bands). Molecular biologic techniques have been used to sequence the hypervariable regions of the immunoglobulin genes expressed by B cells recovered from CSF or CNS tissues of MS cases, usually of recent onset.[76,86] These studies have shown significant restriction of the B-cell repertoire. The search now focuses on what antigen is being recognized by these specific immunoglobulin molecules.

More indirect evidence of antibody participation in the immune response in MS is provided by reports of increased presence of autoantibody-producing B-cell populations (CD5+) and by detection of immune products such as those of the complement cascade and immune complexes that participate in antibody-mediated immune responses.

## Neurobiological Markers

These can be considered in terms of molecules produced by resident cells of the CNS that reflect interaction with the constituents of the immune system and in terms of molecules that reflect the tissue injury or repair process. Again, here one faces the dilemma that CNS tissue cannot be readily sampled; thus, one is dependent on measures of molecules that are shed from the tissues and reach either the CSF or a systemic compartment.

**CNS Immune Interaction-Related Markers.** For such studies, the cell source of the markers being measured is not always certain since, in most cases; the molecules can be produced by both the immune system and the resident CNS cells. The CSF would for the most part seem preferable to blood for conducting such assays. Molecules to be measured are those with which lymphocytes interact during the migration process (chemokines, adhesion molecules), those that are expressed by resident CNS cells in their role as antigen-presenting cells, and those that may serve as targets of immune effector mechanisms (fas, TNF receptor).

**CNS Injury and Repair Markers.** With the evidence that oligodendrocytes and myelin are injured as part of the MS disease process, the CSF (± blood) can be assayed for the presence of products that would reflect such injury. The presence of myelin debris and MBP can be demonstrated in the CSF when there is active tissue destruction in MS cases. Although MBP-like material was found in serum and urine, this material has now been identified as *p*-cresol sulfate. Since myelin regeneration is now also a recognized feature of MS, the search for molecules that are upregulated during the repair process should also be undertaken.

With the recent emphasis on the contribution of axonal injury to neurologic disability in MS, there is a search for axonal products that would be released consequent to such injury. These would be the same candidates as those claimed to be released in other tissue-destructive CNS disorders (for example, neurofilament proteins).

The marked response of astrocytes in the MS disease process (the basis of "sclerosis") suggests that astrocyte-derived molecules could also be detected.

# TECHNOLOGIES AND RESEARCH STRATEGIES

## New Methods in MRI

Magnetic resonance imaging is a nonradioactive, noninvasive way to produce images of internal structures such as the brain. MRI has been an important tool for studying the characteristic white matter lesions of MS.

The varying amounts of water in different structures within the brain produce the light and dark regions of an MRI image.[71] The viscosity, temperature, and general molecular structure of a brain region also affect the MRI signal.[40] Like a photographic flash bulb, contrast agents increase this signal. Older methods used contrast agents as general image enhancers. Now researchers can use contrast agents to selectively enhance visualization of specific tissues or cell types. With this technique, immune cells have been visualized as they traveled to an inflammation site[105] or rejection site of a transplanted organ in the rat (Chien Ho, personal communication). Implanted stem cells or genetically altered cells might be tracked this way, as could the immune cellular involvement in demyelination and remyelination. In the EAE mouse model, this technique could allow researchers to watch immune cells migrate to the CNS long before any obvious damage occurs. With improved methods of targeting, they might be able to determine which immune cells lead the attack on myelin and the remyelination process.

Improvements in MRI equipment and methodology have increased the level of resolution of the images as well as the MRI signal-to-noise ratio. In particular, new ways to use contrast agents have great potential for investigating the early stages of MS.

Another new application for contrast agents uses one of two different methods to "turn on" a contrasting agent only in certain cells. Both rely on a contrast agent, such as gadolinium, that is injected in a caged (chemically neutralized) form into animals. Caged gadolinium cannot do its job as a contrast agent until it is released from its chemical enclosure. In the first method, the cage is made with a sort of hinged door that opens in response to cellular signaling molecules, such as calcium. This method has been used in frog embryos to see cell groups with active calcium signaling (Scott Fraser, personal communication). In the EAE mouse, this technique might highlight cell signaling and biochemical changes that occur in the CNS or in immune cells long before lesions are apparent.

In the second method, an enzyme cuts open the cage and releases gadolinium. Researchers have made frog embryos that produce the necessary enzyme only in certain cells. When the caged gadolinium and the enzyme are in the same cell, gadolinium is released and these cells light up on the MRI image.[52] Researchers can use this technique to probe when and where specific proteins are made.

For each protein there is a piece of DNA, a gene, that is the molecular blueprint for that protein. This blueprint includes the information that tells a cell when it should make the protein. This information is called the promoter. Researchers can take the promoter from one gene, such as the TNF-α promoter, and hook it up to another gene, in this case the gene for the uncaging enzyme. This engineered DNA is then put into a mouse, so that whenever a cell in that mouse makes the TNF-α protein, it will also make the uncaging enzyme. In combination with the caged contrast agent, MRI images from this mouse will show which cells make TNF-α. In an EAE mouse, this technique might provide information about which proteins are made early in diseased animals and which might have a direct effect on lesion formation.

These new MRI techniques hold great promise for increasing our understanding of animal models of MS and, perhaps eventually, the disease itself. Because they are applicable to large fields of research, such as developmental biology and immunology, our knowledge of their advantages and limitations should grow rapidly.

## Genes and Genomics

Available data support the hypothesis that inherited susceptibility to MS involves the interaction of different susceptibility genes, each of which individually contributes a small amount to the overall risk. Whole genome screens confirm the importance of the major histocompatibility complex region in chromosome 6p21 in conferring susceptibility to MS. Susceptibility is likely to be mediated by the MHC class II genes themselves (DR, DQ, or both) and is most likely related to the known function of these molecules in the normal immune response, antigen-binding, and T-cell repertoire determination. The data also show that although the MHC region carries significant susceptibility, much of the genetic effect in MS remains to be explained. By analogy to emerging data on the genetic basis of experimental autoimmune demyelination, it will be of particular interest to identify whether some gene loci are involved in the initial pathogenic events while others influence the development and progression of the disease.

The following genetic approaches should be pursued:

1. Groups and consortia with the appropriate experimental, clinical, and financial resources should be supported to continue the analysis of the

MS genome with larger DNA data sets and dense and informative genetic markers, for example, single nucleotide polymorphisms (SNPs). In all likelihood, the use of phenotypic and demographic variables will assume increasing importance as stratifying elements for genetic studies of MS and in addressing the fundamental question of genotype-phenotype correlation in autoimmune demyelination. These studies will necessarily be linked to the development of novel mathematical formulations designed to identify modest genetic effects, as well as epistatic interactions between multiple genes and interactions between genetic, clinical, and environmental factors.

2. With the advances in deciphering the human genome code and sequences readily available in the public domain, analysis will focus on the detailed analysis of candidate genes, particularly genes located in chromosomal segments linked to MS susceptibility. The problematic "case-control" population-based studies with limited statistical power will be replaced by the analysis of large collections of nuclear or singleton families (the patient and the biological parents or the patient and healthy siblings) using transmission-disequilibrium test (TDT) and Sib-TDT tests of association. For complex disorders such as MS, genomic analysis of multiple candidate genes must be performed on an extremely large group of individuals if small genetic effects are to be detected. Hence, key to the success of the proposed studies will be the availability of rapid, reliable, non-labor-intensive methods for high-throughput polymorphism screening. The inclusion of non-Caucasian patient populations, both in their native environment and after migration, will provide important new insights and clues about MS genetic and clinical heterogeneity.

3. The critical importance of identifying rare families that might have a monogenic variant of MS cannot be overstated; this approach has been extraordinarily fruitful in neurodegenerative diseases such as Alzheimer's disease and Parkinson's disease.

4. Continued analysis of the genes responsible for different forms of demyelinating disease in experimental models such as EAE and Theiler's virus infection is likely to identify syntenic regions in humans that may prove fruitful in MS.

5. Studies with DNA microarrays (DNA chips) to look at the coordinated expression, in both the CNS and the periphery, of ensembles of critical genes encoding cytokines, adhesion molecules, metalloproteinases, molecules involved in apoptosis, and molecules participating in myelin destruction and repair will contribute to our understanding of how these genes influence susceptibility and pathogenesis in MS. As gene chip methodologies mature, there is also the opportunity to perform wider

"whole-genome" analyses of gene expression unbiased by the selection of known candidate genes (see Box 5.1).

6. Gender differences in genetic susceptibility to MS have been well documented. Rigorous studies assessing the potential role of genetic factors in MS sexual dimorphism have not yet been performed. Further, reproductive history in females such as pregnancy and breastfeeding may influence disease pathogenesis. Genomic, clinical, and reproductive information should be combined to investigate potential MS risk factors in large groups of female patients.

---

**BOX 5.1**
**Tracking Gene Activity in Disease: Microarray Technology**

Scientists use genes to figure out what is going on in a cell. Genes are the molecular master switches. The 100,000 or so human genes control everything from how a cell grows to how it responds in times of stress and disease. In the past, researchers have been able to study only a handful of genes at a time. (Imagine trying to navigate in Boston with a road map that shows only two streets.) With microarray technology, scientists can simultaneously keep tabs on thousands of genes. For the first time, researchers can generate detailed genetic profiles of cells. These profiles can give us an integrated picture of gene regulation that can help explain susceptibility to MS and the mechanisms behind myelin destruction and disease progression and even suggest new directions for therapy.

Genes are the functional units in genetic material, or DNA. Each gene is the molecular blueprint for a particular protein. When a gene is turned on (or expressed), it is used as a template to make RNA. This RNA, in turn, serves as the working copy of the blueprint, instructing the cell to build that protein.

Genes are turned on and off in different situations, and their expression patterns provide important clues about what is going on in a cell, tissue, or organism. For example, in the central nervous system of mice with experimental autoimmune encephalomyelitis (EAE), a model for MS, there is increased expression of genes for chemokines.[42] These are small proteins that regulate immune responses. Chemokine expression in the CNS is just one of the many pieces of evidence demonstrating that the immune system plays a role in EAE (and also MS). Microarrays measure the expression patterns of many genes simultaneously.

A microarray, as the name suggests, is a microscopic array of DNA targets. Each target corresponds to a region of a gene. Each of the DNA targets on the array will specifically bind (or hybridize) only to DNA with a complementary sequence. A robot precisely spots the DNA target onto the substrate (for example, a glass microscope slide or membrane). Arrays can contain as many as 300,000 targets on a $1.28\text{-cm}^2$ surface.[49] Researchers commonly use microarray technology to compare gene expression between two samples, for example, RNA from a brain region in an EAE mouse that is in remission versus a mouse that has relapsed. In this case, researchers use each RNA sample as a template to make

*continues*

complementary DNA (cDNA). Incorporated into the cDNA is a fluorescent dye. Using a different dye for each cDNA sample (for example, a red dye for the remission sample and a green dye for the relapsed sample), researchers can visualize the two populations simultaneously.

The combined, fluorescently labeled cDNAs bind, or hybridize, to the target DNA on the array. Following the removal of unbound DNA, the microarray will contain a representation of the relative amounts of RNA from the two samples. Using a laser to excite the fluorescent dyes and a confocal microscope to read the emitted light, researchers can measure the fluorescence at a given DNA target. The ratio of the two fluorescent signals (for example, the amount of red versus green fluorescence) corresponds to the relative amounts of RNA for that target in the two samples. (Some researchers hybridize with one sample, remove the sample, and then hybridize with the second sample, or they compare side-by-side hybridizations on two separate arrays.) It is then up to computers and ever-improving data analysis programs to process these huge amounts of data into a format that is both meaningful and easy to understand.[22,106]

As with any method, it is important to understand both the strengths and the limitations of using microarrays. This technology has given researchers a means to monitor thousands of genes simultaneously. Yet when a scientist contemplates a list of the hundred or so genes that are turned on or off in the relapsing EAE mouse, it is difficult to determine which of these may be important. Also, because sequencing projects have leapt far ahead of the actual annotation of the genome, the function of many of these genes is unknown. Finding the truly significant results will become easier as data analysis improves and as researchers generate and make available more experimental data about gene expression in MS.

Reproducibility is also a concern in microarray studies. RNA is notoriously unstable. If not handled properly, duplicate samples (even those taken from the same batch of tissue) can vary greatly. Well-planned experiments incorporate various controls within the hybridization. (This also allows researchers to compare data from one experiment to the next.) Researchers also routinely confirm microarray results with older methods that look at expression changes in one gene at a time.

Collecting the sample is itself an important issue, especially when, as in the case of MS, researchers are analyzing human RNA. Microarrays use relatively large amounts of RNA, and increased risk of RNA degradation is greater in postmortem samples than in samples collected from living tissue.[11] However, ethical considerations limit the use of fresh human tissue.

Sample homogeneity is another consideration. The brain is made up of many cell types, each of which express different genes. For the sake of accurate comparisons (both within and across experiments), researchers must collect precisely defined samples (for example, through the use of microdissection).[11]

Finally, it is important to consider what microarrays measure. These techniques measure only relative levels of gene expression. Moreover, turning a gene on is just the beginning of the story. The real cellular actors are the proteins. Many proteins, once they are built, are not active until they undergo further processing in the cell, or their actions can change under different cellular conditions. Although microarrays have greatly expanded our view of life in a cell, they still reveal only part of the picture. We will have to wait for such advances as complete genome annotation and protein arrays to capture the entire panorama.

7. A significant number of MS patients are refractory to treatment. Genetic polymorphisms in drug receptors, metabolizing enzymes, transporters, and targets have been linked to interindividual differences in the efficacy and toxicity of many medications. Studies will directly address the question of genetic heterogeneity in MS and the response to immunotherapy by analysis of the correlation between different genotypes and clinical response to therapeutic modalities ("pharmacogenomics").

## REFERENCES

1. Abbott NJ. 2000. Inflammatory mediators and modulation of blood-brain barrier permeability. *Cell Mol Neurobiol.*;20:131-47.
2. Aloisi F, Ria F, Penna G, Adorini L. 1998. Microglia are more efficient than astrocytes in antigen processing and in Th1 but not Th2 cell activation. *J Immunol.*;160:4671-80.
3. Altman JD, Moss PAH, Goulder PJR, et al. 1996. Phenotypic analysis of antigen-specific T lymphocytes. *Science.*;274:94-6.
4. Barres BA, Chun LL, Corey DP. 1989. Glial and neuronal forms of the voltage-dependent sodium channel: characteristics and cell-type distribution. *Neuron.*;2:1375-88.
5. Ben-Nun A, Wekerle H, Cohen IR. 1981. Vaccination against autoimmune encephalomyelitis with T-lymphocyte line cells reactive against myelin basic protein. *Nature.*;292:60-1.
6. Berger T, Weerth S, Kojima K, Linington C, Wekerle H, Lassmann H. 1997. Experimental autoimmune encephalomyelitis: the antigen specificity of T lymphocytes determines the topography of lesions in the central and peripheral nervous system. *Lab Invest.*;76:355-64.
7. Bevan S, Chiu SY, Gray PT, Ritchie JM. 1985. The presence of voltage-gated sodium, potassium and chloride channels in rat cultured astrocytes. *Proc R Soc Lond B Biol Sci.*;225:299-313.
8. Bicknese AR, Sheppard AM, O'Leary DD, Pearlman AL. 1994. Thalamocortical axons extend along a chondroitin sulfate proteoglycan-enriched pathway coincident with the neocortical subplate and distinct from the efferent path. *J Neurosci.*;14:3500-10.
9. Black JA, Dib-Hajj S, Baker D, Newcombe J, Cuzner ML, Waxman SG. 2000. Sensory neuron specific sodium channel SNS is abnormally expressed in the brains of mice with experimental allergic encephalomyelitis and humans with multiple sclerosis. *Proc Natl Acad Sci U S A.*;97:11598-11602.
10. Black JA, Waxman SG, Smith ME. 1987. Macromolecular structure of axonal membrane during acute experimental allergic encephalomyelitis in rat and guinea pig spinal cord. *J Neuropathol Exp Neurol.*;46:167-84.
11. Bowtell DD. 1999. Options available—from start to finish—for obtaining expression data by microarray. *Nat Genet.*;21:25-32.
12. Buonomano DV, Merzenich MM. 1998. Cortical plasticity: from synapses to maps. *Annu Rev Neurosci.*;21:149-86.
13. Calford MB, Tweedale R. 1991. Immediate expansion of receptive fields of neurons in area 3b of macaque monkeys after digit denervation. *Somatosens Mot Res.*;8:249-60.
14. Chambers WW, Liu CN, McCouch GP. 1973. Anatomical and physiological correlates of plasticity in the central nervous system. *Brain Behav Evol.*;8:5-26.
15. Cochran JR, Cameron TO, Stern LJ. 2000. The relationship of MHC-peptide binding and T cell activation probed using chemically defined MHC class II oligomers. *Immunity.*;12:241-50.
16. Cornet A, Bettelli E, Oukka M, et al. 2000. Role of astrocytes in antigen presentation and naive T-cell activation. *J Neuroimmunol.*;106:69-77.

17. Cortese I, Tafi R, Grimaldi LM, Martino G, Nicosia A, Cortese R. 1996. Identification of peptides specific for cerebrospinal fluid antibodies in multiple sclerosis by using phage libraries. *Proc Natl Acad Sci U S A.*;93:11063-7.

18. Davies SJ, Fitch MT, Memberg SP, Hall AK, Raisman G, Silver J. 1997. Regeneration of adult axons in white matter tracts of the central nervous system. *Nature.*;390:680-3.

19. Dembic Z, Haas W, Weiss S, et al. 1986. Transfer of specificity by murine alpha and beta T-cell receptor genes. *Nature.*;320:232-8.

20. Dugandzija-Novakovic S, Koszowski AG, Levinson SR, Shrager P. 1995. Clustering of Na+ channels and node of Ranvier formation in remyelinating axons. *J Neurosci.*;15:492-503.

21. England JD, Gamboni F, Levinson SR, Finger TE. 1990. Changed distribution of sodium channels along demyelinated axons. *Proc Natl Acad Sci U S A.*;87:6777-80.

22. Epstein CB, Butow RA. 2000. Microarray technology—enhanced versatility, persistent challenge. *Curr Opin Biotechnol.*;11:36-41.

23. Ferguson B, Matyszak MK, Esiri MM, Perry VH. 1997. Axonal damage in acute multiple sclerosis lesions. *Brain.*;120:393-9.

24. Fern R, Ransom BR, Stys PK, Waxman SG. 1993. Pharmacological protection of CNS white matter during anoxia: actions of phenytoin, carbamazepine and diazepam. *J Pharmacol Exp Ther.*;266:1549-55.

25. Fern R, Ransom BR, Waxman SG. 1995. Voltage-gated calcium channels in CNS white matter: role in anoxic injury. *J Neurophysiol.*;74:369-77.

26. Fern R, Waxman SG, Ransom BR. 1995. Endogenous GABA attenuates CNS white matter dysfunction following anoxia. *J Neurosci.*;15:699-708.

27. Fitch MT, Silver J. 1997. Glial cell extracellular matrix: boundaries for axon growth in development and regeneration. *Cell Tissue Res.*;290:379-84.

28. Flugel A, Willem M, Berkowicz T, Wekerle H. 1999. Gene transfer into CD4+ T lymphocytes: green fluorescent protein-engineered, encephalitogenic T cells illuminate brain autoimmune responses. *Nat Med.*;5:843-7.

29. Foster RE, Whalen CC, Waxman SG. 1980. Reorganization of the axon membrane in demyelinated peripheral nerve fibers: morphological evidence. *Science.*;210:661-3.

30. Genain CP, Cannella B, Hauser SL, Raine CS. 1999. Identification of autoantibodies associated with myelin damage in multiple sclerosis. *Nat Med.*;5:170-5.

31. Genain CP, Lee-Parritz D, Nguyen MH, et al. 1994. In healthy primates, circulating autoreactive T cells mediate autoimmune disease. *J Clin Invest.*;94:1339-45.

32. George EB, Glass JD, Griffin JW. 1995. Axotomy-induced axonal degeneration is mediated by calcium influx through ion-specific channels. *J Neurosci.*;15:6445-52.

33. Glabinski AR, Ransohoff RM. 1999. Sentries at the gate: chemokines and the blood-brain barrier. *J Neurovirol.*;5:623-34.

34. Goverman J. 1999. Tolerance and autoimmunity in TCR transgenic mice specific for myelin basic protein. *Immunol Rev.*;169.

35. Gray P, Ritchie J. 1985. Ion channels in Schwann and glial cells. *Trends Neurosci.*;8:411-15.

36. Hammond SR, English DR, McLeod JG. 2000. The age-range of risk of developing multiple sclerosis: evidence from a migrant population in Australia. *Brain.*;123 :968-74.

37. Hebb DO. *The Organization of Behavior: a Neuropsychological Theory.* New York, NY: Wiley; 1949.

38. Hemmer B, Vergelli M, Pinilla C, Houghten R, Martin R. 1998. Probing degeneracy in T-cell recognition using peptide combinatorial libraries. *Immunol Today.*;19:163-8.

39. Hesselgesser J, Horuk R. 1999. Chemokine and chemokine receptor expression in the central nervous system. *J Neurovirol.*;5:13-26.

40. Jacobs RE, Ahrens ET, Meade TJ, Fraser SE. 1999. Looking deeper into vertebrate development. *Trends Cell Biol.*;9:73-6.

41. Karpus WJ, Lukacs NW, McRae BL, Strieter RM, Kunkel SL, Miller SD. 1995. An important role for the chemokine macrophage inflammatory protein-1 alpha in the pathogenesis of the T cell-mediated autoimmune disease, experimental autoimmune encephalomyelitis. *J Immunol.*;155:5003-10.

42. Kennedy KJ, Karpus WJ. 1999. Role of chemokines in the regulation of Th1/Th2 and autoimmune encephalomyelitis. *J Clin Immunol.*;19:273-9.

43. Koh DR, Fung-Leung WP, Ho A, Gray D, Acha-Orbea H, Mak TW. 1992. Less mortality but more relapses in experimental allergic encephalomyelitis in CD8-/- mice. *Science.*;256:1210-3.

44. Kossut M, Juliano SL. 1999. Anatomical correlates of representational map reorganization induced by partial vibrissectomy in the barrel cortex of adult mice. *Neuroscience.*;92:807-17.

45. Kramer R, Zhang Y, Gehrmann J, Gold R, Thoenen H, Wekerle H. 1995. Gene transfer through the blood-nerve barrier: NGF-engineered neuritogenic T lymphocytes attenuate experimental autoimmune neuritis. *Nat Med.*;1:1162-6.

46. Krogsgaard M, Wucherpfennig KW, Canella B, et al. 2000. Visualization of myelin basic protein (MBP) T cell epitopes in multiple sclerosis lesions using a monoclonal antibody specific for the human histocompatibility leukocyte antigen (HLA)-DR2-MBP 85-99 complex. *J Exp Med.*;191:1395-412.

47. Li S, Stys PK. 2000. Mechanisms of ionotropic glutamate receptor-mediated excitotoxicity in isolated spinal cord white matter. *J Neurosci.*;20:1190-8.

48. Linington C, Bradl M, Lassmann H, Brunner C, Vass K. 1988. Augmentation of demyelination in rat acute allergic encephalomyelitis by circulating mouse monoclonal antibodies directed against a myelin/oligodendrocyte glycoprotein. *Am J Pathol.*;130:443-54.

49. Lipshutz RJ, Fodor SP, Gingeras TR, Lockhart DJ. 1999. High density synthetic oligonucleotide arrays. *Nat Genet.*;21:20-4.

50. Litzenburger T, Fassler R, Bauer J, et al. 1998. B lymphocytes producing demyelinating autoantibodies: development and function in gene-targeted transgenic mice. *J Exp Med.*;188:169-80.

51. Lodge PA, Johnson C, Sriram S. 1996. Frequency of MBP and MBP peptide-reactive T cells in the HPRT mutant T-cell population of MS patients. *Neurology.*;46:1410-5.

52. Louie AY, Huber MM, Ahrens ET, et al. 2000. In vivo visualization of gene expression using magnetic resonance imaging. *Nat Biotechnol.*;18:321-5.

53. Lukes A, Mun-Bryce S, Lukes M, Rosenberg GA. 1999. Extracellular matrix degradation by metalloproteinases and central nervous system diseases. *Mol Neurobiol.*;19:267-84.

54. Luo L, Salunga RC, Guo H, et al. 1999. Gene expression profiles of laser-captured adjacent neuronal subtypes. *Nat Med.*;5:117-22.

55. Madsen LS, Andersson EC, Jansson L, et al. 1999. A humanized model for multiple sclerosis using HLA-DR2 and a human T-cell receptor. *Nat Genet.*;23:343-7.

56. Malenka RC, Nicoll RA. 1999. Long-term potentiation—a decade of progress? *Science.*;285:1870-4.

57. Malipiero U, Heuss C, Schlapbach R, Tschopp J, Gerber U, Fontana A. 1999. Involvement of the N-methyl-D-aspartate receptor in neuronal cell death induced by cytotoxic T cell-derived secretory granules. *Eur J Immunol.*;29:3053-62.

58. Martin R, Jaraquemada D, Flerlage M, et al. 1990. Fine specificity and HLA restriction of myelin basic protein-specific cytotoxic T cell lines from multiple sclerosis patients and healthy individuals. *J Immunol.*;145:540-8.

59. Mathisen PM, Yu M, Johnson JM, Drazba JA, Tuohy VK. 1997. Treatment of experimental autoimmune encephalomyelitis with genetically modified memory T cells. *J Exp Med.*;186:159-64.

60. McDonald WI, Miller DH, Barnes D. 1992. The pathological evolution of multiple sclerosis. *Neuropathol Appl Neurobiol.*;18:319-34.

61. Medana IM, Gallimore A, Oxenius A, Martinic MMA, Wekerle H, Neumann H. 2000. MHC class I-restricted killing of neurons by virus specific CD8+ T lymphocytes is effected through the Fas/FasL, but not the perforin pathway. *Eur.J.Immunol.*;30:3623-3633.

62. MeinL E, Hoch RM, Dornmair K, et al. 1997. Encephalitogenic potential of myelin basic protein-specific T cells isolated from normal rhesus macaques. *Am J Pathol.*;150:445-53.

63. Merrill EG, Wall PD. 1978. Selective inhibition of distant afferent input to lamina 4 and 5 cells in cat dorsal spinal cord. *J Physiol (Lond).*;278:51P.

64. Mogilner A, Grossman JA, Ribary U, et al. 1993. Somatosensory cortical plasticity in adult humans revealed by magnetoencephalography. *Proc Natl Acad Sci U S A.*;90:3593-7.

65. Moll C, Mourre C, Lazdunski M, Ulrich J. 1991. Increase of sodium channels in demyelinated lesions of multiple sclerosis. *Brain Res.*;556:311-6.

66. Narayanan S, Fu L, Pioro E, et al. 1997. Imaging of axonal damage in multiple sclerosis: spatial distribution of magnetic resonance imaging lesions. *Ann Neurol.*;41:385-91.

67. Neumann H, Wekerle H. 1998. Neuronal control of the immune response in the central nervous system: linking brain immunity to neurodegeneration. *J Neuropathol Exp Neurol.*;57:1-9.

68. Nudo RJ. 1999. Recovery after damage to motor cortical areas. *Curr Opin Neurobiol.*;9:740-7.

69. Olivares-Villagomez D, Wang Y, Lafaille JJ. 1998. Regulatory CD4(+) T cells expressing endogenous T cell receptor chains protect myelin basic protein-specific transgenic mice from spontaneous autoimmune encephalomyelitis. *J Exp Med.*;188:1883-94.

70. Ota K, Matsui M, Milford EL, Mackin GA, Weiner HL, Hafler DA. 1990. T-cell recognition of an immunodominant myelin basic protein epitope in multiple sclerosis. *Nature.*;346:183-7.

71. Paty DW, Moore GR. Magnetic Resonance Imaging Changes as Living Pathology in Multiple Sclerosis. Paty DW, Ebers GC, eds. *Multiple Sclerosis.* Philadelphia, PA: F.A. Davis Company; 1998:328-369.

72. Pette M, Fujita K, Kitze B, et al. 1990. Myelin basic protein-specific T lymphocyte lines from MS patients and healthy individuals. *Neurology.*;40:1770-6.

73. Pitt D, Werner P, Raine CS. 2000. Glutamate excitotoxicity in a model of multiple sclerosis. *Nat Med.*;6:67-70.

74. Pons TP, Garraghty PE, Ommaya AK, Kaas JH, Taub E, Mishkin M. 1991. Massive cortical reorganization after sensory deafferentation in adult macaques [see comments]. *Science.*;252:1857-60.

75. Prat A, Pelletier D, Duquette P, Arnold DL, Antel JP. 2000. Heterogeneity of T-lymphocyte function in primary progressive multiple sclerosis: relation to magnetic resonance imaging lesion volume. *Ann Neurol.*;47:234-7.

76. Qin Y, Duquette P, Zhang Y, Talbot P, Poole R, Antel J. 1998. Clonal expansion and somatic hypermutation of V(H) genes of B cells from cerebrospinal fluid in multiple sclerosis. *J Clin Invest.*;102:1045-50.

77. Ramachandran VS, Rogers-Ramachandran D. 2000. Phantom limbs and neural plasticity. *Arch Neurol.*;57:317-20.

78. Ramachandran VS, Rogers-Ramachandran D, Stewart M. 1992. Perceptual correlates of massive cortical reorganization. *Science.*;258:1159-60.

79. Ramachandran VS, Stewart M, Rogers-Ramachandran DC. 1992. Perceptual correlates of massive cortical reorganization. *Neuroreport.*;3:583-6.

80. Ransom BR, Waxman SG, Davis PK. 1990. Anoxic injury of CNS white matter: protective effect of ketamine. *Neurology.*;40:1399-403.

81. Rioult-Pedotti MS, Friedman D, Hess G, Donoghue JP. 1998. Strengthening of horizontal cortical connections following skill learning. *Nat Neurosci.*;1:230-4.

82. Rodi DJ, Makowski L. 1999. Phage-display technology—finding a needle in a vast molecular haystack. *Curr Opin Biotechnol.*;10:87-93.

83. Rubin LL, Staddon JM. 1999. The cell biology of the blood-brain barrier. *Annu Rev Neurosci.*;22:11-28.

84. Schieber MH, Poliakov AV. 1998. Partial inactivation of the primary motor cortex hand area: effects on individuated finger movements. *J Neurosci.*;18:9038-54.
85. Shaw MK, Lorens JB, Dhawan A, et al. 1997. Local delivery of interleukin 4 by retrovirus-transduced T lymphocytes ameliorates experimental autoimmune encephalomyelitis. *J Exp Med.*;185:1711-4.
86. Smith-Jensen T, Burgoon MP, Anthony J, Kraus H, Gilden DH, Owens GP. 2000. Comparison of immunoglobulin G heavy-chain sequences in MS and SSPE brains reveals an antigen-driven response. *Neurology.*;54:1227-32.
87. Sontheimer H, Waxman SG. 1992. Ion channels in spinal cord astrocytes in vitro. II. Biophysical and pharmacological analysis of two Na+ current types. *J Neurophysiol.*;68:1001-11.
88. Stein DG. Brain injury and theories of recovery. Goldstein LB, ed. *Restorative Neurology: Advances in Pharmacotherapy for Recovery After Stroke.* Armonk, NY: Futura Publishing Co., Inc.; 1998.
89. Steinman L. 2000. Multiple approaches to multiple sclerosis. *Nat Med.*;6:15-6.
90. Steinman RM, Turley S, Mellman I, Inaba K. 2000. The induction of tolerance by dendritic cells that have captured apoptotic cells. *J Exp Med.*;191:411-6.
91. Stys PK, Sontheimer H, Ransom BR, Waxman SG. 1993. Noninactivating, tetrodotoxin-sensitive Na+ conductance in rat optic nerve axons. *Proc Natl Acad Sci U S A.*;90:6976-80.
92. Stys PK, Waxman SG, Ransom BR. 1992. Ionic mechanisms of anoxic injury in mammalian CNS white matter: role of Na+ channels and Na(+)-Ca2+ exchanger. *J Neurosci.*;12:430-9.
93. Trapp BD, Peterson J, Ransohoff RM, Rudick RA, Mork S, Bo L. 1998. Axonal transection in the lesions of multiple sclerosis. *New Engl J Med.*;338:278-285.
94. Vandenbark AA, Hashim G, Offner H. 1989. Immunization with a synthetic T-cell receptor V-region peptide protects against experimental autoimmune encephalomyelitis. *Nature.*;341:541-4.
95. Waters RS, McCandlish CA. Organization and development of the forepaw representation in forepaw barrel subfield. Jones EG, Diamond IT, eds. *Cerebral Cortex.* New York: Plenum Press; 1995;11.
96. Waubant E, Goodkin D. 2000. Methodological problems in evaluating efficacy of a treatment in multiple sclerosis. *Pathol Biol (Paris).*;48:104-13.
97. Waxman SG. 1978. Prerequisites for conduction in demyelinated fibers. *Neurology.*;28:27-33.
98. Waxman SG. 1982. Membranes, myelin, and the pathophysiology of multiple sclerosis. *N Engl J Med.*;306:1529-33.
99. Waxman SG. 1998. Demyelinating diseases—new pathological insights, new therapeutic targets. *N Engl J Med.*;338:323-5.
100. Wekerle H. 1992. Myelin specific, autoaggressive T cell clones in the normal immune repertoire: their nature and their regulation. *Int Rev Immunol.*;9:231-41.
101. Wekerle H, Linington C, Lassmann H, Meyermann R. 1986. Cellular immune reactivity within the CNS. *Trends Neurosci.*;9:271.
102. Werring DJ, Bullmore ET, Toosy AT, et al. 2000. Recovery from optic neuritis is associated with a change in the distribution of cerebral response to visual stimulation: a functional magnetic resonance imaging study. *J Neurol Neurosurg Psychiatry.*;68:441-9.
103. Wilson DB, Pinilla C, Wilson DH, et al. 1999. Immunogenicity. I. Use of peptide libraries to identify epitopes that activate clonotypic CD4+ T cells and induce T cell responses to native peptide ligands. *J Immunol.*;163:6424-34.
104. Yarom Y, Naparstek Y, Lev-Ram V, Holoshitz J, Ben-Nun A, Cohen IR. 1983. Immunospecific inhibition of nerve conduction by T lymphocytes reactive to basic protein of myelin. *Nature.*;303:246-7.
105. Yeh TC, Zhang W, Ildstad ST, Ho C. 1995. In vivo dynamic MRI tracking of rat T-cells labeled with superparamagnetic iron-oxide particles. *Magn Reson Med.*;33:200-8.
106. Zweiger G. 1999. Knowledge discovery in gene-expression-microarray data: mining the information output of the genome. *Trends Biotechnol.*;17:429-436.

# 6

# Future Strategies for MS Therapies

This chapter focuses on the development of therapies that can halt or slow the disease process in multiple sclerosis (MS). Therapies for the relief of specific symptoms are discussed in Chapter 3.

The plethora of potential therapeutic agents and the multiplicity of patterns and stages of disease to which each might be applied will demand tailoring of pivotal clinical trial designs to the specific clinical situation. Such tailoring will involve trial duration, selection of outcome measures, and as a consequence, sample size.

Modification of the course of MS presents opportunities for five types of interventions:

1. *Primary prophylaxis in at-risk individuals.* These trials will be aimed at preventing the appearance of overt disease in two populations of patients: (1) individuals who have presented clinically with an episode of mono-symptomatic demyelinating disease and (2) individuals known to be genetically at risk.
2. *Relapse prevention via immune modulation.* In this category, one would place the recent and ongoing trials of the beta-interferons—those whose primary clinical targets were relapse rate, with secondary outcome measures of magnetic resonance imaging (MRI) progression. In these studies, the interferons, all to a similar degree, decreased relapse rates as well as the number of gadolinium-enhancing lesions. However, glatiramer acetate reduced clinical activity to a similar degree without as profound an effect on the MRI. Thus, different agents might produce similar clinical

results, but with different imaging profiles because each targets a slightly different aspect of the underlying disease pathology.

3. *Relapse limiting.* Current practice is to treat acute relapses with intravenous methylprednisolone. However, no criteria have been adopted that permit uniform designation of the onset and completion of a relapse. The difficulty in this area arises from the fact that relapses can take numerous forms, from monosymptomatic optic neuritis to acute transverse myelitis, and so forth. Nonetheless, if treatments are to be tested for the ability to shorten individual relapses, then criteria for determining precise clinical onset and end of relapse episodes will be required.

4. *Progression altering.* To date, clinical measures of progression of disability have correlated poorly with imaging measures in MS clinical trials. The exception appears to be the estimation of brain atrophy. Studies evaluating the effects of agents on disease progression will have to incorporate measures of brain and spinal cord parenchymal volume as well as more sensitive and reproducible measures of neurological function than those currently in use.

5. *Neuroprotective and restorative.* Chapter 5 discusses the potential of and rationale for the use of various neuroprotective and potentially restorative therapies for MS. Many of the current putative neuroprotective or restorative agents in clinical or pre-clinical research are protein growth factors that must somehow be delivered to the central nervous system (CNS), either directly or across the normally restrictive blood-brain barrier. However, it should be noted that insulin-like growth factor-1 (IGF-1) appears to cross the blood-brain barrier in certain experimental autoimmune encephalomyelitis (EAE) models, so the inflammatory nature of the acute MS lesion might permit the use of such agents in the acute setting. Designs for trials of neuroprotective or glioprotective agents in MS will depend on the nature of the question being asked, as well as the specificities and properties of the agent being tested.

## STRATEGIES FOR DISEASE MODIFICATION

Advances in understanding the molecular neurobiology of myelinated axons, as described in Chapter 2, have revealed much about the contribution of impaired impulse conduction to symptom production in MS. Nonetheless, there is much more to learn about the mechanisms underlying demyelination and axonal injury in MS. What are the precise molecular steps that lead from the initial immunologic assault to the death of oligodendrocytes and the degeneration of axons? Are there steps at which these cascades can be halted? It has recently been suggested that cytokines might play a role in injuring myelinated nerve fibers in MS. More information is needed about which cytokines are involved and which molecular pathways carry out their injurious actions. Cytokines and the toxic levels of nitric oxide (NO) that they produce can be manipulated in a variety of ways and could provide a target for therapeutic interventions in demyelinating disorders.

## Immune-Based Therapy

Antigen-specific tolerance, a method of antigen-specific immunomodulation, relies on administering an MS-related antigen in a manner that induces tolerance, thereby reducing the immune response to that antigen. Myelin basic protein (MBP) acts as a classical encephalitogenic autoantigen in certain EAE models, which has raised hopes for the development of T-cell-based therapies in which MS patients could be vaccinated with targeted portions of the MBP molecule to induce tolerance and prevent further T-cell-mediated attack. However, as reviewed in the "Immunopathology" section of Chapter 2, the human response to MBP is more complex than that in these EAE models. Indeed, MBP does not act as a classic autoantigen in humans, and even among EAE models, it is highly variable. Generally, it appears that the T-cell response against myelin proteins also differs greatly between individual patients, suggesting that immune therapies might have to be individually tailored for different patients.

Another concern of this approach is that the immune response to antigen administration follows an unusual dose-response curve. Although low-dose administration of most drugs is generally the safest course when beginning clinical trials, low-dose administration of antigen can, in fact, sometimes induce unsafe immune responses, whereas high doses can induce tolerance.

### Vaccination

Vaccination, of course, would be an attractive therapeutic avenue. In fact, numerous variants of vaccination have been proposed. These include vaccination with whole myelin-specific T cells,[8,33] with T-cell receptor peptides,[13,107,116] DNA-encoding autoantigens, or T-cell receptor (TCR) sequences.[64,111] Some of these therapies were quite impressive in EAE models when immunization was induced against a *known* target autoantigen (for example, MBP, MOG, or PLP), but at least in the case of TCR vaccination, the therapy failed in human MS. This is already an active area of corporate research, which has thus far has not fulfilled our hopes. Although potentially of significant therapeutic value, the induction of tolerance remains poorly understood, making it difficult to test clinically.

### Suppressor Cells

For the most part, T cells are considered to underlie the immune-mediated attack on myelin, but one class of T cells—suppressor cells—can suppress the activity of pathogenic T cells and might play a protective role in MS.[57] Several types of cells, including CD4 minus and CD8 minus positive suppressor cells have been shown to suppress EAE in some animal models, but the role of suppressor T cells and their potential for therapeutic use in MS are far from clear. CD25+ T cells are closest to the classic suppressor cells, but they are enigmatic and not well characterized in terms of antigen specificity, function, and mechanism of action. Their existence has been postulated on the basis of transfer and depletion studies in vivo (Don Mason, Ethan Shevach), as in the NOD mouse model of insulin-dependent diabetes mellitus (IDDM), in neonatal thymectomy models of multiorgan infiltration (Sakaguchi), and also in T-cell receptor transgenic, "monoclonal" mice (Tonegawa; Lafaille). Evidence for a role of these cells in CNS-specific autoimmune diseases is indirect at best.

## Immunodeviation

Approach potential involves inducing immunodeviation of myelin-specific T cells, that is, shifting the balance of production from Th1 to Th2 cells. This is a crowded field in MS research, as in other putative autoimmune diseases. Several private firms are investigating this strategy, and the committee feels this approach is already receiving adequate attention and is not lacking for encouragement. Further, in the pathogenesis of EAE and MS, there is no clear distinction between "good" Th2 and "bad" Th1 T cells. Both cell types might produce pathogenic inflammation in different situations.

## Genetic Engineering

Another possible innovative therapy would be to use genetically engineered autoimmune T cells. Even though the precise pathological roles of T cells and their autoantigens are unresolved, this line of research has generated many approved or emerging therapies. These include vaccination strategies, which use either attenuated myelin-specific T cells[97][33] or peptides representing myelin-specific T-cell receptors[3] as vaccines to strengthen the body's own regulatory responses against pathogenic T cells (reviewed in 1998 by Zhang et al.).[120] Also under development are "altered peptide" therapies that use peptide analogues of myelin protein segments to induce autoreactive T cells to produce protective, rather than pathogenic, cytokine mediators.[96]

## Neuroprotection

Recent studies have elegantly demonstrated the loss of axons in chronic MS lesions. As discussed elsewhere in this report, the precise mechanisms leading to axonal degeneration in MS are at present unknown. Axons can degenerate as a result of the loss of trophic support of their myelin sheaths. Alternatively, they can be victimized as "innocent bystanders" in the surrounding inflammatory milieu. In addition to the structural loss of axons in MS lesions, axonal dysfunction and conduction block in demyelinated foci also contribute to neurological symptoms in MS patients. Axonal loss occurs early in disease and is possibly the major cause of irreversible neurological impairment.[104] Neuroimaging studies suggest that axonal loss begins as early as the onset of disease.

Axonal damage leads to Wallerian degeneration and the loss of neuronal cell bodies. MRI and computed tomography (CT) scans of MS victims show evidence of widespread atrophy. It is unclear at present whether the loss of axons leads to neuronal cell death in MS. However, accumulated axonal loss and dysfunction, especially in the progressive phase of the disease, underlie the progressive neurodegeneration seen in MS. Thus, therapeutic strategies aimed at preventing neuronal damage might be a key to preventing permanent disability. There are a variety of approaches to anti-inflammatory strategies, remyelination, and the use of specific neuroprotective agents, and these are considered in turn below.

## Anti-inflammatory Strategies

The most obvious "neuroprotective" strategy for the treatment of MS is prevention of the inflammatory lesion that leads to demyelination and oligodendrocyte loss. Anti-inflammatory approaches are discussed elsewhere in this volume. However, it should be noted that in the course of inflammation, cytokines such as tumor necrosis factor-α (TNF-α) and lymphotoxin are produced, and they can be damaging to neurons and glia. Furthermore, the reactive oxygen species, nitrous oxide and glutamate, produced by invading inflammatory cells can be toxic to both oligodendroglia and axons that pass through regions of active demyelination. Therapies aimed at preventing oxidative damage to neurons might, therefore, be effective in minimizing neurological impairment during acute MS attacks.

## Remyelination

Trophic and other interactions between axons and ensheathing glial cells contribute to the structural and functional integrity of axons. Therefore, administration of agents that promote remyelination or ameliorate damage to myelin should also protect neurons. Such strategies might include administration of gliotrophic factors or transplantation of glial precursors or stem cells that repopulate demyelinated regions of the CNS.[112]

Attempts at myelination occur in and around MS lesions.[54,85,92] Especially in recent lesions, an abundance of oligodendrocytes may be found, as well as axons with thin myelin coatings and shortened internodes. This presumably indicates de novo myelin formation as it does in remyelination of peripheral nerves. Lassmann and colleagues have categorized MS lesions into five types, based on the degree of oligodendrocyte destruction and the stage of apparent repair.[54]

Having noted that attempts at myelin repair are not uncommonly found in MS brains, it may be assumed that at some level, this phenomenon is responsible to greater or lesser degree for the recovery of function that occurs after relapses. Thus, the time course and the degree of recovery from individual bouts of demyelination give us some notion of the capacity of the CNS to repair myelin damage. The obvious questions then are why remyelination and recovery are not universal, what factors inhibit remyelination, and what therapeutic options might exist to promote remyelination in the future?

The cell type responsible for initiating the process of remyelination in MS plaques is at present unknown. Mature oligodendrocytes are incapable of mitosis and migration.[44] However, it appears from animal models that there is a pool of progenitor cells available that can, under appropriate circumstances and in the absence of continued immune attack, regenerate myelinating oligodendrocytes.[11,28] However, it would also appear that this pool of potential oligodendrocyte precursors is small and rapidly depleted.[45]

There appear to be two potential strategies for promoting myelin replacement in MS. While both are conceptually appealing, they have their potential drawbacks as well. One strategy might be to attempt to alter the cellular environment of the CNS so that it becomes more permissive, instead of inhibitory, to myelination by providing factors that promote the proliferation, migration, and maturation of oligodendrocytes. Oligodendrocyte precursors appear to originate from the O-2A precursor cell, so named because it gives rise to both oligodendrocytes and astrocytes.

Several protein growth factors are involved in the maturational sequence of oligodendrocytes. Current evidence suggests that initial proliferation of oligodendrocyte precursors is driven by basic fibroblast growth factor (bFGF). Platelet-derived growth factor (PDGF) is also involved in the growth of oligodendrocyte precursors, as well as in migration. The intracellular signaling pathways activated by these growth factors include at least two members of the mitogen-activated protein kinase (MAPK) family as well as pp70 S6 kinase.[11] Activation of cyclic AMP[5] or the PDGF antagonist, trapidil,[85] blocks growth factor-induced proliferation of oligodendrocyte precursors. Withdrawal of PDGF and FGF results in differentiation of oligodendrocyte precursors into mature oligodendrocytes.[5] Insulin-like growth factors 1 and 2 appear to be survival factors for mature oligodendrocytes; transforming growth factor-beta (TGFβ) is also involved in the differentiation of oligodendrocytes, as is the neurotrophic factor neurotrophin-3.

The complexity inherent in enhancing the gliogenic milieu of the CNS can be readily appreciated. The proliferation, migration, and differentiation of progenitor cells into mature, myelinating oligodendroglial cells require a precisely timed sequence of growth signals that, for the treatment of patients, must be delivered to multiple lesions disseminated in space and time, inherently differing in their states of demyelination and remyelination. Furthermore, the success of such a strategy depends on the availability of an endogenous pool of progenitor cells ready to be induced to divide, migrate, and mature into functional myelinating oligodendrocytes. Finally, the newly formed myelinating cells must be protected from further immune attack.

An alternative strategy might be to supply the diseased MS brain with cells that would develop into mature oligodendrocytes, perhaps in conjunction with a source of the requisite growth factors. Many of the same caveats apply to such transplantation strategies as attempts to promote regeneration of endogenous myelinating cells. In addition, the potential for both immune rejection and malignant transformation of transplanted cells must be overcome.

## Specific Neuroprotective Agents

Damaged neurons in the CNS attempt to repair themselves. These attempts are usually not successful and, as indicated previously, can lead to maladaptive effects. An important component of restoration of function, especially in a disease such as MS in which axons are damaged, must include the possibility of axonal repair. Several conditions interfere with attempts at axonal regrowth after lesions develop. These include the presence of a glial scar (depending on the site of the lesion), the lack of neurotrophic factors that support growth, or the presence of inhibitory molecules that impede axonal growth. One of the more promising approaches to encourage axonal growth is the administration of growth-supporting molecules, particularly specific growth factors.

As noted above, axonal transection in areas of demyelination can lead to Wallerian degeneration and neuronal cell loss. Thus, agents that induce protective reactions in neurons or enhance axonal sprouting might preserve or promote recovery of neuronal function. Application of such strategies is not, however, without its challenges. Recent clinical trials of neurotrophic factors for the treatment of amyotrophic lateral sclerosis (ALS), which is a relatively simple, monophasic degenerative disorder of the motor system, have so far failed to produce positive results. Neurotrophic factors are large protein molecules. For therapeutic use, these complex molecules are synthesized in bacteria or cultured animal cells from which they can be purified and then administered by injection. To the best of our knowledge, systemically administered neurotrophic factors do not cross the blood-brain barrier. For the treatment of MS, it would seem that they must be administered directly into the CNS, either in soluble form via an implanted pump or using some novel cellular means of delivery such as transformed cells or direct gene therapy approaches. Small-molecule agonists and enhancers or inducers of neurotrophic activity are in development.

Specificity is the final challenge of using neurotrophic factors to treat degenerative disorders, including MS. Many neurotrophic factors act only on certain cell types within the CNS. For example, the receptor for nerve growth factor

(NGF) appears localized to only basal forebrain cholinergic neurons and a few other cell types in the brain; receptors for the related trophic factor, brain derived neurotrophic factor (BDNF) are widespread throughout the cortex and subcortical structures. Neuronal damage in MS, however, affects axons belonging to multiple cell types, not all of which will necessarily respond to the same neurotrophic factors. In addition to having trophic actions on neurons, a number of neurotrophic factors, including neurotrophin-3 (NT-3), ciliary neurotrophic factor, and IGF-1, exert effects on glia. Many of the "neuroprotective" agents today are protein growth factors.

**Neurotrophins.** The neurotrophins are a family of related 22-kDa proteins that are crucial for the survival and differentiation of neurons during development and in response to injury. They include nerve growth factor (NGF), brain-derived neurotrophic factor (BDNF), neurotrophin-3 (NT-3), and neurotrophin 4/5 (NT-4/5).[59] Originally discovered because of their ability to promote neuronal survival in vitro, the neurotrophins have been found to participate in many aspects of neuronal function, including plasticity, neurotransmitter synthesis and release and regulation of cytoskeletal proteins, receptor proteins, and so forth. The specificity of action of the neurotrophins is dictated by the distribution of their receptors. Neurotrophins bind to two populations of cellular receptors. The so-called low-affinity neurotrophin receptor (p75LNGFR) belongs to the TNF family and binds all members of the family with varying affinities. In some systems, occupancy of this receptor by a cognate ligand can prevent apoptotic cell death. The "high-affinity" receptors for the neurotrophins belong to the Trk family of tyrosine kinase receptors. The three members of this family TrkA, TrkB, and TrkC bind NGF, BDNF, NT4/5, and NT-3, respectively. NT-3 is somewhat "promiscuous" because it can bind to and signal through TrkA as well as TrkC.

Neurotrophins can be produced by inflammatory cells. Both activated lymphocytes[9] and glia[49] possess neurotrophin receptors and can produce neurotrophins. Different cytokines stimulate different patterns of neurotrophin expression. Beta-interferon stimulates NGF production by astrocytes;[14] activated lymphocytes and monocytes can produce BDNF.[9,46] Thus, the neurotrophins appear to be expressed in the milieu of the MS lesion, perhaps as part of the reparative or restorative response.

Neurotrophic factors can protect and rescue neurons in a large number of experimental models. Of particular relevance to MS is the demonstrated ability of BDNF and NT-3, in particular, to promote regeneration of long tracts in the spinal cord.[117]

Neurotrophins are also involved in the development and maintenance of glia, including oligodendroglia. NT-3 stimulates the proliferation of oligodendrocyte progenitors in vitro, and both NT-3 and NGF enhance the survival of differentiated oligodendrocytes in culture.[20] NGF receptors are found on mature human oligodendrocytes.[51] Intracranial injection of NT-3 appears to cause an increase in the proliferation of oligodendrocyte precursors and an inhibition of proteases involved in cell death signaling.[48]

The role of the neurotrophins in demyelinating diseases is presently unclear. Levels of NGF are increased in the CSF of MS patients,[55] in the optic nerve of MS patients,[73] and in the brains of animals with EAE.[72] However, it is not known whether the increase in NGF is due to its release from inflammatory cells or whether it is part of a protective response of the CNS. There is no information available concerning the regulation of BDNF or NT-3 in animal or human demyelinating disease. Exogenous NGF can prevent autoimmune demyelination in marmosets.[110] Whether this is due to inhibition of the immune attack or elicitation of protective responses in oligodendrocytes remains to be determined.

BDNF has been studied in clinical trials in ALS, although the initial results suggested that the doses studied might have been too low.[7] Subsequent studies are examining the safety and efficacy of BDNF administered either at systemic doses higher than those studied in the original trial or intrathecally. These studies are in progress at the time of this writing. Nerve growth factor and NT-3 have both been studied in peripheral neuropathy patients, but not in CNS disorders.

**Neuropoietic Cytokines.** Neuropoietic cytokines are the family of neural growth factors that act on both the nervous and the hematopoietic or immune systems, and which include ciliary neurotrophic factor (CNTF). CNTF is further a member of the interleukin-6 (IL-6) family of cytokines. It was originally isolated from ocular tissues as a protein factor that supports the survival of ciliary ganglion neurons in cell cultures and from the cytoplasm of myelinating Schwann cells of peripheral nerves. It has neuroprotective properties in a number of in vitro and in vivo systems, including models of motor neuron disease and spinal cord injury. CNTF appears to protect oligodendrocytes from TNF-induced cell death in vitro.[21,65] CNTF has been studied in clinical trials of patients with ALS by both subcutaneous and intrathecal routes of administration.[2,83] When administered subcutaneously, CNTF did not affect the course of disease in ALS patients, and the stability of the pharmaceutical formulation limited its use via the intrathecal route.

**Other Growth Factors.** Glial cell line-derived neurotrophic factor (GDNF) is a member of the TGF-$\beta$ family of growth factors. GDNF was originally discovered based on its ability to support the survival of embryonic dopamine neurons in tissue culture. It was subsequently discovered to have effects on several classes of CNS neurons including corticospinal tract cells.[43] GDNF has been studied in clinical trials using intracerebroventricular administration in patients with ALS and Parkinson's disease. These trials were stopped due to the severe side effects of the drug.

Insulin-like growth factor 1 (IGF-1) is a 7.65-kDa polypeptide that has multiple endocrine, metabolic, and neurotrophic actions.[42] It is structurally and functionally related to insulin, and its effects are mediated through a tyrosine kinase receptor of the insulin receptor family. The activity and distribution of IGF-1 are tightly modulated by a group of IGF-specific binding proteins. IGF-1 participates in the development of neurons and glia, and its expression in the developing brain correlates spatially and temporally with the onset of myelination.[56] Myelin content is increased in the brains of mice that overexpress the IGF-1 gene[17] and decreased in IGF-1 knockout animals. The IGF-1 gene is induced in reactive astrocytes by experimental demyelination[47] and in human MS lesions.[31]

In vitro, IGF-1 can protect oligodendrocytes from TNF-induced injury;[119] cellular survival under appropriate conditions can be affected by the balance between IGF and TNF signaling due to cross-talk between postreceptor signal transduction cascades.[108] IGF-1 also modulates the activity of immune-competent cells. Several recent studies have suggested that systemically administered IGF-1 can ameliorate EAE in animals.[60]

IGF-1 has been studied in clinical trials in ALS with inconclusive results.

**"Gliotrophic" Factors.** Oligodendroglial precursor cells respond to several growth factors in the course of their development. Signaling through some of these same pathways appears to be important for remyelination and proliferation of oligodendrocyte progenitor cells in the injured adult CNS as well. IGF-1 has already been mentioned, but it is only one of several growth factors that are important in oligodendroglial function. Some of these molecules can ameliorate the course of EAE. Fibroblast growth factor-2 (FGF-2) and thyroid hormone influence early pluripotential glial precursors to develop into oligodendrocytes. Platelet-derived growth factor controls the migration and proliferation of later-stage oligo precursors (see 1999 review by Rogister et al.[87]). Glial growth factor 2 (GGF-2; neuregulin), a member of the epidermal growth factor family, promotes survival and proliferation of pre-oligodendrocytes, but prevents differentiation to fully mature cells.[16] GGF-2, however, has been reported to delay onset, decrease severity, and reduce relapse rate in a murine EAE model.[67] Yet another neurotrophic factor, ciliary neurotrophic factor (CNTF), has been shown to protect oligodendrocytes from TNF-mediated cell death.[65]

### Augmentation of Local Mechanisms

Neurotrophic factors might be produced in the MS lesion itself. For example, NGF is increased in inflammatory foci and in the CSF of MS patients. Interleukin-1 can stimulate astrocytes to synthesize NGF, which is probably the mechanism through which NGF is increased in inflammatory foci. Therapeutic enhancement of local neurotrophic factor production is a pathway worth exploring.

## Small Molecules

There are many small molecules that can protect neurons. These include glutamate antagonists, neuroimmunophilins, and nitric oxide and are discussed in turn below.

Riluzole is a putative neuroprotective agent that can modestly prolong survival in ALS[74] patients. It is believed to work by blocking neuronal glutamate release and is currently being studied in other neurodegenerative disorders, such as Parkinson's disease and Alzheimer's disease.

Activated macrophages in MS lesions appear to release glutamic acid, as well as other potentially neurotoxic molecules. Neurons possess two types of glutamate receptors, both of which might participate in the neurotoxic effects of glutamate: NMDA and AMPA/kainate receptors. Oligodendrocytes also carry AMPA/kainate receptors. Recent studies have suggested that, like neurons, oligodendroglia might be susceptible to AMPA/kainate receptor-mediated glutamate excitotoxicity.[69] Glutamate antagonists have been found to ameliorate myelin damage in an EAE model.[32,113] AMPA antagonists are currently under study in stroke and neurodegenerative disease trials. Exploration of AMPA antagonism in MS is warranted as both a neuroprotective and a glioprotective strategy.

SR7657A is a small molecule that has been found to enhance and/or mimic the effects of neurotrophins in tissue culture. It is currently being studied in ALS. Thus far, studies of SR7657 on the course of ALS have failed to demonstrate a statistically significant effect of the drug, as measured by the trials' chosen end points.

Neuroimmunophilins are cyclosporin-related molecules that inhibit the signaling pathways that lead to cell death. They have been reported to protect brain dopamine neurons from injury and are currently being tested in early-stage clinical trials in Parkinson's disease.

Nitric oxide is a small, highly reactive molecule that is normally a gas at room temperature. It is synthesized in biological organisms where it exists as a highly lipid-soluble, dissolved nonelectrolyte solute. NO diffuses rapidly in tissues and enters into redux reactions via its unpaired electron. It is less reactive than other free radical species. Under appropriate conditions, NO is synthesized by one of a family of nitric oxide synthase (NOS) enzymes. It reacts with superoxide anion to produce peroxynitrite ($ONOO^-$), a highly reactive substance that can interact with and modify proteins, lipids, and nucleic acids. NO is produced as a neurotransmitter in certain neurons and is also produced by endothelial cells and by active inflammatory cells.[22] The inducible form of nitric oxide synthase (iNOS) has been localized in active MS lesions in human brain specimens.[12] Selective inhibitors of both the neuronal (nNOS) and inducible (non-neuronal, iNOS) enzymes are becoming available[18] and might be another class of neuroprotective and glioprotective agents that merit testing for their therapeutic value in MS.

## Interrupting the Secondary Injury Cascade in Axons

Axons, like neurons, do not always die immediately after an insult. Regeneration ensues after a latent period of hours to days and occurs as a result of a process of "secondary axonal injury." Within gray matter regions of the brain and spinal cord, "excitotoxic" mechanisms trigger this secondary injury cascade. These excitotoxic mechanisms involve the abnormal, exaggerated activation of excitatory postsynaptic receptors, which allow the entry of damaging amounts of calcium into neurons, triggering a destructive cascade of damaging molecular events.

Glutamate is the most common excitatory neurotransmitter within the CNS and appears to play a key role in the excitotoxic process. In contrast to neuronal cell bodies, axons do not express glutamate receptors. Therefore, excitotoxic mechanisms would not be expected to play a major role in triggering the death of axons in white matter. Indeed, glutamate does not injure axons within white matter.[86] Nonetheless, calcium-mediated axonal injury does occur in white matter.[98] A wide variety of cellular insults will cause a sustained influx of sodium via "persistent" or non-inactivating sodium channels. This influx of sodium triggers calcium import via reverse mode operation of the $Na^+$-$Ca^{2+}$ exchanger.[100] The result is a surge of damaging levels of calcium inside the axon. In in vitro experimental models, drugs that block the $Na^+$-$Ca^{2+}$ exchanger or sodium channels can protect axons so that they do not degenerate following injury.[25,99,100] Neurotransmitters and neuromodulators such as $\gamma$-aminobutyric acid (GABA) and adenosine appear to have a modulatory effect on the axonal injury cascade within white matter, and indeed, GABA and adenosine have a neuroprotective effect in white matter where they can preserve axonal function after various insults.[26] Calcium channels also appear to play a role in admitting injurious calcium into axons following some injuries.[29] Blocking calcium channels, as well as sodium channels, thus should be considered in the search for neuroprotective strategies that will preserve axons in MS.

## Delivering Neuroprotective Agents

The various possibilities for delivering neuroprotective agents include direct administration either systemically or directly into the CNS, or "indirectly" via gene therapy in which genes can be introduced that will increase the body's ability to produce more neuroprotective agents.

**Systemic Delivery.** One of the earliest events in the development of an MS lesion is the opening of the blood-brain barrier, which might thus provide a unique window of opportunity to deliver therapeutics to the CNS via systemic delivery. For example, systemically delivered IGF-1 has been found to be protective in EAE models.[114] Studies in primates and in MS patients may be warranted.

**CNS delivery.** Until the last decade or so, direct delivery of drugs into the CNS was too dangerous for human use, but with the emergence of ever-smaller implantable devices and genetically engineered cells, CNS drug delivery is increasingly possible.

Many MS patients have been treated with intrathecal baclofen for spasticity using an implanted pump. Recent clinical trials in ALS with BDNF[82] and CNTF[83] have demonstrated the feasibility of this method for delivering protein therapeutics to the CNS. Penetration to deep structures may be a problem. However, the side-effect profile of intrathecal BDNF, which includes insomnia and other behavioral effects, suggests that active concentrations of the drug are achieved in higher centers.[82]

Studies by Gage and others have demonstrated the potential of transplantation of genetically modified cells to deliver protein trophic factors to the CNS, with promising results. Such an approach has the advantage that multiple agents can be delivered simultaneously through one vehicle. However, like replacement transplantation approaches, the multifocal nature of the MS disease process could make clinical application of this approach problematic.

**Gene Therapy Approaches.** The term "gene therapy" refers to the insertion of specific genetic elements into either intact or diseased cells in the body with the aim of either restoring lost biochemical functions or introducing a molecular compensation for the consequences of a disease process. This may be accomplished by injecting either naked DNA or specially modified "vector" viruses containing the therapeutic genes either systemically or into a restricted location in the body. Gene therapy holds great promise for the treatment of focal or generalized CNS disorders. However, the plethora of protective factors that would have to be invoked for neuroprotective gene therapy of the CNS to be feasible will probably render this approach impractical, at least for the near future.

## Summary of Neuroprotective Strategies

Axons in the MS brain exist in a threatening and destructive milieu, surrounded by toxic cytokines and free radicals, and stripped of their comforting myelin sheaths. Thus, the mechanisms by which axons are damaged in MS might be quite similar to those postulated in other neurodegenerative diseases such as Parkinson's disease. In addition, oligodendroglial cells are likely susceptible to many of the same cytotoxic mechanisms. Several potential therapeutic strategies have been described that could be investigated as neuroprotective approaches in MS.

The ideal neuroprotectant(s) would be able to protect, foster repair, and promote regeneration of all the different types of cells affected in MS and would further have a narrow enough range of function that there would be no undesirable side effects. Unfortunately, this is unrealistic. Few of the agents currently under investigation are specific enough in their action on the cells they affect to avoid undesirable side effects.

In the future, application of neuroprotective or neurorestorative treatments is likely to involve combinations of agents that can be tailored to the stage of the disease. Examples of combination therapy might include the use of an anti-cytokine agent (for example, interferon or glatiramer acetate); an antiexcitotoxic agent, such as an AMPA antagonist (none of which have yet reached the clinic); a mitogenic or differentiating factor for oligodendrocyte precursors, such as IGF, NT-3, GGF-2, or a synthetic small-molecule agonist for one of these growth factors; and an agent that promotes repair or regeneration of central axons, such as BDNF or NT-3. Perhaps these drugs, or others like them, can be administered as "cocktails." More likely, strategies of alternating agents that have different, yet complementary, activities will be adapted from those devised by oncologists.

Finally, the development of neuroprotective and glioprotective treatments will depend on advances in protein drug delivery and high-throughput drug screening. In addition, innovative clinical trial designs and novel outcome measures will be required to screen potential therapies in the clinic.

## CNS Repair and Restoration

### *Strategic Questions About Remissions*

The converse of the concept of relapse prevention, which has driven the most recent round of clinical trials in MS, is the concept of active induction of remission. Remissions, in which there is restoration of neurologic function, such as vision or the ability to walk, that had previously been lost, commonly occur in multiple sclerosis. One potential goal of MS treatment could thus be to try to take therapeutic advantage of the tendency of MS to naturally remit in its early stages in the majority of patients, with the ultimate goal of inducing sustained or even permanent improvement. This concept is not new. For many years, patients have been treated with high-dose intravenous steroids or adrenocorticotropic hormone (ACTH) with the goal of inducing immediate and sustained reversal of acute relapses. The challenges facing remission induction as a therapeutic approach in MS include the fact that some MS patients do not experience remissions and that the transition from relapsing-remitting disease to progressive disease represents an event in the disease course that is not fully understood.

Can we use what we know about the molecular basis for remissions in order to induce them? This question is under study in a small number of laboratories, but our understanding is just in its infancy. More fundamentally, however, the question of the basis for the transition from relapsing-remitting disease to progressive MS also remains unanswered. There are several possible explanations for why MS follows a relapsing-remitting course in some patients.

Axons, as well as myelin and glial cells, are damaged in MS. It is currently believed that axons within the CNS do not regenerate, or regrow, after they degenerate consequent to injury. Thus, one scenario is that irreversible (non-remitting) deficits in MS arise from axonal injury, as opposed to injury to myelin, which either is fundamentally reversible or can be more readily repaired. If axonal injury is, in fact, a basis for the acquisition of irreversible deficits, treatments aimed at reversing disability will have to focus efforts on protecting axons.

A second scenario is that, for some reason, sodium channel plasticity (which is necessary for restoration of impulse conduction in demyelinated axons) might not occur in some demyelinated or degenerating axons. To the extent that molecular plasticity at the channel level permits regeneration of critical channels, deficits might be reversible, but when channel numbers or distributions cannot be reconstituted, conduction fails and permanent disability results. Molecular neuroscience can teach us more about the molecular mechanisms that are responsible for synthesis and deployment of sodium channels in myelinated and demyelinated axons and about ways to manipulate channel distribution along the demyelinated axon therapeutically.

A third scenario is that other mechanisms of plasticity, such as synaptic sprouting or recruitment of previously uninvolved parts of the brain and spinal cord, can compensate for demyelination and even axonal loss early in the disease course, but that these processes become overwhelmed as the burden of disease accumulates, so that they can no longer contribute to recovery. This "threshold" model would focus attention on these mechanisms of plasticity and on strategies for enhancing them so that they are more robust. However, there is a need for information about these mechanisms in MS and about how they can be enhanced or promoted.

### Harnessing Endogenous Neuroplasticity Through Exercise

Several aspects of current thinking about the mechanisms that mediate neuroplasticity are potentially relevant to the restoration of function for people with MS. One interesting concept is the effect of training or exercise. In accordance with the theory that many plastic changes in the CNS are activity dependent, increases or decreases in input to the CNS can result in reorganization of sensory maps and changes in synaptic strength. In experimental and disease states, neurons can be induced to respond to stimuli that were previously not effective in eliciting a response. Similarly, neurons change the efficiency with which they respond to stimuli. Several groups have demonstrated that exercise, or an enriched environment, can improve motor outcomes after cortical lesions.[81] An interesting therapy has been attempted in individuals with impaired limb use due to stroke, by restricting use of the normal limb. Taub and colleagues observed that in both primates and humans, the use of the impaired limb was improved after limiting activity on the normal side.[101] In rats, this type of therapy results in adaptive changes in the motor representation in the spared cortical sites. This overall procedure must be approached with caution, however, since restricting use of the normal limb too quickly after a cortical lesion can also result in persistent motor deficits; this unfortunate result is thought to be due to increases in sensitivity to NMDA toxicity.[80] Although restricting the use of a limb might not be appropriate for people with MS, these observations suggest that achieving a careful balance of excitation and inhibition might substantially enhance appropriate neural responses. It might be possible to reach this goal by appropriately timing a combination of exercise techniques that are known to induce changes in synaptic strength with pharmacotherapy known to alter excitation and inhibition.

## Transplantation

Over several decades, the use of transplantation has emerged as a viable technique for repair of the nervous system. Immature fetal cells are required for transplanted cells to survive and integrate into the host nervous system. These cells have been used in many experimental animal models, as well as in human diseases, such as Parkinson's disease and Huntington's chorea. Although some of the results have been encouraging, the use of fetal cells in human diseases is probably not practical, in large part because of the restricted availability of fetal tissue.

Transplantation offers the opportunity to replace defective or destroyed tissue, cells, or organs with functional ones. A number of potential sources of neural tissue exist. Allotransplantation refers to transplantation from one donor of the same species to another of the same species. Xenotransplantation refers to transplantation of tissue from one species to another. Both are being investigated as potential therapeutic approaches to replace neural tissue destroyed by MS.

The possibility of harvesting animal cells for transplantation into humans is an active area of research. These xenografts could provide either specific replacement cells, such as cell populations that contain a specific neurotransmitter, or immortalized cell lines, such as fibroblasts genetically engineered to produce specific substances, including neurotrophic factors.[39]

Major limitations in transplantation include the requirement for immunosuppressive agents to prevent graft rejection, the toxicity associated with the use of these agents, and difficulty with control of rejection of xenografts even with immunosuppression. Strategies to control rejection, induce tolerance, and enhance xenograft survival have to be developed, and the mechanisms underlying xenoreactivity must be better defined.

## Stem Cells

A mature animal originates from a single cell, which initially has the potential to produce a diverse array of tissues, organs, and cells. That original cell is thus pluripotent, meaning it can give rise to cells of many different types. Certain cells retain this feature throughout the lifetime of an organism and are known collectively as stem cells. They are currently being studied as a possible way of replacing cells that have been destroyed by disease.

The most intensively studied stem cells are the hematopoietic stem cells (HSCs). These stem cells produce at least 11 different cell types, or lineages, including the immune system components (T cells, B cells, NK [natural killer] cells, granulocytes, dendritic cells), microglia of the brain and central nervous system, platelets, and red blood cells (Figure 6.1). Even for HSCs, the mechanisms underlying their regulation, survival, maintenance of pluripotency, and cell fate are still being worked out.

Recently, reports that stem cells from adults can differentiate into developmentally unrelated cell types have offered promise that this ability could be exploited to replace damaged or destroyed neural cells. Intrinsic and extrinsic signals regulate stem cell fate. Although some of these mechanisms have been identified, continuing studies will provide important information to bring this technology closer to clinical application. What a stem cell is, what regulates self-renewal and differentiation, the intrinsic controls of stem cell fate, the microenvironment and its role in regulation, and the control of plasticity are all important unresolved questions.

**Neural Stem Cells.** Another approach to neural repair exploits the observation that the CNS appears to contain multiple cell populations that are capable of self-replication and behave as endogenous stem cells in the adult brain.[6] In certain regions of the brain, these stem cells have been identified and studied for several years, but they were thought to be restricted to repopulating a few specific sites such as the olfactory bulb and the hippocampus.[71] More recently, immature progenitor cells with the potential to participate in neural repair have been identified throughout the forebrain. These are located in the subventricular zone, a region close to the ependymal cells that line the ventricles. Although these cells do not seem to engage independently in neural repair, it might be possible either to isolate and harvest a pluripotential population of stem cells or to induce endogenous self-repair by administering the appropriate growth factors or other substances that will induce these cells to differentiate and repopulate lesioned sites.

Until recently, the concept of a neural stem cell was not considered because the CNS has been regarded as a structure incapable of regeneration. However, a number of prototype neural stem cells have been identified in brain and spinal cord. Neural stem cells can also be derived from embryonic stem cells. Before the full potential of neural stem cells can be realized, we must better understand what controls their proliferation, what tissues they reside in, how the regulation of pluripotency occurs, and how differentiation to daughter cells occurs.

More recently, attention has focused on the potential of stem cells for replacement and repair in the CNS. Very early during embryonic development, true

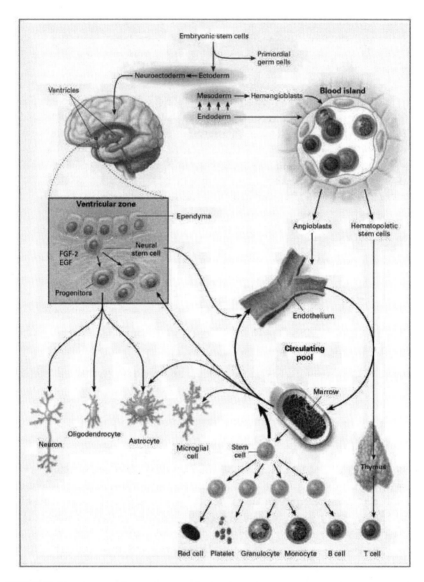

**FIGURE 6.1** Lineage of neural stem cells. In the brain, neural stem cells in the ventricular zone can divide and generate progenitors that proliferate in the subventricular layer, then migrate throughout the brain, where they differentiate into neurons, oligodendrocytes, and astrocytes. Circulating marrow-derived cells can reenter the brain and migrate into the ventricular zone, as well as differentiate into microglial cells and astrocytes. FGF-2 denotes fibroblast growth factor 2; EGF, epithelial growth factor. Reprinted with permission from Moore MA, 1999.[75] Copyright 1999 Massachusetts Medical Society. All rights reserved.

"stem" or primordial cells exist. These are progenitors for all cells in the body. As the organism develops, cells become progressively more committed to their fate as a particular type of cell. During development, different lines of stem cells develop, including those dedicated to the hematopoietic system that produces cells related to blood, bone marrow, and other systems. Other lines of stem cells develop into neurons and glial cells that populate the brain and spinal cord. There are intermediate levels of commitment in the lineage from primordial cells to cells committed to becoming a specific type of neuron or glial cell. Partially committed cells can be tapped at different levels of development to be used as stem cells to repair the nervous system. At this point, most studies investigating neural repair have used cells that are more or less committed to differentiate into either glia or neurons. Several reports have recently suggested, however, that with the right culture conditions, it might be possible to obtain a pluripotent stem cell that can differentiate into either neurally related cells or cells related to the hematopoietic system.[10]

Stem cells taken from embryonic brain are capable of extended self-renewal, but they lose this capacity as they mature. However, the capacity for self-renewal can be retained either by inserting immortalizing genes or by using specific growth factors in the cell culture media that encourage cells to exit the cell cycle and proliferate or return the cells to their immature state. Fetal cells maintained in this way can be transplanted into the CNS where they subsequently develop into both neurons and glial cells. Of particular relevance to MS is the transplantation of precursor stem cells into "shiverer" mice. These mice are missing a portion of the gene that encodes for myelin basic protein and, as a consequence, have poor myelination. When Yandava and colleagues transplanted neural stem cells into the brains of newborn shiverer mice, they migrated widely throughout the brain, and many of them differentiated into oligodendrocytes, producing improved myelination with reduced tremor in the mice.[118] It remains to be shown, however, whether similar transplants in adult animals can produce equally beneficial effects.

Although it is well known that young brains recover from injury more easily and respond better to treatment than adult brains, there are examples of effective transplantation treatment in adult brains. For example, in a model of targeted apoptosis in a specific population of neocortical cells, Snyder and colleagues[94] found that precursor cells were able to selectively repopulate and form appropriate connections in adult brains. They suggest that a number of factors in the microenvironment of both the host and the transplanted cells are required for this kind of transplant to succeed.

Cells from many different sources are being studied, including various animal models, progenitor cells from different regions of immature brain, and cell lines of multiple lineages, including human. Stem cells can also be transfected with viral vectors that allow the delivery of substances capable of inducing neural repair. Various growth factors have been successfully induced in neural stem cells to promote repair in many lesion models. Liu and colleagues grafted cells that were genetically modified to express the growth factor NT-3 into lesioned spinal cords.[61] The transplant cells dispersed for substantial distances within the spinal cord, differentiated into both neurons and glia (probably as a result of environmental cues from the host), and encouraged axonal growth from host axons. Many other studies report positive findings after delivery of growth factors into lesioned spinal cord, including functional improvements in gait.[19,63,84]

**Bone Marrow Transplantation.** The bone marrow is the source of all stem cells responsible for the formation of the blood or hematopoietic system (red blood cells, platelets, immune cells, and white blood cells). Bone marrow transplantation (BMT) and the HSC are associated with a number of autoimmune diseases.[1,52,76,79,103] Bone marrow from disease-prone donors transfers the disease process, and conversely, transplantation of bone marrow from disease-resistant donors into autoimmune recipients reverses the autoimmunity.[37,58,76,77] BMT has therefore been suggested as a potential new strategy to interrupt some autoimmune diseases.

*Animal Experiments Support a Role for HSC in Autoimmunity.* Observations that autoimmunity could be transferred through different types of stem cells in mouse models led investigators to examine clinical correlates. In 1974, Morton and Siegel showed that autoimmunity in New Zealand Black (NZB) mice could be transferred by hematopoietic cells into irradiated disease-resistant recipients[76] Conversely, BMT from disease-resistant donors prevented autoimmunity in NZB mice, an animal model for autoimmune hemolytic anemia.[23,77] Subsequently, disease prevention was reported in two diabetes-prone animal models, the non-obese diabetic (NOD) mouse[37] and the BioBreeding (BB) rat,[78] that had been fully conditioned and transplanted with bone marrow from disease-resistant donors. Mixed chimerism achieved by partial conditioning was sufficient to reverse the autoimmunity in NOD mice and prevent the development of diabetes. Transfer of autoimmunity by BMT has also occurred in other animal models, such as the MRL/lpr (lupus/rheumatologic disorders) mouse, BXSB mouse, and HLAB27 transgenic rat.[15,40,102] Unmodified marrow was administered in the early studies, implicating T cells within the donor inoculum as potential mediators of the effect. Splenocytes or lymph node lymphocytes did not transfer disease, pointing to a role for the HSC itself. When bone marrow from nude mice or bone marrow with reduced T-cell levels from normal allogeneic donors reversed autoimmunity in disease-prone recipients, data in support of a role for the HSC, rather than its progeny (T cells), emerged.[15,35,37,38,52,78,93,102,115] Finally, transplantation of purified HSC from NOD mice into genetically identical disease-resistant recipients transferred the autoimmune state.[36] Therefore, one can hypothesize that the immune dysfunction in autoimmune diseases such as Type 1 diabetes is due to an inherited defect of the pluripotent HSC that is also expressed in their progeny.

van Bekkum recently suggested that autoimmune diseases should be classified as HSC defects.[106]

Bone marrow used for transplantation can be either autologous or allogeneic. In autologous transplants, the recipient serves as his or her own donor. In allogeneic transplants, previously extracted marrow from a different donor provides the stem cells for transplantation to a genetically different recipient. Both types of bone marrow transplantation have an impact upon autoimmune diseases. Further research is needed to understand the mechanisms by which BMT helps to reestablish self-tolerance in the context of autoimmune diseases. Better understanding of this process should significantly improve transplant outcomes. In addition, support of well-developed Phase I pilot studies in which optimal information is obtained about posttransplant outcomes and impact on disease progression should be supported to evaluate the impact of BMT on MS.

*Human Studies Involving Allogeneic Bone Marrow Transplantation.* Recent case reports have confirmed a strong association between the HSC and autoimmunity in humans. BMT has been shown to transfer autoimmunity to disease-free human recipients who underwent BMT to treat leukemia.[34,53,109] Conversely, BMT from disease-resistant donors has reversed the autoimmune process.[68] Seven patients with rheumatoid arthritis who received an allogeneic BMT from disease-free HLA (human leukocyte antigen) identical siblings experienced a dramatic reduction in the severity of the disease, with complete remission in six of the seven patients.[4,41,66,88,89] Other autoimmune diseases including Crohn's colitis,[62] psoriatic arthritis,[24,62] MS, and Type 1 diabetes in the honeymoon period[105] have gone into remission following allogeneic BMT for leukemia. Because life-threatening autoimmune diseases are not controlled by conventional immunosuppressive therapy, BMT is currently being tested in pilot clinical trials as a therapeutic strategy in patients with life-threatening disease. This seminal observation has opened a door for a potentially new strategy to treat autoimmune diseases such as MS. However, a number of challenges have to be better understood and refined through research in this area.

*Limitations of Bone Marrow Transplantation.* The four major limitations of BMT are (1) the toxicity of the conditioning; (2) the requirement for close HLA matching; (3) graft-versus-host disease (GVHD); and (4) failure of engraftment. The toxicity associated with conditioning required in conventional BMT is one of the main limitations that has prevented the widespread application of BMT to nonmalignant diseases, including MS. In fully ablative BMT, the marrow of the recipient is first removed and then replaced by donor marrow, resulting in a fully allogeneic chimeric state. Fully ablative BMT carries a 10 percent mortality risk because of the conditioning process used to make space for the new marrow to become engrafted. If the recipient is only partially conditioned, the result is a mixed chimeric state. The morbidity and mortality associated with partial conditioning are significantly lowered. Strategies to allow engraftment with partial conditioning should be developed. A second major limitation of BMT is the requirement for clone matching. Methods to eliminate this need would make BMT more widely available. The need for clone genetic matching is due to the fact that GVHD is directly correlated to the closeness of genetic matching between donor and recipient. A third major limitation in BMT is GVHD itself. In GVHD, the donor immune system accompanies the HSC. The mature donor T and B cells attack the recipient, destroying the liver, skin, and gastrointestinal tract. Historically, strategies to remove GVHD-producing cells avoided GVHD but resulted in high rates of failures of engraftment. Methods to engineer a BMT that contains the essential cells but not GVHD-producing cells are needed. Research to understand the mechanism of failures, engraftment, GVHD, and graft take will allow this approach to more readily be applied clinically.

In summary, mixed chimerism might be a useful therapeutic approach for MS in two ways: (1) to induce tolerance to neural stem cell transplants and (2) to reverse the underlying autoimmune process. Strategies to apply BMT safely to patients with MS may allow a novel approach for therapeutic intervention. If the risk of the procedure is reduced to a minimum, one could envision intervening to interrupt the autoimmune process at a much earlier time, prior to the development of irreversible complications.

## CHALLENGES IN MS CLINICAL TRIALS

The art of performing clinical trials in MS has been greatly stimulated by the availability of disease-modifying MS drugs—glatiramer acetate and several forms of interferon beta-1b. However, as the field has advanced, new and complex issues have arisen. This section highlights some of these areas, but does not attempt to address the entire universe of clinical therapeutic research in MS. Nor does it review the individual clinical trials of therapeutic agents (for a summary of some of these trials, see Appendix D).

The National Multiple Sclerosis Society has been highly effective in proactively addressing many of these issues through its Advisory Committee on Clinical Trials of New Agents in Multiple Sclerosis and its Clinical Outcomes Assessment Task Force and Task Force on Use of MRI in MS Clinical Trials. These efforts have resulted in (1) a set of guidelines for the conduct of clinical investigations and (2) development of the MS Functional Composite, a brief impairment measure for assessing patient outcomes in clinical trials. These documents have been published in respected clinical neurology journals (see Box 6.1).

The major challenges facing the researcher who plans clinical trials in any area of medicine are the needs to:

* select promising new candidate therapies;
* reject agents that are either potentially harmful or unlikely to prove efficacious, and do so at an early stage in the development process; and

---

**BOX 6.1**
**Published Guidelines for the Conduct of MS Clinical Trials**

Whitaker JN, McFarland HF, Rudge P, Reingold SC. Outcomes assessment in multiple sclerosis clinical trials: a critical analysis. *Multiple Sclerosis* 1995;1:37-47.

Lublin FD, Reingold SC. Defining the clinical course of multiple sclerosis: results of an international survey. *Neurology* 1996;46:907-911.

Miller DH, Albert PS, Barkhof F, et al. Guidelines for the use of magnetic resonance techniques in monitoring the treatment of multiple sclerosis. *Ann Neurol.* 1996;39:6-16.

Rudick R, Antel J, Confavereux C, et al. Clinical outcomes assessment in multiple sclerosis. *Ann Neurol.* 1996;40:469-479.

Whitaker JN, et al. Expanded clinical trials of treatments for multiple sclerosis. *Ann Neurol.* 1996;34:755-756.

Lublin FD, Reingold SC. Guidelines for clinical trials of new therapeutic agents in multiple sclerosis. Relations between study investigators, advisors and sponsors. *Neurology* 1997;48:572-574.

Rudick, R, Antel J, Confavreux C, et al. Recommendations from the National Multiple Sclerosis Society Clinical Outcomes Assessment Task Force. *Ann Neurol.* 1997;42:379-382.

Lublin FD, Reingold SC. Combination therapy for treatment of multiple sclerosis. *Ann Neurol.* 1998;44:7-9.

Fischer JS, Rudick RA, Cutter GR, Reingold SC. The Multiple Sclerosis Functional Composite Measure (MSFC): an integrated approach to MS clinical outcome assessment. *Multiple Sclerosis* 1999;5:244-250.

Goodkin DE, Reingold SC, Sibley W, et al. Guidelines for clinical trials of new therapeutic agents in multiple sclerosis: reporting extended results from Phase III clinical trials. *Ann Neurol* 1999; 46;132-134.

---

- convincingly establish the utility, safety, and efficacy of agents that proceed through the drug development process.

Drug development in MS faces major challenges in a number of these arenas. In addition to challenges that apply to all areas of medicine, MS presents its own challenges. It is a heterogeneous disorder of long duration and—relative to other disabling and life-threatening disorders such as rheumatoid arthritis, diabetes, and cardiovascular diseaseæ its prevalence is low. MS is a difficult disease to study, and the potential market for profit-dependent firms is small relative to the investment needed to produce an approved drug.

Specific challenges to the design of MS clinical trials include the general challenges presented by therapies that alter immune responses, therapies for which there is so much demand that they are applied even before solid clinical data are available; situations in which placebo controls are not appropriate, despite the analytic power they add to a clinical trial; and blinding designs that control for subject and observer biases about expected outcomes. The considerable natural variation in the manifestation of MS also complicates the design and interpretation of clinical trials. In some cases, seemingly reasonable decisions to exclude "atypical patients" from the data analysis or about which diagnostic criteria to use can generate spurious results.[30]

## Need for a Standardized Testing Program

With the plethora of agents becoming available for testing in MS and four approved drugs already on the market, efficient systems are needed to facilitate drug development and comparisons between agents or combinations of treatments. A uniform currency of clinical assessment that incorporates several types of assessments, not all of which may be used in any given trial, is needed. An example is the Airlie House guideline for clinical trials in amyotrophic lateral sclerosis, which were formulated by a working group of the World Federation of Neurology.[32] The authors of this document included academic physicians, pharmaceutical company representatives, and representatives of the Food and Drug Administration (FDA). The Airlie House document provides a menu of evaluations that form the core assessment for most modern ALS trials. The MS Society could contribute by continuing its efforts on behalf of MS clinical trials and convening a similar gathering to consolidate its efforts to this point and help develop standards for future clinical trials.

An ongoing challenge will be to determine what represents a continuum of the spectrum of disease as opposed to unique etiologic or immunopathogenic mechanisms. This is especially complicated because human genetic variation is so extensive.

## Translating Research Results to Treatment Results

A critical underfunded and neglected area for MS is the application of basic research discoveries to the bedside in clinical feasibility (Phase I) studies (see Box 6.2). In the past, hospital centers and universities contributed funds to obtain proof of concept in early testing. In a time of health care reform, this option is no longer available. Funding for well-constructed, high-risk, potentially high-yield clinical trials for exploring feasibility and proof of concept in testing new technologies discovered at an academic center should be considered.

## Need for Controlled Clinical Trials

Another area of concern focuses on those therapies that, although they might provide very real therapeutic benefit, are not being appropriately studied in controlled clinical trials. Allogeneic peripheral blood stem cell therapies currently

---

**BOX 6.2**
**Clinical Trial Phases**

**Phase I**   First studies in people, to evaluate chemical action, appropriate dosage, and safety. Usually enrolls small numbers of participants and typically has no comparison group.

**Phase II**   Provides preliminary information about how well the new drug works and generates more information about safety and benefit. Usually includes comparison group; patients may be assigned to groups by randomization.

**Phase III**   Compares intervention with the current standard or placebo to assess dosage effects, effectiveness, and safety. Almost always uses random allocation to assign treatment. Typically involves many people (hundreds or thousands) but may be smaller.

**Phase IV**   "Postmarketing surveillance" evaluates long-term safety (and sometimes effectiveness) for a given indication, usually after approval for marketing has been granted by FDA.

---

fall under this category. In general, these treatments are not being developed by large pharmaceutical companies but are most often studied in small clinical trials under the auspices of independent researchers. These researchers have neither the funding nor the infrastructure for large, well-controlled, multicenter trials. The resulting publications describe only a handful of experimental patients and do not include control groups. Of danger to the field as a whole is that if controlled, adequately powered trials are not performed soon, the time for clinical trials may pass; clinicians will form an opinion of the treatment based on inadequate trials. Whether the treatment is truly beneficial or not will remain unknown.

The proper choice of control groups is an issue that affects any clinical trial but becomes especially difficult for MS clinical trials as patients gain access to more effective therapies. Asking individuals to forgo effective treatment is an unacceptable option. Yet if a treatment has a modest benefit, this benefit is far more difficult to detect when it is compared with another treatment of modest benefits than when compared to a placebo control. As a result, clinical trials comparing different treatments must be more elaborate; for example, they might test more subjects or for longer periods or collect more data, and will thus be more expensive.

Some modifications of placebo control design might provide viable alternatives for MS studies. So-called *add-on trials* test a new treatment on top of another beneficial treatment. For example, all patients in a clinical trial would receive beta-interferon. On top of this, half of these patients would also receive some novel therapy. As long as the therapies are thought to have significantly different mechanisms of action and toxicity, these trials are relatively straightforward.

Another option is the early-escape placebo-controlled trial, in which control patients are withdrawn from the trial at the first sign of any exacerbation. This technique, of course, relies on a clinically relevant and sensitive method for measuring impairment. An alternative is the randomized withdrawal approach, in which all patients start on a novel therapy and maintain this treatment until they become stabilized. At this point, researchers withdraw treatment randomly from some patients and closely monitor the clinical outcome of both groups. Again, the early-escape approach applies to any patients who worsen in the absence of the treatment.

Active controlled trials, in which two treatments are compared side-by-side, can establish the efficacy of a new treatment through two methods. The first involves demonstrating that a new treatment is more beneficial than an old one. In studies of MS, this approach works well, although as treatments become more and more beneficial, it will become more difficult to find a new treatment that is superior to the old ones even though it may be an effective form of therapy.

The second method involves demonstrating the efficacy of a new drug by showing that it is similar, but not superior, to a known effective treatment. When such similarity is shown, the statistical confidence interval around the estimated difference between the treatments includes the possibility that the new treatment is somewhat inferior. In order to conclude that the new treatment retains some efficacy, it is essential to determine that the amount of potential inferiority of the new treatment is less than the total efficacy of the active control treatment under the conditions studied. However, since trial conditions vary, patient populations are heterogeneous, and data regarding active control therapies in MS are limited, determination of the latter amount can be very difficult or impossible.

### Controlling for Subjective Factors

Two critical elements of clinical trials are (1) the ability to blind both the participants and the observers with respect to treatment so that neither are influenced by their expectations of a treatment's effect (double blinding) and (2) the existence of unbiased, objective measurements of disease severity (objective outcomes measures). Both elements can prove difficult in MS studies. (For a further discussion of the latter factor, see "Outcome Measures in Clinical Trials" below.) Many therapies cause adverse events that can unblind subjects or investigators. In the case of transplantation-based treatments, such as stem cell and bone marrow therapies, blinding would require sham surgeries, which can be unethical or impractical. When a study cannot be blind, it may be possible to reduce bias by having the outcomes assessed by individuals who are blinded to the treatment. It is also particularly desirable in incompletely blinded trials that observers rely on objective end points to avoid subjective bias in interpreting the outcome of the trial.

## Heterogeneous Patient Populations

The great variation in the clinical manifestations of MS presents additional issues in the design of a well-controlled clinical trial. Although MS is inevitably progressive, the rate and pattern of progression are highly variable from person to person. Responsive and unresponsive patient groups, starting with similar clinical or MRI deficits, have not yet been identified, although relapsing-remitting disease (characterized by inflammatory lesions) seems more amenable to immunotherapy than secondary progressive MS (where progression is less related to recurrent inflammation). However, currently used distinctions between relapsing-remitting MS and secondary progressive MS overlap considerably and are not necessarily the optimal distinctions for determining who is likely or unlikely to respond to a given therapy. Identification of disease factors that determine therapeutic response is very important, but difficult.

Some therapies are under development to target subsets of patients based on testing that is not standard in the clinical setting, for example, patients with a specific T-cell receptor subtype or antigen-specific T-cell activity. Several principles are critical in developing such targeted therapies, including the use of validated, standardized outcome measures in the trial, well-defined criteria for participating in a clinical trial and for defining patient subsets, storage of samples from patients for use in validating future tests as methodologies evolve, and finally, giving early consideration to developing a test that will be broadly available clinically should the need arise.

## Response to Withdrawal of Therapy

For any therapy that modulates the immune response, time-course studies are needed. While most MS clinical trials follow patients on a course of treatment for one to three years, few follow these patients after they come off the treatment. For example, could one year of beta-interferon treatment be enough to "reset" the immune response of an individual so that he or she can then stop taking it? Might continued therapy increase long-term toxicity while yielding no additional benefit? These are important questions, yet there is little incentive for pharmaceutical companies to study them, and physicians who have seen their patients improve may not want to risk taking them off the therapy.

## Multiple Agents

Since none of the treatments currently cure MS or halt disease progression entirely, it is important to test multiple agents in combination. Not only are such trials expensive, but they also will be lengthy and require large numbers of patients. Agents of different classes will have to be tested in sequence and in combination. Such trials are best done when the dose range and safety profile of each individual agent to be employed in the trial is known. The potential for adverse drug interactions should be carefully monitored. Separate end points might be required for each agent as appropriate to its individual pharmacological profile. Most importantly, standardized protocols and assessments will have to be devised and agreed upon, including Phase II studies that allow the abandonment of ineffective combinations to avoid unnecessary time, expense, and patient exposure in large, multicenter efficacy trials. At the time of this writing, there are no published reports comparing the efficacy of multiple agents given in combination to their efficacy when given alone. The results of several Phase I studies to test the safety of this approach have been presented at scientific meetings, but so far, none have been published in the peer-reviewed literature.

## Assessment Instruments

The development and validation of efficient, accurate, sensitive and reproducible assessment instruments is critical to the success of clinical trials. As noted in Chapter 4, the MS Society has contributed to this area by promoting the development of the Multiple Sclerosis Functional Composite Measure (MSFC). The MSFC has not yet been prospectively validated in the setting of a multicenter clinical trial. Further development of outcome measures to supplement or replace the Expanded Disability Status Scale (EDSS; see Appendix D) are also needed. Finally, there is a variety of MRI protocols currently available, and it is important to determine which measures can give the most comprehensive assessment of the degree of CNS damage in MS.

**Impairment.** Impairment of neurological function can be measured directly by examination or testing of the patient. Examples of impairment assessments include the Scripps scale, the Functional Systems grading instrument,[50] and so forth. The new MSFC is, in reality, an impairment measure, since it directly quantitates deficits of dexterity, ambulation, and cognitive test performance.

**Disability.** The assessment of disability is complex in a disease as varied as MS. The Kurtzke EDSS is the most widely used disability rating instrument, but it has been criticized for its apparent nonlinearity and insensitivity to change (see discussion in Chapter 4). As currently performed, it does not behave as a continuous outcome measure and does not equally weigh all areas of neurological dysfunction and disability in MS. There is consensus that the EDSS can be improved to yield a more comprehensive clinical disability measure for use in MS clinical trials.

Attempts have been made to apply other, standardized outcome measures such as the Functional Impairment Measure (FIM) to the assessment of clinical outcomes in MS. Application of these scales often suffers from their general nature and lack of specificity for MS-related disabilities.

Clinical investigators in the fields of movement disorders and ALS have developed disease-specific rating instruments that incorporate quantitative or semiquantitative recording of aspects of neurological function together with questionnaire-based assessments of patients' level of function in activities of daily living. Multidimensional ordinal scales such as the Unified Parkinson Disease Rating Scale (UPDRDS), the Unified Huntington Disease Rating Scale (UHDRS) and the Amyotrophic Lateral Sclerosis Rating Scale (ALSRS) have been validated in multicenter studies and found to reflect the progression of disability as well as demonstrating good inter- and intrarater reliability. Protocols have also been developed for the standardized assessment of neural transplant patients. A comparable, comprehensive rating instrument and/or protocol does not yet exist for treatment trials in MS. Attempts to develop and validate comprehensive rating scales are under way. An intriguing pair of instruments is the Symptom Inventory and Performance Scales.[91] However, none of these instruments has yet been tested and validated in the setting of a treatment trial.

**Quality of Life.** The application and validation of quality-of-life measures in MS is an ongoing field of investigation. Generic quality-of-life measures, which have the advantage of being able to permit comparisons of deficits and treatment outcomes across different disease states, often suffer from "floor" effects in the evaluation of aspects of physical functioning of neurological, including MS patients. Recently, an MS-specific quality-of-life measure (the MSQLI), has been developed and validated under the aegis of the Consortium of Multiple Sclerosis Centers and the National MS Society.[27]

## Neuroimaging

The rapid advance in the development and sophistication of magnetic resonance imaging techniques is detailed elsewhere in this volume. Whereas some measures, for example gadolinium enhancement, are most sensitive to acute blood-brain barrier breakdown and inflammation, other measures such as assessments of brain volume or atrophy give a better picture of accumulated tissue loss. The former measure correlates best with acute and even subclinical disease activity; the latter, with long-term disability. Thus, the choice of imaging paradigm for a clinical trial should be selected based on the goals of the trial. A study of a new cytokine-modifying agent might call for assessments of gadolinium-enhancing lesions. A trial of a neuroprotective agent intended to slow or reverse loss of function in patients with progressing disease might instead rely on a measure of brain volume. Additional issues regarding the use of imaging techniques include the timing of imaging relative to treatment administration.

## Electrophysiology

If therapies to aid in remyelination of the CNS in MS are to be developed and tested, the efficiency of remyelination must be assessed. Recently it has been proposed that central conduction times might be useful in this regard,[95] although the lack of positive studies makes validation of this measure in humans difficult at present.

## Outcome Measures in Clinical Trials

The past decade has featured clinical trials that have led to the first approved therapies for MS. The initial definitive trials focused on relapsing-remitting forms of the disease and were combined with MRI studies. One primary end point was clinical relapse rate. Most studies have used relatively standardized definitions of a relapse, although in some trials, efficacy was more apparent where severe relapse rather than overall relapse rate was used as the outcome measure. The sensitivity of MRI to identify the rate of new lesion formation, which is the apparent counterpart to clinical relapse rate, probably makes it less imperative to develop better definitions of relapse.

A more critical issue would seem to be the clinical measures that can be used to assess neurologic disability. Most clinical trials are conducted over periods of one to three years, but the current standard disability scale, the EDSS, changes relatively little over that length of time. (See Chapter 4 for further discussion of problems with the EDSS.) Some, but not all, clinical trials of relapsing-remitting MS showed significant effects of interferons as measured by the EDSS disability scale, which raises the issue of whether the "successful" trials reflected better training of investigators in the use of these measures. An international task force convened by the National MS Society during 1994-1997 recommended use of the MSFC, a modified scale that incorporates measures of ambulation, upper limb function, and cognitive functions (discussed further in Chapter 4 and Box 4.6).[90] Such measures are likely to be especially important in assessing therapies aimed at arresting the more progressive phases of disease or at improving functional capacity. MRI measures of tissue injury are being developed and might serve to support clinical observations regarding disease progression. Clinical studies aimed at functional improvement rely more on clinical measures. It seems unlikely that dramatically improved clinical scales can be developed given the rate of disease progression. Finally, even when the same clinical outcome measures have been used, it is not always statistically valid to compare different clinical trials.

Standardized measures are also needed to demonstrate the effects of clinical therapies on quality of life. There are numerous measures that can be utilized, as discussed in Chapter 4.

## MRI as a Surrogate Outcome Measure

The objective, sensitive, and quantitative changes measured using MRI make it an attractive tool for measuring the outcome of new therapies. This is in distinction to clinical outcome measures that are characteristically insensitive, often poor at reflecting disease activity, and inconsistently defined (for example, different studies define relapse differently). Indeed, the changes seen on MRI, used as a secondary outcome measure a pivotal trial of interferon beta-1b, had an important influence on the approval of this therapy in MS. In 1994, an international group of experts convened by the MS Society concluded that MRI could serve as a primary outcome measure in Phase II or exploratory clinical trials but that it should be used only as a secondary outcome measure in Phase III or pivotal trials.

The recent approval and widespread use of several partially effective therapies for MS have changed the options for testing new therapies and, as a result, interest in using MRI as an outcome measure has intensified. Large, long-term clinical studies conducted over several years raise ethical concerns about the use of placebo controls when approved therapies are already available. Further, the number of untreated patients available for studies will diminish. Also, trials comparing new treatment to active therapies will require larger sample sizes than placebo-controlled studies and will be very expensive. Overall, the MS research community is faced with serious difficulties in testing new and potentially effective therapies thus rendering the ability to conduct trials using small numbers of patients over a shorter duration than previously used in MS pivotal trials of considerable potential merit.

The following discussion of MRI as a surrogate outcome measure is based on a workshop of an international group of MS researchers that was convened jointly by the National Institute of Neurological Disease and Stroke (NINDS) and the National MS Society in November 1999.[70]

## Role of Surrogate Outcome Measures

The issue of surrogacy is complex. In general terms, a surrogate is an outcome other than disability that can reliably predict clinical outcome. An example is the use of blood pressure as a surrogate for heart disease. The concept of surrogacy in MS research has often been misunderstood, and various concepts of surrogacy exist.

**Validated Surrogates.** For an outcome measure to be accepted as a "validated surrogate" measure of treatment efficacy, it must meet the following criteria: First, the surrogate must predict future clinical disease. Second, the effect of treatment on clinical disease must be explained by its effect on the surrogate; the treatment has to affect clinical outcome by working through the surrogate. Third, evidence must exist that treatments of various classes affect the surrogate in the same and predictable manner.

Demonstration of a relationship between a marker and a prognostic outcome in natural history studies is not sufficient to establish the marker as a validated surrogate. Finally, since therapies of different classes must be shown to have a concordant effect on the surrogate as well as on the clinical outcome, evidence from a single class of therapy is not sufficient since other therapies could affect the clinical and surrogate outcomes through different mechanisms.

These stringent criteria make it unlikely that single studies will be sufficient to assess a surrogate marker. Unless treatment differences in clinical outcomes are highly significant, single studies generally lack the precision to provide a robust validation. Interpretation is also difficult if the treatment has multiple mechanisms but the surrogate explores only one. Single studies are more likely to be helpful in excluding useless surrogates than in validating good ones. Meta-analysis of multiple, large studies allows the relationship between the surrogate marker, clinical outcome, and treatment effect to be explored in comparative trials in a more robust manner. Meta-analysis may define the proportion of treatment effect that is explained by the surrogate marker. Collaboration and data sharing between investigators will facilitate validation of surrogate outcome markers.

**Unvalidated Surrogates.** In contrast to the criteria for a validated surrogate, current FDA regulatory guidelines allow for the use, under some conditions, of an unvalidated surrogate. The condition placed on the use of an unvalidated surrogate is that the surrogate outcome must be considered reasonably likely to predict future clinical outcome or disease activity. As discussed below, studies to date that have examined the relationship between MRI measures of disease and clinical disease either in cross section or as future disease have been, with one notable exception, disappointing. Despite this, changes on MRI clearly reflect some of the underlying pathological process in MS, implying that MRI is a reasonable, albeit unvalidated, surrogate. However, serious mistakes have been made in clinical medicine using unvalidated surrogates. For example, it is now clear that CD4 counts do not necessarily predict mortality in AIDS. Thus, the use of an unvalidated surrogate must be viewed with caution by both investigators and regulatory authorities, who must balance the risks against the potential benefits of rapid identification of effective therapies for MS.

It is also important to note that the acceptance of unvalidated surrogates by regulatory authorities in countries other than the United States is less clearly defined. In the European Community, MRI findings in MS trials have, thus far, been given less consideration than in the United States. The use of a surrogate in a clinical trial must be consistent with the guidelines of the countries in which approval for treatment will be sought. Discussion of this issue at an international level is imperative since most pivotal clinical trials are now international studies.

## MRI as an Unvalidated Surrogate Outcome Measure

The use of MRI data as surrogate outcome measures in pivotal trials of new therapies in MS requires an appreciation both of what is being measured and of the potential errors and difficulties. At present, there is insufficient evidence to support any single MRI measure, or combination of measures, as a fully validated surrogate. However, there is evidence to support the concept that various MRI changes reflect changes in the underlying pathology of the disease, and consequently, it has been suggested that under some conditions, MRI changes can be appropriately used as a primary outcome measure in pivotal trials in MS. In other words, the changes in MRI measures can appropriately serve as an unvalidated surrogate for changes in pathology.

If MRI is used as a surrogate outcome, the following potential problems will have to be addressed, and trial designs will have to be devised to minimize the chance of coming to incorrect conclusions.

First, the possibility exists that clinical trials using MRI as an outcome would be of short duration and that an effect could be identified that was temporary and would not translate into persistent clinical effect. This criticism can be countered by incorporating an extension phase that could be used to provide confirmatory clinical data in those studies having a successful early MRI outcome—for example, to include formal Phase IV components to follow-up short-term studies using MRI outcome measures. However, in this setting, lack of comparative control data would be a limitation.

These questions also arise with respect to the nature of MRI as a surrogate outcome and the relationship of the effects of the interventions studied on the appearance of MRI scans and the clinical state of the patients. First, as mentioned above, the justification for using MRI as a surrogate will be based on the belief that MRI reflects the pathology of the disease. Thus, a treatment could produce a change in the pathological process but have little or no effect on clinical disease. Second, trials using surrogate outcome measures will often be of insufficient duration to identify adverse effects of treatment. Extension phases of short trials using MRI as the primary outcome will also be necessary to define the safety profile of a treatment. An additional aspect of this issue relates to defining the risk-benefit ratio of treatments that are established as effective through the use of surrogate MRI outcomes.

Third, a drug could act through mechanisms not easily identified by MRI, which would result in a false-negative study. To minimize this possibility, the decision to use MRI and the choice of imaging paradigm must be made on a case-by-case basis, with careful thought given to the proposed mechanism of action of the new treatment. The MRI protocol might have to be adapted to be compatible with the proposed mechanism of action, for example, serial magnetic resonance spectroscopy (MRS) to evaluate a neuroprotective therapy as opposed to the use of gadolinium enhancement to monitor an anti-inflammatory or anti-cytokine drug effect. It might not be suitable to test some new therapies using currently available MRI outcome measures as the primary assessment.

Fourth, it is possible that a treatment might affect MRI but not be mediated by an action on the underlying pathology reflected by the MRI measure chosen. For example, measures of brain atrophy are thought to reflect tissue loss and to be sensitive to loss of myelin as well as axons. Thus, atrophy is an attractive MRI measure to assess the ability of a therapy to reduce the rate of progression of MS. However, changes in measures of atrophy can also occur through other mechanisms. When acute inflammation subsides, there is some reduction in brain volume. Depending on the relative timing of changes in inflammation and MRI scans, a postinflammation change in brain volume could be misinterpreted as an increase in atrophy. Thus, attention must be given to the sensitivity and specificity of the MRI measure in relationship to the experimental therapy being used.

Finally, careful thought should be given to how MRI data are used as an outcome measure. No single MRI measure is sufficient for evaluating new therapies at every stage of the disease process. Instead, a combination of MRI measures that measure different aspects of lesion development should be used. Various MRI measures are listed in Table 6.1.

**TABLE 6.1** MRI Outcomes for Clinical Trials of New Agents Aimed at Preventing Relapses or Slowing Progression: Recommendations of the November 1999 Workshop Convened by NINDS and the MS Society.

| Process Measured | Imaging Parameter | Clinically Isolated Syndrome | Relapsing-Remitting | Secondary Progressive | Primary Progressive |
|---|---|---|---|---|---|
| **Inflammation** | T2 lesion load | X | X | X | X |
| | Gadolinium enhancing lesions | X | X | X | X |
| **Tissue loss** | T1 hypointense lesions ("black holes") | X | X | X | X |
| | Atrophy-brain volume | X | X | X | X |
| | Spinal cord area | | | X | X |
| **Dysfunctional tissue burden/ biochemical abnormalities** | MR spectroscopy | | | X | X |
| | MTR histograms | | | X | X |
| | Diffusion imaging | | | X | X |
| | T2 decay analysis | | | X | X |
| | T1 relaxation time | | | X | X |

However, many of these techniques are not well validated, and some are difficult to standardize across centers. Further, how various MRI measures would be used to provide a single outcome measure needs to be carefully thought through.

In summary, measures of disease activity provide a robust reflection of the underlying pathobiology of the disease process, and under some conditions, MRI could represent a primary, albeit unvalidated, surrogate outcome in pivotal trials of new therapies for MS. No MRI measure represents a validated surrogate outcome measure using the previously defined criteria; the likelihood that MRI reflects the underlying pathology of the disease implies that if the aim of a treatment is to prevent damage to the brain, then MRI represents an acceptable outcome measure.

Thus, continued follow-up of patients in studies of short duration using MRI as the primary outcome is essential. Further, the decision to use MRI as an outcome measure and the type of outcomes chosen should be made after considering the mechanism of action of the new therapy.

It is critical that the application of MRI as a surrogate outcome measure be done thoughtfully. Additional information on standardization of techniques is necessary. No single MRI measure represents an outcome measure of sufficient predictive value or validation to be used alone. Thus, for each new therapy, the most effective use of the various MRI measures should be carefully considered (see Table 6.1). In general, most investigators seem to feel that multiple MRI measures should be used. The next step in trial design will be to determine the most appropriate use of multiple MRI outcomes to assess the effect of a new therapy. Different MRI measures will be needed at different stages of disease, especially in the relapsing versus progressive phases.

Finally, assessment of MRI outcomes and clinical changes obtained in previous trials must be examined in greater detail, with an emphasis on the degree to which the effect of treatment on the clinical outcome is concordant with MRI outcomes.

Overall, the use of MRI as a surrogate outcome measure is an attractive possibility at a time when clinical trials using conventional clinical outcomes in placebo-controlled studies that require large numbers of patients and a long duration are becoming increasingly problematic. However, the use of MRI as a currently unvalidated surrogate must be approached with caution and with careful thought to the potential errors that could result as well as the possible benefits. The MS research community must next focus on issues of trial design and standardization of imaging techniques. In planning such studies, the ultimate need to validate the surrogate should not be forgotten.

# SHARED RESOURCES

## Data Registries

### *International Multiple Sclerosis Trials Research and Resource Center*

The approval in some countries of up to four treatments that favorably modify the course of multiple sclerosis has created a problem for future clinical trials. Because these agents are only modestly effective, there is a pressing need to develop new, more effective therapies. There is general agreement that double-blind placebo-controlled clinical trials for relapsing-remitting multiple sclerosis, of a size and duration such as have been necessary in the past to demonstrate effectiveness, are no longer ethically justified. Such trials can be justified in certain small clinical subgroups of patients, but their results cannot be assumed to apply to MS patients as a whole. A new approach is needed. In response to this need, the International Federation of Multiple Sclerosis Societies* proposes to set up an International Multiple Sclerosis Trials Research and Resource Center with the primary aim of answering two questions: (1) Is it possible to model the "expected" clinical behavior of multiple sclerosis using clinical, laboratory, and imaging markers of disease in order to determine that "observed behavior" in a treatment trial suggests treatment effectiveness or futility? (2) Does any single MRI measure, or combination of measures, of disease activity have sufficient predictability of future clinical course to be considered a surrogate marker of clinical disease activity?

The center is in an advanced stage of planning. It will be headed by a statistician. Data will be entered from the placebo arms of clinical trials carried out over the past decade, together with data from population-based epidemiological studies. Approval in principle to provide data from these sources has already been given. The center is intended to be an international resource. Access to the data will be open to investigators subject to the approval of hypothesis-driven proposals following peer review. The analyses will be carried out by the staff of the center.

### *A Model for MS Research: Transplant Registries*

As noted elsewhere, clinical trials using cellular transplant protocols are often, by nature, small and institution based rather than being sponsored by corporations and, because of the attendant risks, are often unblinded and uncontrolled. Support, organization, and collation of data from such studies can be greatly facilitated through the use of clinical registries.

---

*In January 2001, the name was change to the Multiple Sclerosis International Federation.

Two associated data registries, the International Bone Marrow Transplant Registry (IBMTR) and the Autologous Blood and Marrow Transplant Registry of North America (ABMTR) provide an exceptionally productive resource for researchers and clinicians. These registries represent a unique example of international cooperation that has greatly benefited the fields of transplantation and cancer treatment. They require considerable investment that is not easily matched, but nonetheless, they offer an insight to the MS community of what might be possible.

The IBMTR and the ABMTR are voluntary, nonprofit organizations of more than 400 institutions in 47 countries that submit data on consecutive blood and marrow transplant recipients to the IBMTR-ABMTR Statistical Center at the Medical College of Wisconsin in Milwaukee. The IBMTR was established in 1972 and the ABMTR in 1990. Together, they maintain databases of comprehensive clinical information for more than 60,000 transplant recipients. These are not donor registries that find donors for patients needing transplants. Rather, they collect information on transplant outcomes. The information gathered by the IBMTR and ABMTR is used to identify trends in transplant use and outcome, to guide physicians and patients in making treatment choices, and to conduct scientific studies of issues pertinent to improving transplant outcomes. Researchers planning clinical trials use the database to aid study design; they are an invaluable resource for estimating effect sizes, targeting appropriate study populations, designing efficient protocols, and determining accrual feasibility. Health care organizations and institutes use the database to better inform policy decisions.

The IBMTR-ABMTR database facilitates analysis of transplant outcomes by focusing on questions that are difficult to answer in randomized trials, including:

- descriptions of transplant results in various disease states and patient groups;
- analysis of prognostic factors;
- comparison of transplant with nontransplant therapy;
- identifying intercenter variability in diagnosis, practice, and outcome;
- developing analytic approaches for evaluating transplant outcome; and
- evaluating costs.

This sort of database is particularly valuable for research on complex and long-term diseases. As with MS treatment outcomes, assessing transplant outcome is complex. Outcomes are influenced by many patient- and disease-related factors such as age, disease stage, and prior treatment, as well as differences in treatment protocols. Ideally, most transplant issues would be addressed by large randomized clinical trials. However, many factors limit the application of randomized trials. Many diseases treated with transplantation are uncommon; single centers might treat only a few patients with a given disorder. This makes randomized trials difficult and also limits the ability to perform nonrandomized trials (Phase II) with sufficient statistical power to detect meaningful effects. Small trials, even when randomized, can give misleading results. Even when randomized trials are performed, enrolled patients often represent only a small proportion of the target population and may not be representative of the larger group. With the participation of many centers in a prospective, observational database, large numbers of subjects representative of the general population can accrue rapidly. This increases the power to detect meaningful changes in outcome and increases the precision with which outcomes can be measured.

It is important to emphasize that studies of observational data from multiple centers do not replace the need for carefully conducted, single-center, Phase I and II studies and single- or multicenter randomized studies. Rather, they offer a complementary approach for addressing issues and can help facilitate trials.

The database serves as an efficient source of information for evaluating new treatments, especially in the preliminary stages of investigation. It also provides information that is unlikely to be extensively pursued in industry-funded clinical trials—for example, long-term effects, continuation of therapy, and different responses to different therapies. In addition, a large, longitudinal database such as the IBMTR-ABMTR is uniquely suited to late and infrequent effects of transplantation—or any other long-term consequence such as accumulated disability in the case of MS.

Since the mid-1990s, HSC transplantation has been used to treat a variety of autoimmune diseases in about 300 patients. Some, but not all, have shown long-lasting improvement, and many issues require further clarification through coordinated clinical trials. The European Bone Marrow Transplant (EBMT) group is working with IBMTR-ABMTR to develop consensus and standardization for data collection related to HSC transplantation in patients with autoimmune disease, as well as guidelines for trials and patient selection.

There are 35 full-time staff dedicated to the registry, including physicians, statisticians, database managers, and a development office for fund raising. The activities of the IBMTR and ABMTR are supervised by more than a dozen volunteer committees that design and conduct studies, develop general policies for use of IBMTR and ABMTR data, review study proposals, and plan and conduct scientific workshops. The success of the registry programs is due, in large part, to the voluntary efforts of the hundreds of physicians, basic scientists, and clinical research associates who contribute their time and expertise.

The annual budget for the IBMTR is about $3 million, with about 60 percent of the funding coming from the National Institutes of Health (Melody Nugent, personal communication). The remaining support comes from corporations, foundation grants, and individual donors. The major expense of the registry is for reimbursement of fully participating centers, who are asked to submit their data in a 75-page form. Institutions can also participate on a limited basis, in which case they submit reports with only 20 items and are not reimbursed for their services. The registry is supported by the Medical College of Wisconsin, the Department of Defense, and the following institutes within the National Institutes of Health (NIH): National Cancer Institute; National Institute of Allergy and Infectious Disease; and National Heart, Lung and Blood Institute.

Comparable data registries for multiple sclerosis would be invaluable. Each of the challenges presented by transplantation is mirrored in those presented by MS. Most importantly, such registries provide a larger data set than would be possible through individual efforts. Although such registries are likely to receive generous federal and industry support, they should be led through collaborative public and nonprofit efforts. An independent, investigator-driven database will likely have more scientific credibility than for-profit ventures and thus ultimately be of greater value to investigators as well as pharmaceutical firms.

The IBMTR-ABMTR includes data on MS patients, but only in the context of transplantation. The most efficient approach for MS research might be to develop a database that would permit comparison with the IBMTR-ABMTR database.

## Human Tissue in MS Research

The scientific value of human tissue is immeasurable. A small amount of diseased human tissue can reveal clues to a disease that no other research strategy can. For MS research, brain tissue is crucial, but this can be obtained only after death or by biopsy. However, brain biopsy for research purposes is generally not possible because of the risk of brain injury to the patient, which means that researchers must rely on postmortem tissue.

In terms of understanding disease mechanisms and developing therapeutic interventions, the most informative tissue would be that of MS patients in the earlier stages of diseases, but these patients are generally young and less likely to die than patients in the later stages of MS. Another complicating factor is that unless brain tissue is processed quickly and according to standard protocols, it degrades to the point where is useful only for relatively crude research techniques, and not for the newer genetic and molecular techniques.

Access to tissues from a wide array of MS patients either with different disease phenotypes or in different phases of the disease not only permits important research on the pathogenesis of the MS disease process, but enables research on the specific causes of neurologic disability, as well as disease heterogeneity. Tissue collection from patients is complex, and cooperative efforts are necessary to achieve sufficient numbers. Some tissues are readily available, such as peripheral blood samples and CSF. Others, such as brain tissue, are not.

Collections of serum and lymphocytes have been built into many natural history and clinical trial studies. Access to such samples has, for the most part, involved collaborations with those who collected the samples. At issue is whether such samples will be stored in optimal condition, which is particularly important with regard to serial samples needed to study the natural cause of disease.

Lymphocyte samples are valuable with regard to both RNA- and DNA-based investigations. RNA would be the basis for evaluating single molecules as well as for use in the emerging DNA microarray technology. DNA is used for the molecular genetic analyses aimed at identifying disease susceptibility genes or genes that modulate disease course. The challenges of collecting, storing, and sharing such resources are dealt with in other sections.

CSF fluid is becoming more difficult to obtain because sampling for diagnostic purposes is done less routinely than in the past. Although private CSF banks continue to exist, most tend to have samples suitable for analysis of the fluid but not for any of the cell constituents that were present (RNA is needed to measure gene expression, but it is highly degradable under normal tissue storage conditions).

### Brain and Tissue Banks

Many brain banks, wherein patients arrange to donate their brains after death, have been established for the advancement of research in a variety of neurological disorders, most commonly Alzheimer's disease. These brain banks have been instrumental in identifying the mechanisms of Alzheimer's disease and should prove equally useful in MS research. However, MS is less prevalent than Alzheimer's disease, and there are fewer available samples. Thus, it is important to be sure that any available tissue is collected using protocols that will optimize its scientific value—for example, by establishing standards for collection, quality control, and collaborations among multiple centers. Finally, brain banks require concerted outreach efforts since this need is not something of which the public is generally aware.

CNS tissue from cases of MS has been collected for many years at many institutions, forming the basis for the classical pathologic descriptions of the disease. As expected, the majority of tissues were collected from long-standing cases. Most of the early disease stage samples represent the most aggressive form of the disease. Samples were not usually preserved in a manner that is ideal for optimal immunohistochemical or molecular analyses. A number of brain banks have been established over the years. Limitations of these collections include the paucity of clinical information available on the cases and the lack of recent modern neuroimaging investigation.

The NIH currently funds 14 brain banks, several of which also receive funding from other sources. Ten of these banks are for research into Alzheimer's disease, and none of them collect tissue from MS patients. The MS Society has funded two brain banks for many years. One is at the Veteran's Administration in California and includes tissue collected from patients with a variety of neurological diseases in addition to MS. The other is in Colorado and collects only tissue from MS patients. According to user surveys conducted by the MS Society, the needs of researchers have been adequately met by these brain banks. There are also MS brain banks in Britain and in the Netherlands. The latter provides services unmatched by any other MS brain bank (Box 6.3). The amount of brain tissue at the British brain bank has been too limited to supply researchers outside

---

**BOX 6.3**
**Netherlands Brain Bank**

The Netherlands Brain Bank was organized in 1985 and, in 1990, established its program related to MS, whose main purpose is to obtain rapid autopsies from which tissues can be used for studies in neuropathology, immunocytochemistry, molecular biology, and tissue culture. The tissues are properly prepared for special studies, and the program has the flexibility to initiate new procedures. Sufficient amounts of all tissues are retained for potential follow-up for future studies.

Thus far, 110 MS autopsies have been performed, averaging 10 to 12 cases per year. The program also emphases obtaining "control" autopsies, of which about 30 or more are performed annually. Only about 10 percent of the rapid autopsy cases performed are for MS; the control cases (20 to 30 percent) are also part of the program. The brain bank also obtains cases of various other neurological diseases, with an emphasis on Alzheimer's disease (30-40 cases per year). Overall, the brain bank team performs 100 to 120 rapid autopsies per year. Of note, the protocols involved in an MS autopsy include MRI pathology studies and lesion dissection, which result in such cases taking three to four times longer (six to seven hours) than many others. The tissues must be analyzed as completely as possible, ideally including assessment of the extent of tissue injury, activity of the disease, and extent of remyelination. Indeed, a key strength of this program is the ability to perform MRI scans in the middle of the night. The MRI-pathology correlation effort of the brain bank is internationally recognized. This effort includes postmortem in situ imaging, as well as imaging of tissue sections. The approach of using MRI-defined lesions to direct the site of neuropathology examination, as well as more traditional MRI correlation with pathologically obvious lesions, is considered very promising.

Because it is part of the larger brain bank, the MS brain bank can share the highly expert staff (secretaries, pathologists, technicians, and undertaker) who are available full-time. Without this type of infrastructure, the rapid response to MS cases could not take place.

There is a well-established program in which patients agree to tissue donation. Donations are organized through direct efforts of the brain bank with the public. The entire staff is attuned to the ethical issues and specific restrictions on tissue access opportunities that exist in the Netherlands.

There is increasing demand on the bank for tissue, and an impressive number of research papers have been published using its materials. A 1999 review of the program indicated that it should be able to deal with any concern *within the Netherlands* regarding access to this national resource. Established users of the bank pay an annual subscription fee of 3000 df ($1,100 U.S.). Commercial companies are charged at higher rates. There is also a "pilot" program for which no charges are made. The brain bank is funded approximately equally by the Dutch MS Society, the hospital in which it operates, and research grants.

Britain, and tissue distribution from the Netherlands brain bank has been largely restricted to European researchers. Finally, some researchers maintain their own brain banks and do not publicly distribute the tissue. Private collections are necessary for researchers who need to tailor tissue collection procedures for specific research techniques.

The issue of access to cases of MS early in the disease course remains an unresolved challenge. Surgical samples are available mainly from cases that represent diagnostic difficulties and cannot be expected to be representative of all early MS cases. These patients can be followed and their subsequent disease course established. They provide an excellent opportunity to correlate neuro-imaging data with tissue analyses. The hope is to establish imaging criteria that will correlate with the suspected different pathologic forms of MS. Serial samples are not likely to be available from these cases. Additional surgical samples may become available if other invasive therapies such as deep brain stimulators come into use to treat some of the disabling symptoms of MS such as tremor.

Combined with the increased demand, the limitations in obtaining MS tissues for research studies suggest a need for international cooperative efforts. Such efforts would include ensuring that all those involved in tissue collection aim to meet the ideals described above with regard to tissue handling. Collected tissue should be preserved to allow as many types of analyses as possible. Specifically, tissue collection and storage protocols that allow for histologic, immunocytochemical, and molecular analyses should be established and consistently followed. Tissues that are to be provided to investigators for biochemical and molecular analyses of disease activity must be carefully evaluated pathologically. Standard criteria for rating disease activity would improve comparisons between different studies. It is also important to have facilities that can respond rapidly when cases of MS become available for postmortem analyses, including the ability to perform immediate pre-autopsy MR scanning and scanning of tissues immediately after collection. Education of MS patients about the value of such programs is also important. As discussed under communication in Chapter 4, it is important that patients and their families participate in the development of informational materials. The protocols of the Amsterdam brain bank offer an instructive model for brain banks in other countries (Box 6.3).

# REFERENCES

1.  Akizuki M, Reeves JP, Steinberg AD. 1978. Expression of autoimmunity by NZB/NZW marrow. *Clin Immunol Immunopathol.*;10:247-50.
2.  ALS CNTF Study Group. 1996. The Amyotrophic Lateral Sclerosis Functional Rating Scale. Assessment of activities of daily living in patients with amyotrophic lateral sclerosis. The ALS CNTF treatment study (ACTS) phase I-II Study Group. *Arch Neurol.*;53:141-7.
3.  Antel JP, Becher B, Owens T. 1996. Immunotherapy for multiple sclerosis: from theory to practice. *Nat Med.*;2:1074-5.

4. Baldwin JL, Storb R, Thomas ED, Mannik M. 1977. Bone marrow transplantation in patients with gold-induced marrow aplasia. *Arthritis Rheum.*;20:1043-8.

5. Baron W, Metz B, Bansal R, Hoekstra D, de Vries H. 2000. PDGF and FGF-2 signaling in oligodendrocyte progenitor cells: regulation of proliferation and differentiation by multiple intracellular signaling pathways. *Mol Cell Neurosci.*;15:314-29.

6. Barres BA. 1999. A new role for glia: generation of neurons! *Cell.*;97:667-70.

7. BDNF Study Group. 1999. A controlled trial of recombinant methionyl human BDNF in ALS: The BDNF Study Group (Phase III). *Neurology.*;52:1427-33.

8. Ben-Nun A, Wekerle H, Cohen IR. 1981. Vaccination against autoimmune encephalomyelitis with T-lymphocyte line cells reactive against myelin basic protein. *Nature.*;292:60-1.

9. Besser M, Wank R. 1999. Cutting edge: clonally restricted production of the neurotrophins brain-derived neurotrophic factor and neurotrophin-3 mRNA by human immune cells and Th1/Th2-polarized expression of their receptors. *J Immunol.*;162:6303-6.

10. Bjornson CR, Rietze RL, Reynolds BA, Magli MC, Vescovi AL. 1999. Turning brain into blood: a hematopoietic fate adopted by adult neural stem cells in vivo. *Science.*;283:534-7.

11. Blakemore WF, Keirstead HS. 1999. The origin of remyelinating cells in the central nervous system. *J Neuroimmunol.*;98:69-76.

12. Bo L, Dawson TM, Wesselingh S, et al. 1994. Induction of nitric oxide synthase in demyelinating regions of multiple sclerosis brains. *Ann Neurol.*;36:778-86.

13. Bourdette DN, Chou YK, Whitham RH, et al. 1998. Immunity to T cell receptor peptides in multiple sclerosis. III. Preferential immunogenicity of complementarity-determining region 2 peptides from disease-associated T cell receptor BV genes. *J Immunol.*;161:1034-44.

14. Boutros T, Croze E, Yong VW. 1997. Interferon-beta is a potent promoter of nerve growth factor production by astrocytes. *J Neurochem.*;69:939-46.

15. Breban M, Hammer RE, Richardson JA, Taurog JD. 1993. Transfer of the inflammatory disease of HLA-B27 transgenic rats by bone marrow engraftment. *J Exp Med.*;178:1607-16.

16. Canoll PD, Musacchio JM, Hardy R, Reynolds R, Marchionni MA, Salzer JL. 1996. GGF/neuregulin is a neuronal signal that promotes the proliferation and survival and inhibits the differentiation of oligodendrocyte progenitors. *Neuron.*;17:229-43.

17. Carson MJ, Behringer RR, Brinster RL, McMorris FA. 1993. Insulin-like growth factor I increases brain growth and central nervous system myelination in transgenic mice. *Neuron.*;10:729-40.

18. Chabrier PE, Demerle-Pallardy C, Auguet M. 1999. Nitric oxide synthases: targets for therapeutic strategies in neurological diseases. *Cell Mol Life Sci.*;55:1029-35.

19. Cheng H, Almstrom S, Gimenez-Llort L, et al. 1997. Gait analysis of adult paraplegic rats after spinal cord repair. *Exp Neurol.*;148:544-57.

20. Cohen RI, Marmur R, Norton WT, Mehler MF, Kessler JA. 1996. Nerve growth factor and neurotrophin-3 differentially regulate the proliferation and survival of developing rat brain oligodendrocytes. *J Neurosci.*;16:6433-42.

21. D'Souza SD, Alinauskas KA, Antel JP. 1996. Ciliary neurotrophic factor selectively protects human oligodendrocytes from tumor necrosis factor-mediated injury. *J Neurosci Res.*;43:289-98.

22. Dawson VL, Dawson TM. 1998. Nitric oxide in neurodegeneration. *Prog Brain Res.*;118:215-229.

23. DeHeer DH, Edgington TS. 1977. Evidence for a B lymphocyte defect underlying the anti-X anti-erythrocyte autoantibody response of NZB mice. *J Immunol.*;118:1858-63.

24. Eedy DJ, Burrows D, Bridges JM, Jones FG. 1990. Clearance of severe psoriasis after allogenic bone marrow transplantation. *BMJ.*;300:908.

25. Fern R, Ransom BR, Stys PK, Waxman SG. 1993. Pharmacological protection of CNS white matter during anoxia: actions of phenytoin, carbamazepine and diazepam. *J Pharmacol Exp Ther.*;266:1549-55.

26. Fern R, Waxman SG, Ransom BR. 1995. Endogenous GABA attenuates CNS white matter dysfunction following anoxia. *J Neurosci.*;15:699-708.

27. Fischer JS, LaRocca NG, Miller DM, Ritvo PG, Andrews H, Paty D. 1999. Recent developments in the assessment of quality of life in multiple sclerosis (MS). *Multiple Sclerosis.*;5:251-9.

28. Gensert JM, Goldman JE. 1997. Endogenous progenitors remyelinate demyelinated axons in the adult CNS. *Neuron.*;19:197-203.

29. George EB, Glass JD, Griffin JW. 1995. Axotomy-induced axonal degeneration is mediated by calcium influx through ion-specific channels. *J Neurosci.*;15:6445-52.

30. Goodin DS. 1999. Perils and pitfalls in the interpretation of clinical trials: a reflection on the recent experience in multiple sclerosis. *Neuroepidemiology.*;18:53-63.

31. Gveric D, Cuzner ML, Newcombe J. 1999. Insulin-like growth factors and binding proteins in multiple sclerosis plaques. *Neuropathol Appl Neurobiol.*;25:215-25.

32. Hammond SR, English DR, McLeod JG. 2000. The age-range of risk of developing multiple sclerosis: evidence from a migrant population in Australia. *Brain.*;123:968-74.

33. Hauben E, Butovsky O, Nevo U, et al. 2000. Passive or active immunization with myelin basic protein promotes recovery from spinal cord contusion. *J Neurosci.*;20:6421-30.

34. Holland FJ, McConnon JK, Volpe R, Saunders EF. 1991. Concordant Graves' disease after bone marrow transplantation: implications for pathogenesis. *J Clin Endocrinol Metab.*;72:837-840.

35. Ikehara S, Good RA, Nakamura T, et al. 1985. Rationale for bone marrow transplantation in the treatment of autoimmune diseases. *Proc Natl Acad Sci U S A.*;82:2483-7.

36. Ikehara S, Kawamura M, Takao F, et al. 1990. Organ-specific and systemic autoimmune diseases originate from defects in hematopoietic stem cells. *Proc Natl Acad Sci U S A.*;87:8341-4.

37. Ikehara S, Ohtsuki H, Good RA, et al. 1985. Prevention of type I diabetes in nonobese diabetic mice by allogenic bone marrow transplantation. *Proc Natl Acad Sci U S A.*;82:7743-7.

38. Ikehara S, Yasumizu R, Inaba M, et al. 1989. Long-term observations of autoimmune-prone mice treated for autoimmune disease by allogeneic bone marrow transplantation. *Proc Natl Acad Sci U S A.*;86:3306-10.

39. Isacson O, Breakefield XO. 1997. Benefits and risks of hosting animal cells in the human brain. *Nat Med.*;3:964-9.

40. Ishida T, Inaba M, Hisha H, et al. 1994. Requirement of donor-derived stromal cells in the bone marrow for successful allogeneic bone marrow transplantation. Complete prevention of recurrence of autoimmune diseases in MRL/MP-Ipr/Ipr mice by transplantation of bone marrow plus bones (stromal cells) from the same donor. *J Immunol.*;152:3119-27.

41. Jacobs P, Vincent MD, Martell RW. 1986. Prolonged remission of severe refractory rheumatoid arthritis following allogeneic bone marrow transplantation for drug-induced aplastic anaemia. *Bone Marrow Transplant.*;1:237-239.

42. Jones JI, Clemmons DR. 1995. Insulin-like growth factors and their binding proteins: biological actions. *Endocr Rev.*;16:3-34.

43. Junger H, Junger WG. 1998. CNTF and GDNF, but not NT-4, support corticospinal motor neuron growth via direct mechanisms. *Neuroreport.*;9:3749-54.

44. Keirstead HS, Blakemore WF. 1997. Identification of post-mitotic oligodendrocytes incapable of remyelination within the demyelinated adult spinal cord. *J Neuropathol Exp Neurol.*;56:1191-201.

45. Keirstead HS, Blakemore WF. 1999. The role of oligodendrocytes and oligodendrocyte progenitors in CNS remyelination. *Adv Exp Med Biol.*;468.

46. Kerschensteiner M, Gallmeier E, Behrens L, et al. 1999. Activated human T cells, B cells, and monocytes produce brain-derived neurotrophic factor in vitro and in inflammatory brain lesions: a neuroprotective role of inflammation? *J Exp Med.*;189:865-70.

47. Komoly S, Hudson LD, Webster HD, Bondy CA. 1992. Insulin-like growth factor I gene expression is induced in astrocytes during experimental demyelination. *Proc Natl Acad Sci U S A.*;89:1894-8.

48. Kumar S, Kahn MA, Dinh L, de Vellis J. 1998. NT-3-mediated TrkC receptor activation promotes proliferation and cell survival of rodent progenitor oligodendrocyte cells in vitro and in vivo. *J Neurosci Res.*;54:754-65.

49. Kumar S, Pena LA, de Vellis J. 1993. CNS glial cells express neurotrophin receptors whose levels are regulated by NGF. *Brain Res Mol Brain Res.*;17:163-8.

50. Kurtzke JF. 1983. Rating neurologic impairment in multiple sclerosis: an expanded disability status scale (EDSS). *Neurology.*;33:1444-52.

51. Ladiwala U, Lachance C, Simoneau SJ, Bhakar A, Barker PA, Antel JP. 1998. p75 neurotrophin receptor expression on adult human oligodendrocytes: signaling without cell death in response to NGF. *J Neurosci.*;18:1297-304.

52. LaFace DM, Peck AB. 1989. Reciprocal allogeneic bone marrow transplantation between NOD mice and diabetes-nonsusceptible mice associated with transfer and prevention of autoimmune diabetes. *Diabetes.*;38:894-901.

53. Lampeter EF, Homberg M, Quabeck K, et al. 1993. Transfer of insulin-dependent diabetes between HLA-identical siblings by bone marrow transplantation. *Lancet.*;341:1243-1244.

54. Lassmann H, Bruck W, Lucchinetti C, Rodriguez M. 1997. Remyelination in multiple sclerosis. *Mult Scler.*;3:133-6.

55. Laudiero LB, Aloe L, Levi-Montalcini R, et al. 1992. Multiple sclerosis patients express increased levels of beta-nerve growth factor in cerebrospinal fluid. *Neurosci Lett.*;147:9-12.

56. Lee WH, Javedan S, Bondy CA. 1992. Coordinate expression of insulin-like growth factor system components by neurons and neuroglia during retinal and cerebellar development. *J Neurosci.*;12:4737-44.

57. Lenz DC, Swanborg RH. 1999. Suppressor cells in demyelinating disease: a new paradigm for the new millennium. *J Neuroimmunol.*;100:53-7.

58. Li H, Kaufman CL, Boggs SS, Johnson PC, Patrene KD, Ildstad ST. 1996. Mixed allogeneic chimerism induced by a sublethal approach prevents autoimmune diabetes and reverses insulitis in nonobese diabetic (NOD) mice. *J Immunol.*;156:380-8.

59. Lindsay RM. 1996. Role of neurotrophins and trk receptors in the development and maintenance of sensory neurons: an overview. *Philos Trans R Soc Lond B Biol Sci.*;351:365-73.

60. Liu X, Yao DL, Webster H. 1995. Insulin-like growth factor I treatment reduces clinical deficits and lesion severity in acute demyelinating experimental autoimmune encephalomyelitis. *Mult Scler.*;1:2-9.

61. Liu Y, Himes BT, Solowska J, et al. 1999. Intraspinal delivery of neurotrophin-3 using neural stem cells genetically modified by recombinant retrovirus. *Exp Neurol.*;158:9-26.

62. Liu Y, Jowitt S. Resolution of immune-mediated diseases following allogeneic bone marrow transplantation for leukemia. *Bone Marrow Transplantation.* 1992;9.

63. Liu Y, Kim D, Himes BT, et al. 1999. Transplants of fibroblasts genetically modified to express BDNF promote regeneration of adult rat rubrospinal axons and recovery of forelimb function. *J Neurosci.*;19:4370-87.

64. Lobell A, Weissert R, Storch MK, et al. 1998. Vaccination with DNA encoding an immunodominant myelin basic protein peptide targeted to Fc of immunoglobulin G suppresses experimental autoimmune encephalomyelitis. *J Exp Med.*;187:1543-8.

65. Louis JC, Magal E, Takayama S, Varon S. 1993. CNTF protection of oligodendrocytes against natural and tumor necrosis factor-induced death. *Science.*;259:689-92.

66. Lowenthal RM, Cohen ML, Atkinson K, Biggs JC. 1993. Apparent cure of rheumatoid arthritis by bone marrow transplantation. *J Rheumatol.*;20:137-140.

67. Marchionni MA, Cannella B, Hoban C, et al. 1999. Neuregulin in neuron/glial interactions in the central nervous system. GGF2 diminishes autoimmune demyelination, promotes oligodendrocyte progenitor expansion, and enhances remyelination. *Adv Exp Med Biol.*;468:283-295.

68. Marmont A. 1995. Immune ablation followed by stem cell rescue: a new radical approach to the treatment of severe autoimmune diseases. *Forum.*;5:24.

69. McDonald JW, Althomsons SP, Hyrc KL, Choi DW, Goldberg MP. 1998. Oligodendrocytes from forebrain are highly vulnerable to AMPA/kainate receptor-mediated excitotoxicity. *Nat Med.*;4:291-7.

70. McFarland H, Barkhof F, Antel J, Miller DH. 2001. The role of MRI as a surrogate outcome measure in MS. *Ann Neurol.*;in press.

71. McKay RD. 1999. Brain stem cells change their identity. *Nat Med.*;5:261-2.

72. Micera A, De Simone R, Aloe L. 1995. Elevated levels of nerve growth factor in the thalamus and spinal cord of rats affected by experimental allergic encephalomyelitis. *Arch Ital Biol.*;133:131-42.

73. Micera A, Lambiase A, Rama P, Aloe L. 1999. Altered nerve growth factor level in the optic nerve of patients affected by multiple sclerosis. *Mult Scler.*;5:389-94.

74. Miller RG, Mitchell JD, Moore DH. 2000. Riluzole for amyotrophic lateral sclerosis (ALS)/ motor neuron disease (MND). *Cochrane Database Syst Rev.*;CD001447.

75. Moore MA. 1999. "Turning brain into blood"—clinical applications of stem-cell research in neurobiology and hematology. *N Engl J Med.*;341:605-7.

76. Morton JI, Siegel BV. 1974. Transplantation of autoimmune potential. I. Development of antinuclear antibodies in H-2 histocompatible recipients of bone marrow from New Zealand Black mice. *Proc Natl Acad Sci U S A.*;71:2162-5.

77. Morton JI, Siegel BV. 1979. Transplantation of autoimmune potential. IV. Reversal of the NZB autoimmune syndrome by bone marrow transplantation. *Transplantation.*;27:133-4.

78. Naji A, Silvers W, Bellgrau D, Anderson A, Plotkin S, Bakker C. Prevention of diabetes in rats by bone marrow transplantation. *Annals of Surgery.* 1981;194:328.

79. Nakamura T, Ikehara S, Good RA, et al. 1985. Abnormal stem cells in autoimmune-prone mice are responsible for premature thymic involution. *Thymus.*;7:151-60.

80. Nicolle MM, Shivers A, Gill TM, Gallagher M. 1997. Hippocampal N-methyl-D-aspartate and kainate binding in response to entorhinal cortex aspiration or 192 IgG-saporin lesions of the basal forebrain. *Neuroscience.*;77:649-59.

81. Nudo RJ. 1999. Recovery after damage to motor cortical areas. *Curr Opin Neurobiol.*;9:740-7.

82. Ochs G, Giess R, Bendszus M, Krone A. 1999. Epi-arachnoidal drug deposit: a rare complication of intrathecal drug therapy. *J Pain Symptom Manage.*;18:229-32.

83. Penn RD, Kroin JS, York MM, Cedarbaum JM. 1997. Intrathecal ciliary neurotrophic factor delivery for treatment of amyotrophic lateral sclerosis (phase I trial). *Neurosurgery.*;40:94-9; discussion 99-100.

84. Rabchevsky AG, Fugaccia I, Turner AF, Blades DA, Mattson MP, Scheff SW. 2000. Basic fibroblast growth factor (bFGF) enhances functional recovery following severe spinal cord injury to the rat. *Exp Neurol.*;164:280-91.

85. Raine CS. 1996. Multiple sclerosis: prospects for remyelination. *Mult Scler.*;2:195-7.

86. Ransom BR, Waxman SG, Davis PK. 1990. Anoxic injury of CNS white matter: protective effect of ketamine. *Neurology.*;40:1399-403.

87. Rogister B, Ben-Hur T, Dubois-Dalcq M. 1999. From neural stem cells to myelinating oligodendrocytes. *Mol Cell Neurosci.*;14:287-300.

88. Rose NR, Bona C. 1993. Defining criteria for autoimmune diseases (Witebsky's postulates revisited). *Immunol Today.*;14:426-430.

89. Roubenoff R, Jones RJ, Karp JE, Stevens MB. 1987. Remission of rheumatoid arthritis with the successful treatment of acute myelogenous leukemia with cytosine arabinoside, daunorubicin, and m-AMSA. *Arthritis Rheum.*;30:1187-1190.

90. Rudick R, Antel J, Confavreux C, et al. 1997. Recommendations from the National Multiple Sclerosis Society Clinical Outcomes Assessment Task Force. *Ann Neurol.*;42:379-82.

91. Schwartz CE, Vollmer T, Lee H. 1999. Reliability and validity of two self-report measures of impairment and disability for MS. North American Research Consortium on Multiple Sclerosis Outcomes Study Group. *Neurology.*;52:63-70.

92. Scolding NJ, Franklin RJ. 1997. Remyelination in demyelinating disease. *Baillieres Clin Neurol.*;6:525-48.

93. Serreze DV, Leiter EH, Worthen SM, Shultz LD. 1988. NOD marrow stem cells adoptively transfer diabetes to resistant (NOD x NON)F1 mice. *Diabetes.*;37:252-5.

94. Snyder EY, Macklis JD. 1995-1996. Multipotent neural progenitor or stem-like cells may be uniquely suited for therapy for some neurodegenerative conditions. *Clin Neurosci.*;3:310-6.

95. Stangel M, Boegner F, Klatt CH, Hofmeister C, Seyfert S. 2000. Placebo controlled pilot trial to study the remyelinating potential of intravenous immunoglobulins in multiple sclerosis. *J Neurol Neurosurg Psychiatry.*;68:89-92.

96. Steinman L. 2000. Despite epitope spreading in the pathogenesis of autoimmune disease, highly restricted approaches to immune therapy may still succeed [with a hedge on this bet]. *J Autoimmun.*;14:278-82.

97. Stinissen P, Raus J, Zhang J. 1997. Autoimmune pathogenesis of multiple sclerosis: role of autoreactive T lymphocytes and new immunotherapeutic strategies. *Crit Rev Immunol.*;17:33-75.

98. Stys PK, Ransom BR, Waxman SG, Davis PK. 1990. Role of extracellular calcium in anoxic injury of mammalian central white matter. *Proc Natl Acad Sci U S A.*;87:4212-6.

99. Stys PK, Sontheimer H, Ransom BR, Waxman SG. 1993. Noninactivating, tetrodotoxin-sensitive Na+ conductance in rat optic nerve axons. *Proc Natl Acad Sci U S A.*;90:6976-80.

100. Stys PK, Waxman SG, Ransom BR. 1992. Ionic mechanisms of anoxic injury in mammalian CNS white matter: role of Na+ channels and Na(+)-Ca2+ exchanger. *J Neurosci.*;12:430-9.

101. Taub E, Uswatte G, Pidikiti R. 1999. Constraint-Induced Movement Therapy: a new family of techniques with broad application to physical rehabilitation—a clinical review. *J Rehabil Res Dev.*;36:237-51.

102. Theofilopoulos AN, Balderas RS, Gozes Y, et al. 1985. Association of lpr gene with graft-vs.-host disease-like syndrome. *J Exp Med.*;162:1-18.

103. Theofilopoulos AN, Dixon FJ. 1985. Murine models of systemic lupus erythematosus. *Adv Immunol.*;37:269-390.

104. Trapp BD, Ransohoff RM, Fisher E, Rudick RA. 1999. Neurodegeneration in multiple sclerosis: relationship to neurological disability. *The Neuroscientist.*;5:48-57.

105. Tyndall A. 1997. Hematopoietic stem cell transplantation in rheumatic diseases other than systemic sclerosis and systemic lupus erythematosus. *J Rheumatol Suppl.*;48.

106. van Bekkum DW. 1993. BMT in experimental autoimmune diseases. *Bone Marrow Transplant.*;11:183-7.

107. Vandenbark AA, Chou YK, Whitham R, et al. 1996. Treatment of multiple sclerosis with T-cell receptor peptides: results of a double-blind pilot trial. *Nat Med.*;2:1109-15.

108. Venters HD, Tang Q, Liu Q, VanHoy RW, Dantzer R, Kelley KW. 1999. A new mechanism of neurodegeneration: a proinflammatory cytokine inhibits receptor signaling by a survival peptide. *Proc Natl Acad Sci U S A.*;96:9879-84.

109. Vialettes B, Maraninchi D, San Marco MP, et al. 1993. Autoimmune polyendocrine failure—type 1 (insulin-dependent) diabetes mellitus and hypothyroidism—after allogeneic bone marrow transplantation in a patient with lymphoblastic leukaemia. *Diabetologia.*;36:541-546.

110. Villoslada P, Hauser SL, Bartke I, et al. 2000. Human nerve growth factor protects common marmosets against autoimmune encephalomyelitis by switching the balance of T helper cell type 1 and 2 cytokines within the central nervous system. *J Exp Med.*;191:1799-806.

111. Waisman A, Ruiz PJ, Hirschberg DL, et al. 1996. Suppressive vaccination with DNA encoding a variable region gene of the T-cell receptor prevents autoimmune encephalomyelitis and activates Th2 immunity. *Nat Med.*;2:899-905.

112. Warrington AE, Asakura K, Bieber AJ, et al. 2000. Human monoclonal antibodies reactive to oligodendrocytes promote remyelination in a model of multiple sclerosis. *Proc Natl Acad Sci U S A.*;97:6820-6825.

113. Waubant E, Goodkin D. 2000. Methodological problems in evaluating efficacy of a treatment in multiple sclerosis. *Pathol Biol (Paris).*;48:104-13.

114. Webster HD. 1997. Growth factors and myelin regeneration in multiple sclerosis. *Mult Scler.*;3:113-20.

115. Wicker LS, Miller BJ, Chai A, Terada M, Mullen Y. 1988. Expression of genetically determined diabetes and insulitis in the nonobese diabetic (NOD) mouse at the level of bone marrow-derived cells. Transfer of diabetes and insulitis to nondiabetic (NOD X B10) F1 mice with bone marrow cells from NOD mice. *J Exp Med.*;167:1801-10.

116. Wilson DB, Golding AB, Smith RA, et al. 1997. Results of a phase I clinical trial of a T-cell receptor peptide vaccine in patients with multiple sclerosis. I. Analysis of T-cell receptor utilization in CSF cell populations. *J Neuroimmunol.*;76:15-28.

117. Xu XM, Guenard V, Kleitman N, Aebischer P, Bunge MB. 1995. A combination of BDNF and NT-3 promotes supraspinal axonal regeneration into Schwann cell grafts in adult rat thoracic spinal cord. *Exp Neurol.*;134:261-72.

118. Yandava BD, Billinghurst LL, Snyder EY. 1999. "Global" cell replacement is feasible via neural stem cell transplantation: evidence from the dysmyelinated shiverer mouse brain. *Proc Natl Acad Sci U S A.*;96:7029-34.

119. Ye P, D'Ercole AJ. 1999. Insulin-like growth factor I protects oligodendrocytes from tumor necrosis factor-alpha-induced injury. *Endocrinology.*;140:3063-72.

120. Zhang J, Stinissen P, Medaer R, Truyen L, Raus J. T-cell vaccination for the treatment of multiple sclerosis. In Zhang J, ed. *Immunotherapy in Neuroimmunologic Diseases.* London, England: Martin Dunitz; 1998.

# 7

# Building and Supporting
# the Research Enterprise

The foundations of scientific progress are laid in the building and mainte-nance of the research enterprise. In simplest terms, this means getting the "right" people in the "right" places, and that is the essential role of research managers. For biomedical research, this encompasses five key domains: [13]

1. Research funding
2. Human resources
3. Infrastructure
4. Clinical trials
5. Biotechnology and pharmaceutical firms

The drive to end the devastating effects of multiple sclerosis (MS) rests on building and sustaining these key domains of biomedical research, which are discussed in turn below. The accompanying box provides a snapshot of the Na-tional Multiple Sclerosis Society's research programs (Box 7.1).

## RESEARCH FUNDING

According to one analysis that compared funding levels at the National Institutes of Health (NIH) to the total burden of specific diseases, MS funding is higher than might be expected (Figure 7.1).[8] In terms of funding from private health foundations that target specific diseases, MS research is also relatively well supported, at least in the United States. The research budget of the MS

## BOX 7.1
## National Multiple Sclerosis Society Research Programs

The society is the largest private sponsor of MS research in the world. Support for basic and clinical research is provided in the form of research grants and contracts, training programs, faculty awards, pilot project grants, workshop support, and other award programs including targeted, society-initiated projects.

Most research program money is spent on full research grants (averaging $114,000 per year), followed by postdoctoral fellowships (averaging $32,000 per year). The top area of research emphasis is immunology, followed by glial biology (study of myelin-making cells and other support cells of the brain that do not conduct nerve signals) and infectious triggers. Some 42 percent of all newly funded research projects focus on humans or human tissues; the remaining funds support fundamental research.

In the spring 1999 review cycle, annual research grant awards ranged from $70,960 to $251,855, averaging about $114,000. These awards include no more than 10 percent indirect costs. The society's research awards exceed those of other major voluntary health agencies. For example, the American Diabetes Association gives a maximum of $100,000 (including indirect costs) per year for research grants. The American Cancer Society gives a maximum stipend of $32,000 per year for postdoctoral fellowships. By contrast, National Institutes of Health research grants currently average $255,000 annually, including indirect costs, which can exceed 50 percent of total direct costs.

In fiscal year 1998 (October 1, 1997-September 30, 1998), research and related expenses accounted for 18 percent of combined chapter and home office expenses and 37 percent of expenses of the home office. During FY 1999, the society supported more research than in any previous year—expending $22.5 million (unaudited) for all research programs and support activities, including some 333 new and ongoing MS research projects.

Applications are reviewed and funded in two cycles per year. Research grant proposals are reviewed in the fall and spring; fellowships are reviewed once each year in the spring (for July 1 startups); pilot projects are reviewed and approved on a year-round, ad hoc basis; and health care delivery and policy (HCDP) contracts are reviewed once each year in the spring (for July 1 startups). Funding decisions are made within five months of the deadline for applications, awards are made three months later, adding up to at least eight months from submission of application to receipt of award. The comparable cycle at the National Institutes of Health is nine to ten months.

Of 300 projects reviewed for all programs during FY 1999, 129 (43 percent) were found meritorious and approved for funding. Successful applicants are required to submit annual and final reports detailing progress toward their research aims and fiscal reports of their award money expenditures.

When needed, the society convenes special task forces of experts in a particular field to explore new possibilities in MS research and to make recommendations for steps to stimulate research in these areas. Recent examples include the 1996 Task Force on Clinical Trial Outcome Measures, the 1997 Database Advisory Panel; and in 1998, the Task Force on Gender in MS and Autoimmunity, the

*continues*

Task Force on Combination Therapy, and the Task Force on Clinico-Pathological Correlates of the MS Lesion.

In 1987, the society formalized a program to attract proposals in management, care, and rehabilitation. These research grants are of one to five years' duration. In 1988, an HCDP research program was developed to fund studies on access, quality and funding of health care and quality of life for people with MS and/or family members. In FY 1996, HCDP research began to focus on large contracts addressing society-established priorities.

Research to find the cause of MS and its cure is only one of several roles of the National MS Society. The society also supports professional and public education, legislative advocacy, information referral, and programs to help people with MS cope with their disease.

The society counts on the voluntary services of members of six advisory panels and numerous task forces to help determine which projects are worthy of support. One panel, the Research Programs Advisory Committee, provides oversight and helps direct the society's overall research programs. This senior committee is an international panel that includes top basic and clinical MS researchers and lay leaders who are members of the society's National Board of Directors.

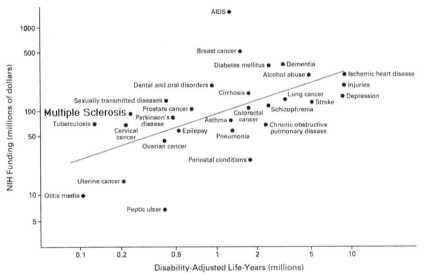

**FIGURE 7.1** Relationship between NIH disease-specific research funding in 1996 and disability-adjusted life-years for 29 conditions. The axes are drawn to logarithmic scale. The line represents funding predicted on the basis of a linear regression with disability-adjusted life-years as the explanatory variable. A disability-adjusted life-year is a summary measure of population health status that represents the burden of disease in the form of lost years of healthy life due to either disability or premature death. SOURCE: Gross et al., 1999.[8] Copyright 1999 Massachusetts Medical Society. All rights reserved. Reprinted with permission.

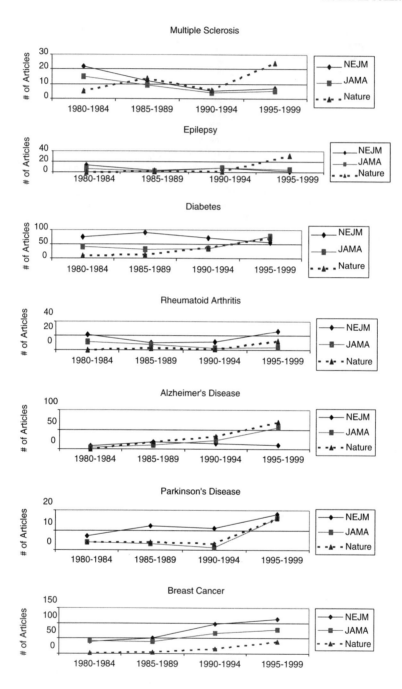

**FIGURE 7.2a** Summary of publications in general medical journals.

Society is within the range of similar foundations in the United States (Table 7.1), and MS research is also relatively well funded in Great Britain.[2] In sum, it appears that the overall funding levels for MS research are at least comparable to those for other chronic diseases, but it would be a mistake to conclude from total funding levels that funding for MS research is as good as or better than can be expected. The vitality of the MS research enterprise also depends on the distribution of these funds. Are they distributed in a manner that optimizes the generation of the most critical information about MS? The ideal distribution of research monies is more than a matter of simply funding the best research proposals. It also involves recruiting researchers that will generate the most innovative and productive research strategies and, likewise, establishing programs that will yield the most useful information. Such programs might range from grants awarded to individual investigators to international collaborative networks in which investigators establish common research protocols and outcome measures.

Measuring the productivity of a research discipline is anathema to many scientists, yet that is what a committee attempted to do for the field of immunology in 1999 for a joint committee of the National Academy of Sciences, National Academy of Engineering, and Institute of Medicine.[13] (This request was in response to the passage of a congressional act in 1993 requiring that federal agencies develop performance measurements.) As the immunology review committee noted, although precise measurement is not possible, general conclusions can be drawn. Publication rates offer a snapshot of productivity. A review of publications from 1985 to 1999 on MS, epilepsy, diabetes, rheumatoid arthritis, Alzheimer's disease, Parkinson's disease, and breast cancer showed that MS is the only one of these that has consistently declined in terms of number of publica-

**TABLE 7.1** Research Budgets of Selected Health Organizations in 1998

| Organization | Total Revenue | Net Assets | Total Expenditures | Research Budget | % of Budget Spent on Research |
|---|---|---|---|---|---|
| Alzheimer's Association | 48.2 | 34.2 | 46.7 | 12.8 | 27 |
| American Diabetes Association | 125.1 | 49.6 | 122.9 | 19.6 | 16 |
| Arthritis Foundation | 114.1 | 141.9 | 103.1 | 24.2 | 23 |
| March of Dimes | 181.3 | 43.0 | 174.7 | 35.6 | 20 |
| Muscular Dystrophy Association | 135.0 | 113.2 | 112.5 | 24.6 | 22 |
| National Multiple Sclerosis Society | 59.3 | 23.8 | 52.6 | 19.6 | 37 |
| National Parkinson Foundation | 16.5 | 12.1 | 16.6 | 4.0 | 24 |
| Huntington's Disease Society of America | 3.7 | 1.7 | 3.7 | 1.0 | 27 |

NOTE: Data in this table are based on annual reports for each organization and have been confirmed by each of the organizations listed.

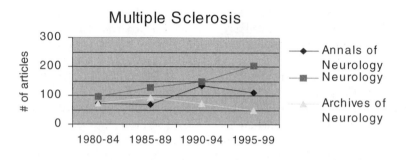

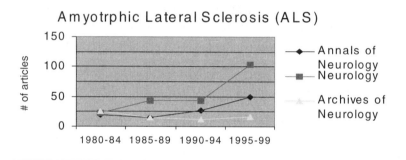

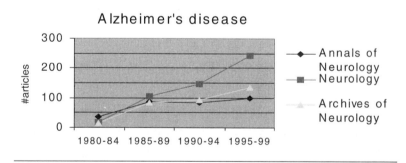

**FIGURE 7.2b**  Summary of publications in neurology journals.

tions (Figure 7.2a). Compared to epilepsy, diabetes, rheumatoid arthritis, Alzheimer's disease, Parkinson's disease, and breast cancer, publications on MS showed the greatest downward trend in the *New England Journal of Medicine* and the *Journal of the American Medical Association*. Except for publications on rheumatoid arthritis, which declined and then rebounded, publications on the

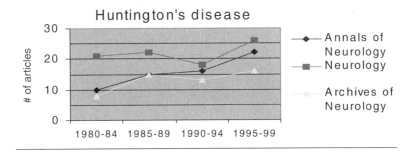

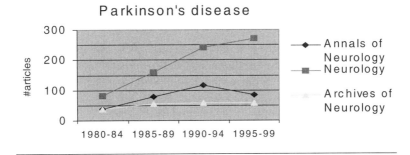

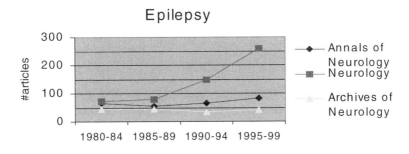

**FIGURE 7.2b** *(Continued).*

other diseases steadily increased or generally remained constant. The trend for MS publications was somewhat stronger in the *Nature* journals in the mid-1990s, after showing one of the strongest declines in the late 1980s.

As with the general medical journals, the publication rates of MS research articles in neurology journals tend to lag behind those of other neurological disorders (Figure 7.2b). Compared to articles on ALS, Alzheimer's disease, Parkinson's disease, epilepsy, and Huntington's disease, MS research articles ranked the lowest overall in terms of average percent increase in numbers of articles published from 1980 to 1999. Among the six neurological diseases compared, the average percent increase of MS articles ranked 5th in *Neurology*, 5th in *Annals of Neurology*, and 6th in *Archives of General Neurology*. (Note that these comparison are based on counting the number of articles in which a particular disease was mentioned in the title of the article, thus a few relevant articles might not have been included, but this is unlikely to cause a systematic bias in ranking of overall publication rates.)

## Research Centers

There has been great interest in redirecting funds that might otherwise go to individual investigators to fund large multilaboratory centers. Indeed, the MS Society funded several centers in the 1970s and 1980s, but stopped in 1983. At the time, interest in MS research was increasing across the country, and after careful review, the Society concluded that the concentration of funds in such centers was hindering the development of MS research in other laboratories. The British MS Society also decided not to continue funding MS research centers.

Multisite research centers are ideal for certain types of research, such as clinical research requiring larger numbers of patients than can be readily enrolled in a single region, large epidemiological trials, or studies that require scarce or expensive resources such as magnetic resonance imaging (MRI) scanners or brain banks. However, centers offer less advantage for other types of research, particularly exploratory research, which is often the most innovative. For example, the early-stage, proof-of-concept clinical trials that led to the development of stem cell transplantation would not likely have been conducted in an MS research center.

The traditional model of research funding is to establish a funding program, wait for applicants, and then select the best. NIH now advertises its grant programs far more widely than in the past, but the advertising is still predominantly in a broadcast format and is not directed at specific individuals or institutions. This is also the model that has historically prevailed at many private health-research foundations, including the MS Society, but there are other models.

Public institutions are constrained by the need to provide equal access to research funds for all qualified citizens and are thus generally subjected to a variety of regulations, with their attendant administrative costs. Private foundations are not subject to such constraints and have more opportunities to adopt creative strategies in pursuit of their missions. For example, the Hereditary Disease Foundation has reaped great benefits through its departure from the "broadcast-and-wait" funding strategy. It has been very aggressive in identifying key researchers that have the appropriate techniques or outlook to contribute to the foundation's mission, and has offered them research grants with an emphasis on bringing in young people and setting them up with established scientists.

Another approach is to "superfund" a new center devoted to multidisciplinary research on a particular disease. Examples of this include the Davis Center for research on diabetes in Denver and the CaP CURE center for research on prostate cancer. A critical element in both of these examples is a link to an already-existing world-class research facility and a program that can attract top researchers. Such centers should emphasize inclusion of a broad range of research perspectives, training, and community-wide resource sharing and the nurturing of sustainable relationships among the organizations and investigators involved.

Funding of MS centers of excellence has been tried. The downside is the sequestering of large amounts of resources, the creation of a research community divided into "haves" and "have nots," and the creation of conservative insider groups. Centers can also be inimical to the entrepreneurial and creative spirit.

### Promoting Innovation

There are two important contributors to research innovation—ideas and programs. Innovation rarely rests on the strength of an individual. Indeed, industries or firms that are consistently innovative typically support an innovative culture, as opposed to employing a few key individuals. This suggests the importance of actively fostering innovation in MS research. In the past, the MS research community suffered from a reputation as overly insular, even stodgy. Even if this is not accurate, such perceptions can deter investigators who feel they would be unlikely to thrive in such a community.

Reflecting a deeply held belief among the research community, a 1994 report evaluating cancer research in the United States stated: "Real progress and new ideas in cancer research usually comes from unexpected and unpredictable directions."[15] The 1994 report evaluating cancer research in the United States noted that "excessive targeting of specific areas for research can be counterproductive. It can distract scientists, disrupt research programs, and divert funds from more productive lines of research."

Innovation starts with new ideas or new perspectives on old ideas and is perhaps most likely to come from people who have been exposed to ideas and techniques from outside the field of MS research. This highlights the importance of recruitment, not only to sustain the scientific work force, but also for the infusion of new ideas.

## HUMAN RESOURCES

Someone once said that if you want to ruin your reputation, go into MS research.
Jacqueline Friedman[17]
*The Scientist*

Human resources require continual renewal. A research field that fails to attract innovative, productive researchers is a stagnant field. Although data are not available, many people in the field of MS have the impression that too few people have entered the field in recent years. The committee agreed that recruitment of new MS researchers must remain a high priority.

The keys to building human resources are recruitment and retention, and since retention of researchers in their particular disciplines is so high, recruitment is the most important component to consider for the MS research enterprise. Researchers are recruited as they enter their research training—either in medical school or graduate school or as postdoctoral fellows. Alternatively, they are recruited in mid-career after having worked in other research areas. In terms of programs to recruit and support MS researchers, there are distinct advantages and disadvantages to recruiting new versus established researchers. New researchers are relatively inexpensive to support, but as investments they are relatively risky because they have yet to prove themselves and will have a higher attrition rate than established researchers. Established researchers, on the other hand, are more expensive to support but are already successful and provide cross-fertilization by applying knowledge and perspectives from their previous research areas to MS. Recruitment of new versus established researchers is considered separately below.

## Recruitment of New Investigators

Although the committee was not in a position to analyze trends in the quality of applications for postdoctoral fellowships in MS research, it is possible to look at the interest level as reflected in the trends in numbers of applications. More applications not only indicate a higher rate of recruitment to a research field, they also provide a larger pool from which to choose the best applicants.

A 1996 survey by the MS Society of its postdoctoral fellowship program indicated that 88 percent of all former society fellows had been successful in obtaining full grant funding during their subsequent careers, and more than half reported that MS research was still their primary career activity. Whether this was a net gain or loss in terms of recruitment depends on whether these fellows were already committed to MS research and how many entered the field as opposed to left it. A moderate level of field switching is probably the ideal, because of the benefits of cross-fertilization of perspectives and techniques.

During the last decade, the number of Ph.D.s awarded in the natural sciences increased by about 20 percent, with an even greater rise in the number of postdoctoral appointments (Figure 7.3). During this same period, applications to the MS Society for postdoctoral fellowships declined by about 20 percent (Figure 7.4). At first glance, one might conclude from this that young scientists are losing interest in MS as a research area, but the situation is more complicated. For one, this trend is not unique to MS. The Arthritis Foundation, Juvenile Diabetes Foundation, and American Cancer Society all saw declines in applications after 1995, as did the NIH. The amount of the awards from these societies ($26,000 to $32,000 per year) is comparable to that of NIH fellowships. It should be noted

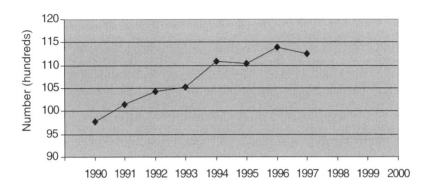

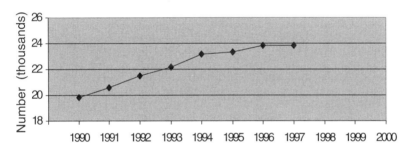

**FIGURE 7.3** Ph.D. and postdoctoral fellowship trends (1997 is the last year for which these data are available). SOURCE: NSF Science and Engineering Indicators 2000.[14]

that applicants to the MS Society did show a different trend than those applying to the other societies in that applications declined from 1990 to 1995 when they were increasing elsewhere, indicating that at least during this period MS post-doctoral fellowships were not seen as an attractive option.

Although it has been suggested that postdoctoral application rates might have declined at private foundations because applicants' success rates were increasing at NIH, the fact that postdoctoral applications also declined at NIH suggests another explanation. One possibility is the poor job market for academic scientists that discouraged many Ph.D.s from pursuing research careers.[11] In addition, the total numbers of applicants for postdoctoral fellowships at the MS

Society each year is considerably lower than that for the other private foundations for which the committee collected data (Figure 7.4).

Finally, the recruitment of health care researchers deserves particular attention. In 2000, the Health Care Delivery and Policy Research Program Committee of the National MS Society voted to discontinue the Ph.D. fellowship program because the few applications they received were consistently too weak to merit funding. Whether this reflects too little advertising or the nature of the fellowship is unclear, but both possibilities should be considered. Alternatively, it might be more effective to recruit health care researchers at different career stages, perhaps at mid-career. One possibility might be a one-year fellowship program organized in collaboration with health care foundations that target different, but relevant, diseases. If several societies funded one to two fellows per year, those fellows could form a cohort that would, ideally, stimulate health services research for all chronic and debilitating diseases. Another alternative might be to work with the Robert Wood Johnson Clinical Scholars Program in an effort to encourage more applicants with an interest in MS research. This multidisciplinary training program is designed to allow young physicians who are committed to clinical medicine to acquire new skills and training in the nonbiological sciences important to medical care systems. Indeed, the Robert Wood Johnson Clinical Scholars Program for physicians might also offer a model for its converse—multidisciplinary programs in which survey scientists, health economists, psychologists, clinical epidemiologists, nurses, and social workers receive training to enhance their collaborations with physicians.

## Recruitment Strategies

The recruitment package might be enhanced relatively inexpensively by providing an optional travel allowance to permit a fellow to spend time in the laboratory of another MS Society grantee. A strategy to stimulate recruitment into the MS field would be to encourage more junior-level applicants. Applications could be relatively simple and reviewed more frequently, or on an expedited basis, and the fellowship could offer successful applicants more options, such as greater freedom of movement between laboratories or institutions and the option of taking the fellowship with them to a beginning faculty position.

Increased recruitment might be accomplished in a variety of ways, such as by directly contacting promising Ph.D. and M.D./Ph.D. students, by advertising in journals and at meetings that students outside the MS field would attend, and by encouraging people who might not consider themselves "MS researchers" to apply.

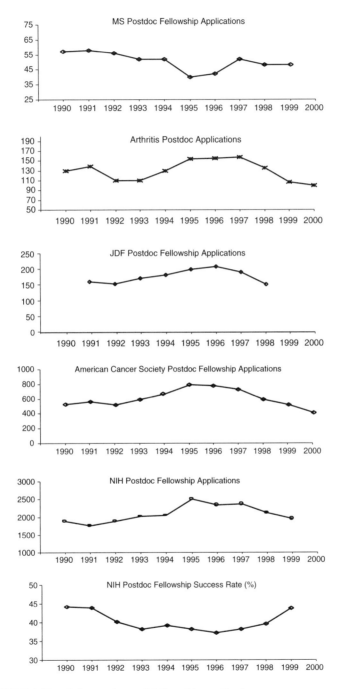

**FIGURE 7.4** Trends in postdoctoral fellowship applications.

## Declining Numbers of Physician-Researchers

For the long-term, medical schools and teaching hospitals, the NIH, health-related foundations, and the pharmaceutical industry need to examine the successful models for training health services researchers, patient oriented researchers, and clinical trials researchers and support the dissemination of those models.

American Association of Medical Colleges, 2000, p.vii[1]

The declining role of physicians has been a persistent concern for the last quarter of a century. In a series of reports first published in 1975 and as recently as 2000, 11 National Research Council committees have called for increased efforts to recruit physicians into research.[12] (The National Research Council is the operating arm of the National Academy of Sciences.) A number of training and career development programs for physician-researchers have been established over the years, but the decline in the proportion of clinicians doing research has continued. While clearly an issue for MS research, declining numbers of physician-researchers pose problems for all areas of medical research. The committee believes that policy and program changes in medical training and research *as a whole* are most likely to benefit MS research.

Physicians face strong disincentives to enter research where salaries are substantially lower than in medical practice and the time available for research—at least, in the United States—is increasingly limited by the competitive health care market.[12] Physicians also typically face enormous debt burden upon graduation from medical school as they consider a career in research. In 1997, the average burden of debt for U.S. medical school graduates was $64,000.[12] However, debt repayment programs, although attractive, are uncommon, limited, and expensive (reviewed in 2000 by the Institute of Medicine).[9] The problem of debt is probably best solved at the federal government level, rather than by individual organizations such as the MS Society. The society could, of course, contribute by encouraging the efforts of larger organizations, such as the Association of American Medical Colleges, whose mission is to serve medical education and research as a whole. The committee does not recommend that individual MS societies establish medical debt repayment programs.

## Recruitment of Established Investigators: Cross-Fertilization

The strong ties of the MS Society to the research community, including the high level of integration at the international level, are among its great strengths. However, concerted efforts should be made to stimulate enduring cross-pollination among biomedical research areas.

In the past, the National Multiple Sclerosis Society has provided small amounts of funding (for example, $100,000) to researchers in established laboratories, but the committee felt that this was relatively ineffective because it was too little to encourage them to pursue MS research. A number of other private health foundations, such as Huntington's, CaP CURE, and the Amyotrophic Lateral Sclerosis Association, have been successful in persuading specific investigators to join their mission by offering them attractive packages for funded research. Simply inviting individuals to apply for grants, however, is unlikely to be effective. Indeed, in the past, when the MS Society has invited specific individuals to apply for research funding, their grants generally have not passed peer review. This suggests the need for either a different recruitment strategy or a system other than peer review for quality control, at least when specific individuals have been recruited.

Another facet of cross-pollination is the collaboration between clinical and basic scientists. Although there are many researchers who combine skills in clinical and basic science, there is a conspicuous lack of basic scientists pursuing MS research, particularly in the neurosciences. This could be actively encouraged by organizing symposia in conjunction with the annual scientific meetings of other medical and basic science organizations, such as the Society for Neuroscience where MS research has received considerably less attention than other neurological diseases. Another means of stimulating more exchange between researchers and clinicians could be to provide funding for minisabbaticals in which basic scientists could work with clinicians for one- to two-month visits.

## INFRASTRUCTURE

Infrastructure refers to equipment and databases, as well as administrative capabilities such as staff who can coordinate collaborations, run centers, and provide statistical guidance and analysis.

The United Kingdom MS Society played a pivotal role in the application of MRI by funding the Queen's Square facility. The MRI facility at the Canadian MS Center in Montreal, Quebec was fortuitously enabled as an unintended consequence of health coverage policy in that province. However, neuroimaging facilities are expensive. Rather than funding the purchase or development of equipment, it would be most cost-effective to fund individual investigators to spend time at sites where the development of novel technologies is under way. There they might learn to apply the technology to MS research while advising and refining to foster cutting-edge developments.

Data registries and tissue banks are other important elements of infrastructure. The Amsterdam Brain Bank and the International Bone Marrow Transplant Registry, discussed in Chapter 6, are examples of an outstanding tissue bank and patient data registry, respectively.

# CLINICAL TRIALS

## Challenges to Clinical Trials: Limited Patient Pool

According to the U.S. National Cancer Institute, only 2 to 3 percent of cancer patients are ever enrolled in clinical trials.[6] If enrollment rates in MS were comparable to those of cancer trials, there would be approximately 5,000 to 10,000 MS patients enrolled in clinical trials in the United States. Given a moderately sized clinical trial of 500 subjects, it could soon become difficult to find patients who had not already participated in a trial. Another complication is enrolling patients who are not already being treated with disease-modifying therapies. In the United States, approximately 110,000 MS patients are currently taking one of those therapies—close to one-third of all patients in the country (Nicholas LaRocca, personal communication).

Compared to clinical trials for drugs that are tested to treat acute conditions in the general population, MS trials are particularly challenging. Because MS is chronic, the treatments must show long-term effects, and because MS symptoms so often wax and wane, improvements in patients' condition must be shown to be statistically greater than the improvements that occur without therapeutic intervention.

In addition, MS imposes its own disincentives to participation in clinical trials. Because it is a chronic disease in which patients can remain symptom free or experience only mild symptoms for years, they might be less willing to assume the risk of a clinical trial than others, such as cancer patients, who have little reasonable hope that their health will improve without intervention. Another deterrent is that unlike cancer patients, many MS patients live for many years with severe disability and their lack of mobility is a deterrent to their participation in a clinical trial.

Participants themselves or their surrogates in patient advocacy groups have traditionally had relatively little involvement in recruiting trial participants. Yet this tradition has been successfully broken in several cases. For example, the National Breast Cancer Coalition, a patients' advocacy group, successfully intervened to improve patient accrual for a pivotal trial of Herceptin for breast cancer.\* Michael Milken, the founder of CaP CURE, is another example. His appearance on Larry King's nationally televised talk-show was very successful in raising funds for prostate cancer research. A member of this committee was similarly successful after appearing on television with Montel Williams, an African-American talk-show host who was recently diagnosed with MS. Before his television appearance with Montel Williams, he had been unable to recruit enough African Americans for a genetic study of non-Caucasians, but a few days after

---

\*Herceptin was approved by the U.S. Food and Drug Administration in 1998 and was the first biological drug for the treatment of metastatic breast cancer.

that he found himself with hundreds of subjects. People with MS are in a unique position to help others with the disease, and their willingness to assist in the enrollment of patients in clinical trials could be an important asset.

## Sponsorship of Clinical Trials

Although academic medical centers were once considered the main citadels of clinical research, most clinical studies that bring new drugs from bench to bedside are now led by pharmaceutical companies.[3] In the United States, 70 percent of the money for clinical drug trials in the U.S. comes from industry rather than the federal government.[5]

Until recently, the pharmaceutical industry needed academic physicians to perform drug trials because the industry lacked the in-house expertise and the academic medical centers had better access to patients as subjects for trials. Pharmaceutical firms, frustrated with the slow pace of academic medical centers (in particular, with the slow reviews of industry proposals by academic research offices and institutional review boards), have increasingly turned to contract research organizations and site management organizations to design, execute, and analyze their clinical trials.[3,16] In 1991, 80 percent of industry money for clinical trials went to academic medial centers. By 1998, this figure had dropped to 40 percent.[7]

Most investigators (and this was the sentiment among committee members) prefer that design, implementation, data analysis, and publication be controlled by academic medial centers and investigators. Many feel that clinical trials in academic centers are less likely to be compromised by conflicts between the desire to maximize scientific progress and the financial considerations of pharmaceutical firms. Yet with the rise of contract research organizations and the decline in "market share" of clinical trials in academic health centers, the control of clinical trials within academic centers is increasingly less common.

## BIOTECHNOLOGY AND PHARMACEUTICAL FIRMS

As mentioned, most clinical studies that bring new drugs from the laboratory to the medicine chest are financed by pharmaceutical companies, not by government funding agencies or private foundations. Research strategies aimed at treating or curing diseases will thus fail if they do not establish informed partnerships with the sector that can deliver research results to patients. Although drug development generally begins in the realm of the research community, it bears fruit only in the realm of the marketplace. These realms are necessary partners, but they are molded by different contingencies.

Although private firms and the academic research community might share the goal of curing and treating disease, their survival depends on distinctly different currencies. Private firms survive by their ability to make profits. The coin of this realm is approval of new therapies. In a free-market economy, only those firms that produce profits will survive to produce medically valuable therapies. In contrast, the coin of the academic realm is publication in scientific journals. Producing profits often conflicts with full disclosure of scientific research, and it is almost axiomatic that access to data is an area of great contention in academic-industry collaborations.

## From Research to Medications

Before a drug reaches the medicine chest, it must be approved for human use. In the United States, this approval comes from the Food and Drug Administration (FDA), which regulates human testing and the introduction of new drugs into the marketplace. In addition, because the U.S. market represents such a large share of the global economy, FDA regulations also influence drug development around the world. Drug approval is based on the results of clinical trials, which means that the FDA, in effect, sets the standards for clinical research. At times, these standards have been challenged as being so rigid that they impede progress and the development of critically needed medications. Although it has happened only rarely, the FDA has occasionally permitted early and expedited drug approvals where there were otherwise no existing therapeutic options. The most effective recent challenges have come from AIDS patient advocate groups who succeeded in relaxing standards for promising, but unproven medications for HIV/AIDS. In obtaining expedited drug approvals for both cancer and AIDS therapeutics, it was the affected populations that were the most effective advocates, and only those associated with long-established health organizations. Neither researchers nor research funders played a significant role.

People with MS face a somewhat similar situation, but they have not established a political organization to accelerate the development of therapeutic options as have other patient advocacy groups, such as those for breast cancer, Parkinson's disease, and AIDS. The committee neither encourages nor discourages this option but notes that patient advocates can be highly effective in stimulating the availability of therapeutic options, in terms of using their political will both to modify FDA decisions and to increase research support for particular diseases.

## MS Drugs Are Orphans

One critical element in encouraging development of therapeutic options for people with MS is the existence of specific revenue-generating incentives for private firms. One such incentive is orphan drug status. The Orphan Drug Act of 1983 provides incentives to manufacturers to develop drugs to treat "orphan diseases." An orphan disease, as defined in an amendment to the act, is one that affects 200,000 or fewer people in the United States.* The act's most important incentive is a period of exclusive marketing protection of seven years, during which FDA is prohibited from approving the same drug for the same indication.[5,6] If a disease affects more than 200,000 people, the manufacturer sometimes subdivides the patient population into smaller units to qualify. For example, a drug for the treatment of Parkinson's disease is not likely to receive an orphan designation because its prevalence exceeds 200,000, but orphan designation has been accorded to drugs for subsets of Parkinson's patients, such as those suffering from early-morning motor dysfunction in the late stages of the disease.

## The Catalytic Effect of Drug Approval

The first approval of a drug for a disease is a catalytic event in that it stimulates both academic researchers and companies to enter a field that they might have previously seen as unready for therapeutic advances. It can also create the optimism for expanded investment in research, from both the public and the private sectors. The impact of development and approval of the first disease-modifying drugs for MS might thus be much more far-reaching than their specific benefits to patients. If the history of research in other diseases is any guide, there should be a substantial surge in interest for research and development of MS therapeutics. Although early and expedited drug approval might be controversial, the stimulatory effect of encouraging follow-on research and development is worth considering.

# HEALTH CARE RESEARCH

The MS Society created its Health Care Delivery and Policy Research (HCDPR) program in 1988. Since then it has grown from a small grant program to a modest contract program to a more ambitious contract program. The HCDPR program accounts for about 5 percent of the total MS Society research budget, although there are several grants funded outside this program that also include health services research.

The American Cancer Society has an extramural research budget of $171 million, of which approximately 5 percent is devoted to health services research.[10] This figures compares favorably to public spending in health services research in the United States, which is proportionately much less than it is for biomedical research. The 1999 research budget for the Agency for Health Research and Quality (AHRQ), the primary funding agency that supports health services re-

---

*FDA can grant orphan designation to a drug intended for a condition that affects a larger population if the manufacturer's estimated expenses are unlikely to be recovered by sales in the United States. (Public Law 98-551).

search in the United States, was $140 million, slightly less than 1 percent of the $14.8 billion NIH research budget. It is important to understand, however, that these numbers provide only rough approximations, because the lines distinguishing health services research from traditional clinical research are often indistinct. Nonetheless, it is reasonable to conclude that proportionately more health services research is supported through private foundations than by federal agencies.

There are not many applicants. A 1999 request for proposals (RFPs) on quality indicators for health care in MS and another RFP on access to health care for MS among rural populations care generated only 2 applications each. Only two applications were submitted for dissertation fellowships. It would be useful to determine whether this is because the pool of applicants is so small or because qualified applicants are either unaware of or uninterested in the opportunities.

## ROLE OF VOLUNTARY HEALTH ORGANIZATIONS

The role of philanthropic funding in strengthening health research is vital in that it carries the unique capacity to invest in innovative and creative risk-taking projects.

Enriqueta Bond, president
Burroughs Wellcome Fund

Gaps and opportunities that currently exist that could be filled by foundations include training physicians and Ph.D. researchers to adapt to changing needs; support for emerging field and interdisciplinary research; support for risky research; speeding research from bench to bedside; behavioral research; public understanding of science and communication; and new partnerships.[4]

"The federal research grant administration process, encompassing the peer review process, has become cumbersome, inefficient, and an impediment to scientific excellence. Investigators spend as much as 30 percent of their time preparing lengthy grant applications, responding to regulations, and preparing administrative documentation. Although some time and expense are necessary, the current system siphons excessive dollars and time into efforts that do nothing to promote progress against cancer."[15] (Note that this quote was not intended as a criticism of peer review, which the report noted was a great strength of the federal research grant administration process.)

Unlike federal agencies, private research foundations are not encumbered by the obligations of a public agency, which allows them considerably more freedom to adopt flexible policies. They can also to some degree piggyback onto policies established by the federal government—for example, policies for the appropriate care and use of animals in research, trainee programs for the ethical conduct of research, and intellectual property agreements. Private foundations can more readily develop expedited grant review, and select individual investiga-

## BOX 7.2
## CaP CURE: An Innovative Approach to Accelerating Research

CaP CURE was founded in 1993 to develop a scientific strategy that would accelerate the development of effective therapies for prostate cancer and get help to the men who need it. It is now the world's largest private source of prostate cancer research funding, and it has provided more than $65 million in support for over 450 projects in the past six years. CaP CURE has worked together with survivors, scientists, and advocates to establish a system that encourages collaboration, reduces bureaucracy, and speeds the process of discovery. CaP CURE reaches out to private industry, the patient advocacy community, and government research institutions. These partnerships provide a model to accelerate progress in developing treatments for specific diseases.

Research is funded through competitive awards, based on the peer-review model used at NIH and similar to that used by the MS Society. In addition, CaP CURE has established a fast-track grant review and award process as a central feature of its mission. Applications are limited to five pages in length, and awards are made within 90 days of the deadline for applications. The approach appears to have paid off. Applications for competitive awards have increased nearly sixfold, from 86 to 570, in the last five years. Moreover, in 1993, only 10 percent of the research awards had near-term clinical application, compared with more than 70 percent in 1997. Significant results are claimed: at least 80 CaP CURE-sponsored projects, ranging from gene therapy to therapies targeting the androgen receptor, are now making their way into clinical trials. In 1998, CaP CURE introduced young investigator awards to provide stable, four-year funding for outstanding young physician-scientists attracted to the prostate cancer field.

The CaP CURE Therapy Consortium, which consists of three teams of scientists, is dedicated to rapidly incorporating discoveries. Physicians in the consortium work at 11 medical centers across the United States, testing new treatments for men with advanced prostate cancer. The consortium creates new clinical trials, recruits participants, shares results, and attracts pharmaceutical and biotechnology sponsors. CaP CURE consortium researchers face vastly fewer administrative hurdles than government-sponsored cooperative groups do, which means that they can evaluate exciting therapeutic agents with much less delay. Researchers associated with CaP CURE cite the greater involvement of patients in clinical trials and the network of clinicians engaged in the clinical trial as important factors in the recently accelerated progress of prostate cancer research, also claiming that CaP CURE has significantly shortened the time required to develop new treatments. Kenneth Pienta, M.D., of the University of Michigan Comprehensive Cancer Center notes, "In the past when I would design a new therapy, it would take me two years to test it in my own clinic. Now with the consortium, we can test these things in six months."

CaP CURE has been working with computer engineers from Oracle Corporation to develop a database that will allow scientists at each individual institution to compare and analyze findings at trials across the country. As with most clinical research, data are presently stored and tabulated at each individual institution (but see description of the IBMTR-ABMTR transplantation database in Chapter 6). CaP CURE has brought a spirit of innovation to a field that, in the past, has been criticized for discouraging new thinking.

SOURCE: Stokstad, 1999,[18] www.capcure.org (World Wide Web, accessed 12/1/2000).

tors for research support. Compared to a public agency, they generally have more opportunity to take proactive and flexible approaches to research support. CaP CURE, the organization founded to promote the development of therapies for prostate cancer, offers but one example of an innovative approach (Box 7.2).

# REFERENCES

1. Association of American Medical Colleges. *For the Health of the Public: Ensuring the Future of Clinical Research. Report of the AAMC Task Force on Clinical Research.* Washington, DC: Association of American Medical Colleges; 2000;1.
2. Association of Medical Research Charities. *The Association of Medical Research Charities Handbook 2000.* Leicestershire, UK: Chartwell Press Ltd.; 1999.
3. Bodenheimer T. 2000. Uneasy alliance—clinical investigators and the pharmaceutical industry. *N Engl J Med.*;342:1539-1544.
4. Bond EC, Peck MG, Scott M. The future of philanthropic support for medical/health research. How to Fund Science: the Future of Medical Research: A Workshop. February 14-16, 1999. The Aspen Institute, Wye, Maryland: American Association for the Advancement of Science. Retrieved 5/26/99 from the World Wide Web: http//www.fundingfirst.; 1999.
5. Centerwatch. *An Industry in Evolution.* Boston: Centerwatch; 1999.
6. Gelband H. Institute of Medicine. *A Report on the Sponsors of Cancer Treatment Clinical Trials and Their Approval and Monitoring Mechanisms.* Washington, D.C.: National Academy Press; 1999.
7. Getz KA. *AMCs Rekindling Clinical Research Partnerships With Industry.* Boston: Centerwatch; 1999.
8. Gross CP, Anderson GF, Powe NR. 1999. The relation between funding by the National Institutes of Health and the burden of disease. *N Engl J Med.*;340:1881-7.
9. Institute of Medicine. Pellmar TC, Eisenberg L, editors. *Bridging Disciplines in the Brain, Behavioral, and Clinical Sciences.* Washington, DC: National Academy Press; 2000.
10. Institute of Medicine and National Research Council. Hewitt M, Simone JV, eds. *Ensuring Quality Cancer Care.* Washington, DC: National Academy Press; 1999.
11. National Research Council. *Trends in the Early Careers of Life Scientists.* Washington, D.C.: National Academy Press; 1998.
12. National Research Council. *Addressing the Nation's Changing Needs for Biomedical and Behavioral Scientists.* Washington, DC: National Academy Press; 2000.
13. National Research Council. COSEPUP. *Experiments in International Benchmarking of US Research Fields.* Washington, DC: National Academy Press; 2000.
14. National Science Board. *Science and Engineering Indicators 2000.* Arlington, VA: National Science Foundation; 2000.
15. NCAB Subcommittee to Evaluate the National Cancer Program. *Cancer at a Crossroads: A Report to Congress for the Nation.* Bethesda, MD: National Cancer Institute; 1994.
16. Spilker B. *The Future of Pharmaceutical Funding. How to Fund Science: the Future of Medical Research: A Workshop. February 14-16, 1999.* The Aspen Institute, Wye, Maryland: American Association for the Advancement of Science. Retrieved 5/26/99 from the World Wide Web: http//www.fundingfirst.; 1999.
17. Steinberg D. 2000. Does multiple sclerosis have a herpesvirus connection? HHV-6 seems to play a role, but the mechanism is far from clear. *The Scientist.*;14:16.
18. Stokstad E. 1999. From junk bond king to cancer crusader. *Science.*;283:1100-1103.

# 8

# Recommendations

The ultimate goal of research in multiple sclerosis (MS) is the development of interventions that can improve the lives of those living with MS and prevent or cure MS. However, understanding of the MS disease process is not yet sufficient to predict which therapeutic strategies will be most effective. While the new disease-modifying drugs are a major leap forward, they are not a cure, nor are they effective for all patients. MS remains a mysterious disease with no known pathogen or even known determinants of its severity and course. Basic research provides a crucial foundation for innovative approaches to the discovery of effective therapies.

This chapter summarizes the recommendations that the committee believes have the greatest potential to facilitate broad advances in MS research. The committee was not asked to review specific programs of the National Multiple Sclerosis Society (the MS Society), but instead conducted its review more broadly to identify promising research strategies and opportunities for advancing MS research on a variety of fronts.

The committee did not suggest how the MS Society or others should prioritize the recommendations listed below. Prioritization of the recommendations requires programmatic decisions that will have to balance scientific opportunity with organizational goals. The choices, such as what balance to strike between patient services and research support, or between research on underlying disease mechanism and research to improve the lives of people with MS, go beyond strictly scientific questions and exceed the charge to the committee. Answers to those questions depend on the organization's mission and how it interprets that mission and should be determined by the directors, members, and constituents.

The committee feels that each of the research strategies listed below should be actively supported. However, which among them should take priority at any one time should be determined by a mix of scientific opportunity and institutional concerns, which will be different for different organizations, be they federal research sponsors or charitable health organizations. The most productive research strategies for an organization such as the MS Society will be influenced by the activities (or lack thereof) of the relevant federal agencies such as the National Institutes of Health, Agency for Healthcare Research and Quality, Veteran's Administration, and the National Institute on Disability and Rehabilitation Research, as well as those of other private organizations that sponsor research relevant to MS.

This chapter does not include numerous other committee recommendations that cover specific aspects of MS-related research, especially the recommendations dealing with specific symptoms or alternative medicine. These areas of research are covered individually in the pertinent chapters. The recommendations below are for research areas that the committee believes hold the greatest promise for developing treatments that can prevent or cure MS and for improving the lives of people with MS. They are organized into specific recommendations for the following:

- research to understand the basic disease mechanisms, and specifically, the cellular and molecular events of MS;

- tools for research and diagnosis;

- research on new therapeutic approaches;

- research toward improving the lives of people with MS; and

- programs to promote progress in MS research.

## ETIOLOGY AND PATHOGENESIS

RECOMMENDATION 1: **Research on the pathological changes underlying the natural course of MS should be emphasized, because it provides the key to predicting disease course in individual patients, understanding the physiological basis of MS, and a basis for developing improved therapeutic approaches.**

Unpredictability imposes a particularly acute burden on people with MS. They have no way of knowing when a relapse will occur, how impaired they will be, or whether they will recover from the relapse. Yet it is now clear that disease activity precedes relapses. Understanding these pathological changes is the first step toward predicting—at least in the short term—disease progression in individual patients.

Research on the natural course of MS would include defining the relationship between cellular and molecular changes and the progression of disability, as well as determining the physiological basis for different clinical manifestations of MS. Changes in gene expression should be analyzed in individual cell types, particularly those in and at the borders of lesions. Such information will also improve the ability to develop more refined diagnostic tools, provide benchmarks against which to measure the effect of therapeutic interventions, and provide the scientific basis for new therapeutic approaches.

Research on pathological changes occurring early in the disease should be particularly emphasized. This should also include the development of improved diagnostic criteria (most likely, criteria based on neuroimaging) that allow early and more accurate diagnosis of MS. If aggressive treatment is to be instituted at the onset of disease, early and accurate diagnosis is essential.

RECOMMENDATION 2: **Research should be pursued to identify how neurons are damaged in MS, how this damage can be prevented, and how oligodendrocytes and astrocytes are involved in damage and repair processes.**

Specific needs for research on neurons include the following:

- investigations into the molecular pathophysiology of axonal injury in MS—what is the response of the neuronal cell body to demyelination and to degeneration of axons in MS?

- delineation of the relationship of axonal injury to demyelination and inflammation, to the role of cytokines, and to the role of cell and anti-body-mediated immune mechanisms;

- delineation of the detailed nature of the secondary injury cascade that underlies calcium-mediated damage of axons within white matter;

- improved understanding of the molecular mechanisms underlying restoration of conduction in demyelinated axons, with particular attention to identification of the sodium channel subtype(s) involved in conduction in chronically demyelinated axons, and identification and characterization of the promoter regions of the sodium channels that support impulse conduction in myelinated and demyelinated axons; and

- identification of promoters and inhibitors of axon regeneration.

Specific needs for research on oligodendroctyes include identification of:

- the role of oligodendrocytes in the trophic support of axons and neurons;

- the role of oligodendrocytes in maintaining the distribution of sodium channels in axons;

- the mechanisms that disable and destroy oligodendrocytes in MS;

- how and to what extent progenitor cells are induced to become oligodendrocytes that remyelinate axons; and

- the relationship between demyelination, injury to axons, and neuropathic pain in MS, and demyelination and axon injury in appropriate animal models.

Specific needs for research on astrocytes include the following:

- *Astrocytes as antigen-presenting cells.* To what extent do astrocytes participate in the immunopathogenesis of MS? Is there an underlying disorder of astrocyte function in MS?

- *Astrocytes as producers* of cytokines, chemokines or other molecules that influence blood-brain barrier permeability, immune cells, or myelin. Astrocyte response to neurotrophins should also be studied.

- *Astrocytes as scarring cells.* Do scarring astrocytes inhibit remyelination or regeneration of axons in MS? If so, can this process be controlled?

- *Astrocytes as regulators of axonal conduction.* The possible role of astrocytes as producers of sodium channels that are transferred to demyelinated axons should be explored.

- *Astrocytes as homeostatic regulators of the neuronal microenvironment.* It is now well known that astrocytes can regulate the levels of biologically important ions, neurotransmitters, and related molecules in the healthy nervous system. Better understanding of this role of astrocytes in MS is needed.

Specific needs for research on interaction between neural and immune cells include:

- more complete delineation of the mechanisms by which the immune system contributes to demyelination and remyelination;

- interaction of T cells and antibodies with axons and neuron cell bodies;

- identification of the humoral factors that increase the permeability of the blood-brain barrier, thereby allowing the trafficking of immune cells through the brain; and

- evidence that immune cells destroy oligodendrocytes through the excitatory amino acids acting through the AMPA/kainate receptors that are known to mediate cell death in a variety of circumstances should be clearly established and extended.

RECOMMENDATION 3: **The genes that underlie genetic susceptibility to MS should be identified, because genetic information offers such a powerful tool to elucidate fundamental disease processes and prognosis, and to develop new therapeutic approaches.**

Compelling data indicate that MS is a complex genetic disorder. The identification of susceptibility genes for MS represents a significant challenge but also a major opportunity to elucidate the fundamental disease process. Genetic discoveries are likely to contribute to a better understanding of heterogeneity, clinical course, prognosis, and response to therapy. Even the discovery of a new gene with a very small genetic effect on MS could have major implications for the development of entirely new therapies. The committee believes that an aggressive effort in human genetics is essential.

The critical importance of identifying rare families with monogenic variants of MS cannot be overstated; this approach has been extraordinarily fruitful in neurodegenerative diseases such as Alzheimer's disease and Parkinson's disease.

The following genetic research strategies should be emphasized:

- **The major histocompatibility complex (MHC) region in chromosome 6p21 should be targeted.** The available data support the hypothesis that inherited susceptibility to MS involves the interaction of different susceptibility genes, each of which individually contributes to the overall risk. Whole-genome screens confirm the importance of the MHC genes in conferring susceptibility. Susceptibility is likely to be mediated by the MHC class II genes themselves (DR, DQ, or both) and is most likely related to the known function of these molecules in the normal immune response, antigen binding, and T-cell repertoire determination. The MHC region contains more than 250 genes, and despite the common assumption that DR2 is an MS susceptibility gene, because of marked linkage disequilibrium (or fixity of certain haplotypes) it has not been possible to determine with certainty which gene or genes are in fact responsible. The entire MHC region has now been sequenced, and it should be possible to better define the genetic role of the MHC in MS.

- **New statistical approaches should be developed to identify small genetic effects.** Data show that although the MHC region contains significant susceptibility, much of the genetic effect in MS remains to be explained. It is likely that the non-MHC genes are all genes of small effect that contribute to susceptibility in an additive or synergistic fashion. In all likelihood, the use of phenotypic and demographic variables will assume increasing importance as stratifying elements for genetic studies of MS and as a means of addressing the fundamental question of genotype-phenotype correlation in autoimmune demyelination. These studies will necessarily be linked to the development of novel mathematical formulations designed to identify modest genetic effects, as well as interactions between multiple genes and interactions between genetic, clinical, and environmental factors.

- **Methods for rapid, high-throughput screening of genetic polymorphisms should be used.** With the advances in deciphering the human genome code and sequences readily available in the public domain, future work should focus on the detailed analysis of candidate genes, in particular genes located in chromosomal segments linked to MS susceptibility or to susceptibility to demyelination in animal models.

- **"Case-control" population-based studies with limited statistical power should be replaced with the analysis of large collections.** These collections should include nuclear or singleton families (the patient and the biological parents or the patient and healthy siblings) using transmission-disequilibrium tests (TDT) and Sib-TDT tests of association.

For complex disorders such as MS, genomic analysis of multiple candidate genes must be performed on an extremely large group of individuals if small genetic effects are to be detected. The key to the success of such studies will be the availability of rapid, reliable, non-labor-intensive methods for high-throughput polymorphism screening and a collaborative network.

- **Groups and consortia with the appropriate experimental, clinical, and financial resources should be supported to continue analysis of the MS genome.** Larger DNA databases and dense and informative genetic markers—for example, single nucleotide polymorphisms (SNPs)—will be important to translate the basic understanding that genes are involved in MS into knowledge that can be used to facilitate the development of new therapeutic approaches and to provide more information for patients and physicians about risks associated with MS.

- **The inclusion of non-Caucasian patient populations, both in their native environment and after migration, will provide important new insights and clues about MS genetic and clinical heterogeneity.** When MS occurs in non-Caucasians it is likely to provide more genetic information against a "non-MS" genetic background than against the Caucasian "MS-susceptible" background. Haplotypes of linked genes are often different in different ethnic or racial groups. When linkage studies identify a genetic region harboring an MS susceptibility gene, there are often 70 to 100 genes within that region. Many of those genes are polymorphic, and common polymorphisms detected in different haplotypes and from different ethnic groups provide powerful clues to the location of the disease gene. Examples of genetically complex disorders in which this approach of transracial genotyping has been successful include narcolepsy and insulin-dependent diabetes mellitus.

- **Genomic, clinical, and endocrinologic information should be combined to investigate potential MS risk factors in large groups of female patients.** Although sex differences in genetic susceptibility to MS have been well documented, rigorous studies assessing the potential role of sex-linked genetic factors in MS have not yet been performed. Further, changes in hormonal status associated with menstrual cycles, pregnancy, breastfeeding, and menopause might influence disease activity and should be investigated.

- **Studies should directly address the question of genetic heterogeneity in MS and the response to immunotherapy by analysis of the correlation between different genotypes and clinical response to therapeutic modalities ("pharmacogenomics").** A significant number of MS patients do not respond to the available disease-modifying treatments. Genetic polymorphisms in drug receptors, metabolizing enzymes, transporters, and targets have been linked to individual differences in the efficacy and toxicity of many medications.

RECOMMENDATION 4: Because the discovery of an MS pathogen would likely provide the single most important clue for identifying effective treatments, this search must remain a high priority, but should be conducted using powerful new and efficient methods.

Conventional tissue culture approaches to the isolation of pathogens in MS have consistently failed to find any convincing result, possibly because the pathogen does not grow in the tissue or media used. Newer approaches should be used, such as those that involve the identification of genomic information relevant to the pathogen and those that have the potential to reveal a broader range of pathogens than are detectable in culture. The methods include polymerase chain reaction (PCR), representational difference analysis, and sequence screening using the host immune response (described below). These powerful new methods have not yet been applied to investigations of MS tissues in any concerted and organized way, and their use should be a high priority.

Discovery of a trigger for the first MS event would likely provide the single most important clue for identifying a cure and a means of prevention. This event might precede clinically observable symptoms and might be different from the events that drive subsequent autoimmune attacks. Thus, despite the long and thus far unsuccessful search, research to identify the trigger event(s) of MS must remain a high priority.

- Representational difference analysis (RDA), one method of differential sequence analysis, has recently been used successfully to identify a new pathogenic herpesvirus in Kaposi's sarcoma. RDA employs PCR to amplify DNA fragments that are present in the diseased tissue, but not in healthy tissue from the same patient. The identification of even a small amount of sequence information may be sufficient to characterize the agent.

- DNA microarrays, also known as DNA chips, can be used to reveal the coordinated expression of ensembles of critical genes. Different tissues can be probed to reveal which genes are activated by different candidate pathogens, or which genes are activated during tissue destruction or repair. This information will also provide important clues as to how these genes influence susceptibility and pathogenesis in MS. As gene chip methodologies mature, there is also the opportunity to perform wider whole-genome analyses of gene expression, unbiased by selection of known candidate genes.

- Phage display libraries can be used to screen for the antigenic target of oligoclonal immunoglobulin G (IgG). The antigenic targets of the oligoclonal IgG might be a consequence of immunodysregulation rather than its cause, but knowledge of the target might guide the development of new therapies.

- Other methods can be used to probe the antigenic targets of T cells that are present in the MS brain, although these results might be more difficult to interpret than when antibody is used.

RECOMMENDATION 5: **Research to identify the cascade of immune system events that culminates in the destruction of myelin should remain a priority.**

The most striking pathology in MS is the immune system's attack and destruction of the body's own myelin sheath. What causes the immune system to attack myelin is unknown. Although myelin basic protein (MBP) might trigger a particularly vigorous autoimmune response, it is not the only autoantigen, nor does it account for the full autoimmune response. Any brain protein is a potential autoantigen, although an autoimmune reaction to different proteins would have variable consequences. Two critical foci for research in the immunopathology of MS include:

1. identification of the most important triggers for autoimmune responses in MS; and

2. increased understanding of pathogenic immune cells.

One of the first pathological processes leading to MS attacks is thought to be activation of autoreactive T lymphocytes and their migration into the central nervous system (CNS) where they release cytokines that induce B cells to differentiate into antibody-secreting cells.[2,3] However, T cells and the inflammatory molecules they secrete are not the only players. Many cells and molecules of the immune system—likely unleashed by T-cell activation—appear to participate in demyelination. The entire cascade of immune system events eventually culminates in myelin destruction. The key features of this cascade are not fully understood, including the precise ordering of events, the precise antigens targeted by T cells, and the precise contributions of B lymphocytes and other cells of the immune system.

Specific goals in research on pathogenic immune cells include the following:

- identification of pathogenic T-cell clones using animal models that incorporate human-related genes and potential autoantigens and methods such as PCR, microarray assays, and phage display that do not rely on the ability of pathogens to grow in cell cultures;

- characterization of the disappearance, reappearance, and persistence of autoreactive T lymphocytes over time;

- identification of the blood-borne substances and cellular mediators that stimulate the migration of T cells and permit their passage across the blood-brain barrier and into the CNS; and

- elucidation of the involvement of B cells in immune-mediated attack on the central nervous system.

## TOOLS FOR RESEARCH AND DIAGNOSIS

RECOMMENDATION 6: **The power of neuroimaging as a tool for basic research and for clinical assessment should be taken advantage of more extensively.**

Neuroimaging is an invaluable adjunct to the history and clinical exam for evaluating the effects of therapeutic intervention. Research should emphasize the application of various accepted and evolving neuroimaging techniques to understanding the evolution of MS lesions from pre- or asymptomatic stages through the progression to permanent tissue alteration or recovery from disability.

Examples of the application of various techniques to understanding the MS disease process include the following:

- magnetic transfer imaging (MTI), which provides an overall index of brain tissue destruction;

- magnetic resonance spectroscopy (MRS), which provides an index of neuronal destruction, to study the evolution of early changes in normal-appearing white matter and to evaluate neurochemical change at various stages of the disease process;

- gadolinium enhancement and contrast intensification of MRI to probe the evolution of inflammatory and blood-brain barrier changes;

- diffusion tensor imaging, which can detect subtle pathological changes not apparent on conventional magnetic resonance imaging (MRI) and might thereby allow detection of pathological change in white matter tracts, including demyelination and loss of axons;

- quantitative volumetric analyses of tissue destruction including the presence of "black holes" and atrophy;

- functional MRI (fMRI) and positron emission tomography (PET) to evaluate changes in brain activity during active and recovering stages of MS and to analyze how these changes contribute to recovery; and

- further development and validation of the use of spinal cord imaging to increase diagnostic sensitivity.

The committee also encourages the development of newer imaging modalities, such as:

- high field-strength MRI to improve image resolution; and

- specific labeling techniques that will allow the visualization of individual cellular *populations* (lymphocytes, glia, and specific neuronal populations) and *processes* (demyelination, remyelination, or neuroplastic changes).

RECOMMENDATION 7: **Animal models should be developed that more faithfully mirror the features of MS and permit the analysis of how specific molecules and cells contribute to the disease process.**

An animal model for a particular disease or condition can provide the understanding to design therapies based on biological knowledge, rather than shotgun testing. For example, mouse models with targeted mutations in the cystic fibrosis gene are providing a means for testing gene therapy delivered by aerosol into the lungs. Characterization of mouse models of various dwarfing syndromes, cloning of mutated genes, and parallel comparative genetic mapping and cloning of genes for similar human syndromes have led to an understanding of various human dwarfing conditions.

Generation of a reliable animal model of MS has been a long-standing goal in MS research. Current animal models of MS express diseases like experimental allergic encephalomyelitis (EAE) or virus-induced demyelination. Although the models that are presently available have yielded a tremendous amount of information relevant to MS, better animal models can be developed. Key advantages of current animal models include the fact that the initiating trigger is known, the exact time of the initiating event is known, a great deal is known about the genetics and the immune system in the case of rodents, and finally, the availability of animal mutants with "knockouts" of genes for particular arms of the immune system or those that carry a transgene perturbing a protein that is relevant to MS.

A key disadvantage to available models is that they do not replicate the cellular or molecular pathology of MS. Some types of EAE, for example, produce brisk demyelination, whereas others produce little demyelination. In addition, these models are not very tractable for studies of the electrophysiology and biophysics of neuronal function, a serious limitation in a disease such as MS in which symptoms and signs arise from impaired nerve function.

Information gleaned from research studies of animal models could guide investigations into MS in the following ways:

- Continued analysis of the genes responsible for different forms of demyelinating disease in experimental models such as EAE and Theiler's virus infection are likely to permit identification of the human chromosomal regions that contain the counterparts to these genes (syntenic regions). The possible role of the human genes in susceptibility to MS could then be probed.

- Preclinical testing of CNS repair strategies (for example, cell transplant, growth factors, gene therapy) and optimal methods of CNS gene delivery can be carried out.

- New methods for diagnosis of inflammatory demyelination, such as neuroimaging or spinal fluid evaluation, can be developed or refined in animal models.

- Redundant EAE animal models can be developed that incorporate human-related genes and potential autoantigens, and new methodologies can be used to investigate animal models of MS. For example, investigations that involve mice with an inducible knockout of a specific arm of the immune system (for example, CD4+ T cells) may be of value. In the case of virus-induced demyelinating diseases, this approach will allow one to dissect the role of the immune system in virus clearance early after infection from its role in mediating the demyelinating disease late after infection.

- Human virus-induced demyelinating disease and animal models of virus-induced demyelinating disease can be investigated for clues to the pathogenesis of MS. There are several advantages to investigating these disease processes: the initiating trigger for these diseases (that is, the virus infection) is known, and in many cases, the immune system appears to play a role in the pathology, as is the case with MS. In addition, a great deal is known about the immune system in rats and mice, and a wide variety of genetic models are readily available.

## THERAPEUTICS

RECOMMENDATION 8: **Strategies for protection and repair of neural cells, including the use of neuroprotective factors as well as stem cells, hold great promise for the treatment of MS and should be a major research priority.**

Specific neuroprotective strategies to be investigated include:

- elucidation of the pathways leading to cell death in the central nervous system;

- identification of neuroprotective and repair strategies that will reduce or repair axonal injury;

- development of therapeutic approaches that will induce restoration of conduction in demyelinated axons, for example, by inducing expression of appropriate densities of the appropriate subtype(s) of sodium channels among them;

- development of approaches to stimulate re-growth of damaged axons; and

- development of systems for the delivery of neuroprotective and repair factors to the central nervous system.

An effective delivery system is an essential link in the development of neuroprotective or restorative therapies. Thus, the development of such delivery tools, for example, cells that have been genetically engineered to produce specific neuroprotective factors, or molecular packaging systems, is a high priority.

Specific goals to identify the cellular and molecular pathways that control the death of myelin-forming oligodendrocytes include identification of the following:

- therapeutic strategies that can protect oligodendrocytes from immune attack;

- strategies to activate endogenous oligodendrocyte precursor cells to promote remyelination (endogenous stem cells); and

- strategies for the transplantation of myelin-forming cells into the demyelinated CNS; this includes using precursor cells or genetically engineered cells (exogenous stem cells).

The last two strategies must be considered in the context of specific features of MS. For example, newly formed myelin might be destroyed through the same immune response that destroyed the original myelin.

RECOMMENDATION 9: **New, more effective therapeutic approaches to symptom management should be pursued, including those directed at neuropathic pain and sensory disturbances.**

- The pathophysiology of pain and paresthesia in MS is not understood. Although neuronal hyperexcitability appears to underlie these symptoms, it is not known why it occurs in MS. The cellular and molecular basis for neuronal hyperexcitability in MS should be investigated.

- Molecular targets should be identified, for example, inappropriately expressed ion channels that cause abnormal impulse trafficking in MS. After identification of such targets, pharmacological methods can be developed for regulating the activity of these critical molecules.

- The impact of electrical activity within neurons and of exercise and physical therapy should be investigated in regard to disease progression and functional capacities. This will require the development of better tools to measure function.

RECOMMENDATION 10: **In the absence of any fully effective therapies, integrated approaches for the delivery of currently available therapeutic agents should be investigated.**

Since there are, as yet, no treatments that cure MS or halt disease progression entirely, it is important to develop integrated approaches to testing those agents that can at least modify the course of the disease. Such trials are expensive and lengthy, and they require large numbers of patients. Agents of different classes will have to be tested in sequence and in combination. Such trials are also best done when the dose range and safety profile of each individual agent to be employed in the trial are known, and the potential for adverse drug interactions should be carefully monitored. Separate end points might be required for each agent as appropriate to its individual pharmacological profile. Most importantly, standardized protocols and assessments will have to be devised and agreed upon, including Phase II studies that will allow abandonment of ineffective combinations before incurring the time, expense, and exposure to risk that are inherent in large, multicenter efficacy trials.

Specific considerations include:

1. timing of initiation of treatment in regard to clinical course;

2. use of combination regimens:

   • appropriate dosing of single agents;

   • use of appropriate combinations, such as interferon and glatiramer acetate, and interferon and cytostatic drugs;

   • use of chemotherapy regimens as a model approach; and

   • sequencing or cycling of different agents; and

3. improved classification of disease stage to permit the selection of agents or combinations of agents that are most appropriate for each disease stage.

RECOMMENDATION 11: **Better strategies should be developed to extract the maximum possible scientific value from MS clinical trials.**

The committee noted that many of the pivotal MS clinical trials on disease-modifying therapies were terminated early, usually because of predetermined stopping rules and, thereby, unique opportunities to obtain critical data were lost. The MS Trials Research and Resource Center that is being organized by the International Federation of MS Societies* is an example of the sort of project that should increase the potential scientific value of MS clinical trials.

Other suggestions for increasing the efficiency of clinical trials include the following:

• Alternatives to placebo-controlled studies should be investigated. Despite their scientific power, randomized placebo-controlled clinical trials are not always practical or ethical. Withholding effective treatment from a patient enrolled in the placebo arm of a clinical trial could be unethical.

• Clinical trials should be designed in close collaboration with immunologists, virologists, geneticists, and neuroimaging experts.

• Clinical research in MS should move toward adopting the inclusion of a brief and concise measure of health status. Such a measure not only

---

*In January 2001, the name was changed to Multiple Sclerosis International Federation.

would provide a direct measure of health outcome, but also would increase the likelihood of detecting unanticipated side effects.

- A data registry of patients taking disease-modifying drugs should be established that would allow for the detection of long-term effects and provide the basis for an understanding of individual variations in response to those therapies. The data should include neuroimaging-based information and should be accessible for reanalysis as a baseline for serial studies. At the same time, the confidentiality of individual patient records must be protected.

- The number of patients available for clinical trials is limited and should be managed in an organized fashion. As increasing numbers of early-stage patients are on disease-modifying therapies (beta-interferons or glatiramer acetate), increasingly fewer will be available for clinical trials that rely on previously untreated patients.

## HEALTH STATUS AND QUALITY OF LIFE

RECOMMENDATION 12: Health status assessment methods for people with MS should be further developed and validated to increase the reliability and power of clinical trials and to improve individual patient care.

Quantifying health status, including functional status and quality of life, for persons with MS is essential for several reasons. Given the chronicity and uncertain course of MS, tracking its impact over time can assist with care of individual patients by suggesting near-term prognoses and the need for various interventions. Tabulating these findings across individuals offers insight into the burden of MS-related disability within populations, information increasingly used to set research, health, and social policy priorities. Longitudinal studies of the trajectory of functioning and quality of life should help to define the natural history of the disease and expand understanding of the variations in its clinical course and patterns of progression. Finally, functional status and quality of life are critical end points in measuring the effectiveness of therapy, both for clinical trials and for routine patient care.

Clinical neurology should move toward adopting as a standard of care a concise measurement of health status that includes quality-of-life measures, as well as impairment and disability measures. This could serve as the basis for communication between physicians and other caregivers and for increasing the efficiency and thoroughness of consultations between patients and physicians, particularly if filled out by patients before meeting with the physician. If long-term records of such data were maintained in a data registry, they would also provide much needed insights into the natural course of the illness. Individual records would provide information about patient health that would not normally be collected in a routine clinical exam.

The development and validation of new impairment and disability measures should continue to be supported. Validation of the MS Functional Composite Scale should continue, particularly to measure its sensitivity to changes in patient condition over time.

RECOMMENDATION **13: Research strategies aimed at improving the ability of people with MS to adapt and function should be developed in partnership with research practitioners, managers, and patients; toward this end, a series of forums to identify the most pressing needs experienced by people with MS should be convened.**

The goal of such forums would be to define research needed to identify ways to help people with MS adapt to their illness and enhance their ability to function. There is such a small body of empirical research on this topic that the committee was not able to specify the most appropriate research strategies. Rather, the committee recommends that the MS Society work in partnership with people with MS to guide the development of specific research strategies that will identify the most effective approaches toward improving their everyday lives. A series of forums could provide the needed perspective to defining those research strategies and should include the following constituencies:

- patients and their families;

- health care providers;

- allied heath professionals, such as physical therapists, occupational therapists, and social workers;

- health services researchers, including survey scientists and clinical epidemiologists;

- social scientists, including sociologists, anthropologists, and psychologists; and

- representatives of organizations of patients with other disorders that present some of the same challenges faced by people with MS.

Specific individuals should be identified, including those whose work focuses on related issues outside the field of MS. Since the research community that deals with these issues is small and has so many fewer funding resources than biomedicine, it is essential to look more broadly for resources. The needs of people with other chronic, debilitating diseases have much in common with those of people with MS. The MS Society might work with other relevant societies and government funding agencies to identify the most important research questions with the goal of improving the lives of people with chronic and debilitating diseases.

New strategies are needed to improve dissemination of the latest research information and to develop the best methods of informing patients so they can take full advantage of treatment options and available assistance. This includes developing a better understanding of the most effective timing, settings, and modes of delivering information. Some information is important to deliver at the time of diagnosis (for example what to expect in the next few years, how to ensure health care); other information is only of interest to patients much later in the disease course (for example, how to obtain and choose a wheelchair). How, when, and where information is communicated needs to be considered. Certain information is best imparted by a health care provider during a private, scheduled visit; other information is best gained in a group setting. Some information has to be processed and molded to fit individual needs, and this is often accomplished more effectively in the back-and-forth exchange of a group setting. Uses of computers, including the Internet and chat groups, should be researched.

Specific research needs include:

- research to better understand the best approaches to making decisions about patient care in the face of uncertainty, with emphasis on addressing needs expressed by the patient;

- research on ways to help people with MS adapt to the illness and enhance ability to function;

- research to define the optimal models of care at different disease stages— this should include the impact of managed health care and policies of national health care plans; and

- research to define protocols for appropriate health care referrals. These should be useful for all health care providers, but especially primary care physicians and nurses who are not MS specialists and who would benefit from guidance about when to refer patients to occupational or physical therapy or when to recommend assistive technology.

## RESEARCH ENTERPRISE

In order to stimulate and support MS research, there is a need to broaden the community of MS researchers, to recruit more neuroscientists to MS research, and to increase exchange between clinical and basic MS researchers. New approaches gained from outside the realm of the MS scientific community are worth considering.

RECOMMENDATION 14: New researchers should be actively recruited
to work in MS, and training programs should be designed to foster
productive interactions with established investigators both within
and outside the MS research community.

MS defies disciplinary boundaries. Understanding the biological mechanisms
that underlie the disease and developing effective therapies rest on contributions
from immunology, microbiology, genetics, genomics, neuroscience, and other
fields. For instance, any therapies directed at neural repair will be effective only
if they are not thwarted by the underlying immune-mediated attack. Conversely,
while immune-based therapies might slow or halt the further advance of disease,
they are relatively unlikely to offer much in terms of repair. Even if all demyelinating attacks could be stopped overnight, there are still thousands of people with
MS who could potentially benefit from neural repair therapies.

In the last few decades there has been a tremendous influx of talented researchers into the field of neuroscience. Yet committee members observed that
this burgeoning pool of researchers has not been drawn to MS research in the
same numbers as they have to other neurological diseases. Contemporary neuroscientists bring an appreciation of nervous system functioning across the breadth
of cell and molecular biology, and the committee feels that specific efforts should
be made to encourage greater integration of neuroscience researchers into the
multidisciplinary MS research community.

To bring new researchers into MS, it is not enough to rely on people who
have already shown an interest in it. Active outreach is necessary. Promising
researchers from all relevant disciplines should be sought and encouraged to
participate in the fight against MS. Funding new researchers is of little value
without the ability to sustain the investment. Attracting new researchers should
be balanced with reasonable expectations that successful researchers can continue. In the 1990s, more Ph.D.s were awarded than could be employed in research. During such periods, recruitment efforts by private research foundations
might be more productive if they were to shift the balance of their recruitment
efforts toward reducing support for training Ph.D. students and increasing support for postdoctoral fellows.

RECOMMENDATION 15: Concerted efforts should be made to stimulate
enduring interdisciplinary collaborations among researchers in the
biological and non-biological sciences relevant to MS and to recruit
researchers from other fields into MS research.

Concerted efforts should be made to stimulate enduring cross-pollination
among researchers in the biological and non-biological sciences. It is not enough
to bring in researchers from other fields to participate in isolated workshops.
While this can provide fruitful injection of new ideas, it does not go far enough to
ensure cross-pollination. Sustained interactions that promote productive collaborations or the development of new ideas need to be fostered.

The committee felt that giving a small amount of funding (for example, $100,000) to an established laboratory, which has been done in the past, is not enough to encourage researchers to pursue MS research. Programs to encourage cross-pollination should be proactive. Individual researchers should be targeted. This has been tried successfully by a number of other private health foundations (for example, the Hereditary Disease Foundation, CaP CURE, and the Amyotrophic Lateral Sclerosis Association).

There is still too little cross-talk between clinical and basic scientists. One means of stimulating more exchange between basic researchers and clinicians would be to provide funding for minisabbaticals in which basic scientists could work with clinicians for one- to two-month visits. Although there are many researchers who combine skills in clinical and basic science, there is a major need for basic scientists, particularly in the neurosciences, who have an interest in pursuing MS research. This should be actively encouraged by organizing symposia at scientific meetings, such as those of the Society for Neuroscience, where MS research has received relatively little attention.

RECOMMENDATION **16: Programs to increase research efficiency should be developed, including collaborations to enable expensive large-scale projects (for example, clinical trials, genome screens) and to organize collection of scarce resources (for example, human tissue).**

The committee recommends that MS societies consider exploring less conventional approaches such as those tried by other health care foundations. The societies should consider leading an effort to identify and develop successful models of collaboration. Although the MS societies cannot fund many clinical trials, they might be able to work as a catalyst to facilitate more effective, far-reaching clinical trials, for example, by bringing together the right people.

This would also include the development of data registries that would apply to natural history studies and long-term therapeutic evaluations.

RECOMMENDATION **17: New strategies should be developed to encourage more integration among the different disciplines that support and conduct research relevant to improving the quality of life for people with MS.**

This would include research on the instruments used to assess quality of life, employment issues, personal independence, and the identification of optimal models of caring for people with MS. Research in these areas has too often proceeded in parallel paths with little apparent recognition of the work of others. For example, many articles about the psychosocial aspects of MS are published in nursing, psychology, physiotherapy, and neurology journals, and yet they often fail to cite articles on the same topic published outside their professional disciplines.

Because the health policy research field is relatively small and research funds are limited, partnerships should be developed among MS societies and other voluntary health research organizations supporting research on diseases that confront patients with similar challenges. Although each of these diseases has some unique features, for the most part, the research techniques, patients' needs, and even the investigators themselves overlap across different diseases, particularly chronic, debilitating diseases. Examples of such diseases include rheumatoid arthritis, diabetes, Parkinson's disease, Alzheimer's disease, and amyotrophic lateral sclerosis (ALS). Much of the research on quality-of-life issues for any of these diseases is likely to be relevant to people with MS. Indeed the development of partnerships among the related health care organizations should benefit a far greater number of patients than each could serve alone. Partnerships could take a variety of forms from collaborative development and funding of requests for proposals (RFPs) to collaborations in convening symposia and workshops.

The committee does not believe that research in health care is optimally served by contracts. However, in recent years, the National MS Society has emphasized the use of contracts for directed research in health care, a strategy it adopted in response to the generally poor quality of the grant applications they had received in past years. While contracts can provide for the collection of useful data, they also bypass the greatest source of creativity—the individual investigator. Committee members noted that otherwise qualified people have chosen not to apply because they find the contracts intellectually confining or conceptually incompatible with their perspectives. Thus, the most innovative researchers might be the least likely to apply, which is troubling since the pool of qualified applicants is already small compared to biomedical researchers. The committee endorses the 2000 decision of the Health Care Delivery and Policy Research Committee of the National MS Society to adopt a more open framework allowing potential applicants more latitude to propose their own ideas. This represents a middle-ground between targeted research and open-ended investigator-initiated proposals.

RECOMMENDATION 18: To protect against investing research resources on false leads, there should be an organizational structure to promote efficient testing of new claims for MS pathogens and disease markers.

Over the years, various viruses, bacteria, and toxins have been proposed as possible causes of MS. None of them have withstood the scrutiny of careful research, although, in a few cases, they have not been ruled out as causes. Although erroneous claims in MS research are relatively rare—there have been fewer than five in the last five years—their effects can be far-reaching. In some cases, erroneous claims have misdirected research, resulting in a substantial but unproductive investment in time and money. These erroneous claims have also led to the treatment of patients with inappropriate, expensive, and potentially harmful therapies. For example, the claim that metal toxicity causes MS induced some patients to have teeth extracted and amalgam fillings removed. New claims of MS pathogens, when appropriate, should be resolved as quickly as possible.

The MS societies are the most likely organizations to undertake efforts to test the validity of a newly proposed pathogen on an ad hoc basis. Following a potentially credible claim implicating a particular pathogen in MS, the society could oversee a project whereby the investigator making the claim, as well as an expert in the particular pathogen, could review clinical samples. A similar approach could be made in response to other claims related to the diagnosis or the treatment of MS in situations in which a quick confirmation of the results would be of importance to MS patients or the neurological and scientific communities. This approach should reduce costs to patients, researchers, and even the MS Society. The key elements of such a program would be evaluation of credible claims that are judged to have the potential for influencing research strategies or treatments, rapid response, and the generation of replicate data sets necessary to establish reliability of claims.

If the validation experiments were conducted in established laboratories equipped with the necessary expertise and research tools, the costs should be relatively low. These could be supported by a direct payment or small grant supplement provided in advance to investigators who agree to participate in such a program. It might also be possible to offer the possibility of confirming such path-breaking claims prior to their initial publication in order to increase the immediate impact of the discoveries or spare investigators embarrassment should their data be incorrect.

The Amyotrophic Lateral Sclerosis Association has recently tried such an approach in response to a report of enteroviral RNA found in gray matter tissue of the spinal cord of patients with ALS.[1] The association provided funds to the author of that paper to replicate the study and expand it. The same blinded samples will also be sent to the Enterovirus Section of the National Center for Infectious Diseases, part of the Centers for Disease Control and Prevention, for independent verification.

# REFERENCES

1. Berger MM, Kopp N, Vital C, Redl B, Aymard M, Lina B. 2000. Detection and cellular localization of enterovirus RNA sequences in spinal cord of patients with ALS. *Neurology.*;54:20-5.
2. Hohlfeld R. 1999. Therapeutic strategies in multiple sclerosis. I. Immunotherapy. *Philos Trans R Soc Lond B Biol Sci.*;354:1697-710.
3. Lassmann H. 1999. The pathology of multiple sclerosis and its evolution. *Philos Trans R Soc Lond B Biol Sci.*;354:1635-40.

# Appendixes

# Appendix A

# Committee and Staff Biographies

## COMMITTEE

**Richard B. Johnston, Jr., (Chair)** is currently Professor of Pediatrics at National Jewish Medical and Research Center and University of Colorado School of Medicine. Until January 1999, he was Medical Director of the March of Dimes Birth Defects Foundation and Chief of the Section of Immunology in the Department of Pediatrics at Yale University School of Medicine. Among his previous appointments is the position of Chairman of Pediatrics, University of Pennsylvania. He is a member of the Association of American Physicians and the Institute of Medicine and a Fellow of the American Association for the Advancement of Science. His publications include work on immune diseases in children and mechanisms of host defense and inflammation. Dr. Johnston is a past president of the Society for Pediatric Research and the American Pediatric Society.

Dr. Johnston is a member of the Board on Health Promotion and Disease Prevention of the IOM and has chaired four IOM committees, including the Committee for Assessment of Asthma and Indoor Quality and the Vaccine Safety Committee. He has served on several other IOM committees, including the Committee to Review Adverse Consequences of Pertussis and Rubella Vaccines and the Immunology Benchmarking Guidance Group.

**Jack P. Antel** is a clinical neurologist involved in a major multiple sclerosis research and treatment center at the Montreal Neurological Institute and Hospital. He is a Professor at McGill University where he has served as Chairman of the Department of Neurology and Neurosurgery. He has served on editorial boards for numerous neurological journals and on advisory boards for such organizations as the National Multiple Sclerosis Society, the American Neurological Association, and the Multiple Sclerosis Society of Canada. Prior to his work at McGill, Dr. Antel was Professor of Neurology at the University of Chicago. His interests include interactions between the immune and central nervous systems and inflammatory demyelinating disorders, including multiple sclerosis.

**Samuel Broder** is the Executive Vice President of Celera Genomics, whose mission it is to become the definitive source of genomic and information. He is the former director of the National Cancer Institute at NIH and worked there for 23 years as an investigator and administrator. Dr. Broder is a Fellow of the American College of Physicians, a member of the Institute of Medicine, American Society for Clinical Investigation, Association of American Physicians, American Association of Immunologists, and the Clinical Immunology Society and serves on the editorial advisory boards of numerous journals. His expertise includes research management in government and industry, the development of anti-retroviral drugs, and cancer biology. Dr. Broder served on the IOM Forum on Drug Development.

**Jesse M. Cedarbaum** is Vice President of Clinical Affairs at Regeneron Pharmaceuticals, Inc., and Clinical Associate Professor of Neurology at Mount Sinai Medical School. His expertise includes clinical research, biostatistics, regulatory affairs, clinical pharmacology and pharmacokinetics and toxicology. His areas of clinical research interests and activities have included Parkinson's disease, amyotrophic lateral sclerosis, peripheral neuropathy, and retinal degenerative disorders. Prior to joining Regeneron in 1990, Dr. Cedarbaum was Director of the Parkinson's Disease and Movement Disorder program at New York Hospital-Cornell Medical Center in New York, and the Burke Rehabilitation Center in White Plains, NY, and Associate Clinical Professor of Neurology at Cornell Medical School from 1983 to 1990. Dr. Cedarbaum received his B.A. and M.A. from Stanford University and his M.D. from Yale Medical School.

**Patricia K. Coyle** is Professor of Neurology and Director of the Stony Brook Multiple Sclerosis Comprehensive Care Center at SUNY Stony Brook. Her areas of expertise include neurologic infectious disease, in particular Lyme disease and multiple sclerosis. She is actively engaged in multiple sclerosis therapeutic trials and studies to elucidate neurologic Lyme disease. She is a member of many committees of the American Academy of Neurology, American Neurological Association and National Multiple Sclerosis Society, and has been an expert adviser to the Food and Drug Administration.

**Stephen L. Hauser** has served as Chairman and Betty Anker Fife Professor of Department of Neurology at the University of California, San Francisco since

1992. Dr. Hauser's research has focused on the immunologic and genetic aspects of multiple sclerosis. He is a fellow of the American Academy of Arts and Sciences and the American Associations of Physicians, is past President of the Medical Staff at UCSF, and serves as an editor of the medical textbook Harrison's Principles of Internal Medicine. Dr. Hauser was elected to the Institute of Medicine in 1999.

**Lisa I. Iezzoni** is Professor of Medicine at Harvard Medical School and Co-Director of Research in the Division of General Medicine and Primary Care, Department of Medicine, Beth Israel Deaconess Medical Center in Boston. She has conducted numerous studies for the Health Care Financing Administration, the Agency for Health Care Policy and Research, and private foundations on a variety of topics, including the use of clinical data to predict hospitalization costs and patient outcomes, comparing severity of illness across teaching and non-teaching hospitals, evaluating the utility of severity information for quality assessment, and using information from hospital data systems to predict patient clinical and functional outcomes and satisfaction with care. A 1996 recipient of The Robert Wood Johnson Investigator Award in Health Policy Research, she is studying disability policy and its implications for patients' lives. Dr. Iezzoni is on the editorial boards of major medical and health services research journals, and she serves on the National Committee on Vital Statistics. Dr. Iezzoni served on the IOM Committee to Advise the National Library of Medicine on Information Center Services, and the Committee on the Role of Institutional Review Boards in Health Services Research Data Privacy Protection, and was elected to the Institute of Medicine in 2000.

**Suzanne T. Ildstad** is Director of the Institute for Cellular Therapeutics and Professor of Surgery, Department of Surgery at the University of Louisville. With Dr. David Sachs, she established the model for mixed hematopoietic stem cell chimerism. After a pediatric surgery/transplant surgery fellowship in Cincinnati, Dr. Ildstad joined the faculty at the University of Pittsburgh. Her research on mixed chimerism to induce tolerance to organ allografts and treat nonmalignant diseases such as sickle cell anemia and autoimmune disorders is currently being applied clinically in six Food and Drug Administration (FDA) approved Phase I trials. Dr. Ildstad holds several patents related to her research in expanding bone marrow transplantation to treat nonmalignant diseases by optimizing the risk-benefit ratio through graft engineering and partial conditioning. She is the founding scientist of Chimeric Therapies, Inc., a biotechnology company focused on bone marrow graft engineering, and she serves on the board of directors of the company. Dr. Ildstad has been a member of the Institute of Medicine since 1997 and served on the IOM Committee on Organ Procurement and Transplantation.

**Sharon L. Juliano** is Professor of Anatomy and Cell Biology and Neuroscience at the Uniformed Services University of the Health Sciences. She has been a guest researcher at the NIMH and the INSERM in Creteil, France, served on a number of Advisory Committees for the NIH and Society for Neuroscience, won several research related awards, and is a member of editorial boards. Her research focuses on the development and plasticity of neocortex and the role of radial glia and Cajal Retzius cells in neuronal migration. She also studies the influence of neuronal migration on subsequent formation and processing within the cerebral cortex and the role of specific neurotrophins in neocortical plasticity.

**Donald L. Price** is Professor of Pathology, Neurology and Neuroscience and Director of the Division of Neuropathology at Johns Hopkins School of Medicine. Trained in neurology, neuropathology, and cell/molecular biology, Dr. Price's principle research interests are in the mechanisms of human neurodegenerative diseases, like Alzheimer's disease and amyotrophic lateral sclerosis (ALS). He and his collegues at Johns Hopkins have used transgenic strategies to introduce mutant genes into mice to reproduce the clinical, pathological, and biochemical phenotypes of AD, ALS, parkinsonism, and trinucleotide repeat expansion diseases in mice. These mice are being used to understand the pathogenic processes leading to these disorders. In addition, the Hopkins group has knocked out key genes/products relevant to these illnesses, work that has provided insights into therapeutic targets. Strategies effective in mice can be brought to clinical trials. He was elected to the Institute of Medicine in 1998, and is President-Elect of the Society for Neuroscience.

**Raymond P. Roos** is Professor and Chairman of the Department of Neurology at the University of Chicago. His main clinical interests are multiple sclerosis, CNS viral infections, and neurodegenerative disease. A basic goal of his studies is to use molecular techniques to better understand the pathogenesis of these diseases. He is interested in the pathogenesis of unconventional viral infections of the central nervous system, molecular determinants of neurovirulence and persistence of experimental viral infections in animals, and virus vectors in central nervous system gene delivery for use as neurobiological research tools and as a means for gene therapy.

**Alan J. Thompson** is Professor of Clinical Neurology and Neurorehabilitation in the Department of Clinical Neurology, Institute of Neurology, Queen Square, London, Medical Director of the NeuroRehabilitation Unit and Research and Development Director at the National Hospital for Neurology and Neurosurgery, Queen Square, London (affiliated with the University College of London). He is National Medical Advisor to the MS Society of Great Britain, President of ECTRIMS (European Committee for Treatment and Research in Multiple Sclerosis), European editor of the journal *Multiple Sclerosis*, and past-President of RIMS (Rehabilitation in Multiple Sclerosis). His main research interests are in the mechanisms underlying disability in neurological disorders, including multiple sclerosis and spinal cord disease. He is currently applying MR techniques to look at mechanisms underlying disability and recovery in MS. He has also been active in the application of outcome measures and the evaluation of rehabilitation in neurological disorders.

**Stephen G. Waxman** is Professor and Chair of the Department of Neurology at Yale Medical School. He also holds appointments as Professor of Neurobiology and Pharmacology at Yale University; Neurologist-in-Chief at Yale-New Haven Hospital; and Director of the Neuroscience Research Center, Department of Veterans Affairs Medical Center, West Haven. Dr. Waxman serves as co-director of the Yale London collaboration in nervous system repair. He has served on numerous scientific advisory committees including the Advisory Boards of the American Paralysis Association, Veterans Administration, the Spinal Cord Research Foundation, the Board of Scientific Counselors of NINDS, and on the Board of Neuroscience and Behavioral Health of the IOM. Dr. Waxman has published more than 300 scientific papers, has authored two books, and has edited five books on neuroscience. He is editor of The Neuroscientist, and serves on the editorial boards of over a dozen scientific journals. Dr. Waxman was elected to the IOM in 1996, and serves on the IOM's Board on Neuroscience and Behavioral Health.

**Hartmut Wekerle** is Director of the Max Planck Institute for Neurobiology, and Chairman of the Biological Medical Section. He was formerly the head of the Clinical Research Unit for Multiple Sclerosis. Dr. Wekerle has served on the advisory boards of research organizations such as the European Committee for Multiple Sclerosis, the European Charcot Foundation for Multiple Sclerosis Research, the International Federation of MS Societies, the German Multiple Sclerosis Society, the Italian Multiple Sclerosis Association, the UK National MS Society, and the Robert Koch Minerva Center for Research in Autoimmune Diseases. He has served on the editorial boards of such journals as *Multiple Sclerosis, Brain Pathology, European Journal of Immunology,* and *Journal of Autoimmunity.* His research focuses on functional interactions between nervous and immune systems, including pathogenic autoimmune responses against neural, modulation of neuronal function by immune mediators, and neuronal control of immune reactivity.

## STAFF

**Janet E. Joy** is a Senior Program Officer in the Division on Neuroscience and Behavioral Health of the Institute of Medicine at the National Academies where she has been since 1994. She has served as study director for Academy reports on intellectual property rights in molecular biology, resource management, and medical uses of marijuana. Before coming to work at the National Academies she conducted research in neural control of biological rhythms.

**John A. Rockwell** is a Research Assistant in the Division on Neuroscience and Behavioral Health. He has been with the Institute of Medicine since 1999. He has a B.S. in Kinesiology from the College of William and Mary, and an M.S. in Human Nutrition, Foods and Exercise from Virginia Tech. John's master's thesis assessed the effects of short-term energy restriction on muscle fuel stores and exercise performance.

**Amelia B. Mathis** is a Project Assistant/Senior Secretary in the Division on Neuroscience and Behavioral Health. She has 6 years of experience working at the National Academies and the Institute of Medicine. She has provided support on several Institute of Medicine projects, and her main responsibility is to handle logistical arrangements for meetings and travel for committee members and staff.

# Appendix B

# List of Expert Consultants

**Dedra S. Buchwald**
Associate Professor and Director
Chronic Fatigue Clinic
University of Washington Department
  of Medicine

**Howard L. Fields**
Professor of Neurology and
  Physiology
University of California at San
  Francisco

**Robert W. Hamill**
Chair, Neurology Department
University of Vermont

**David E. Krebs**
Professor and Director
MGH Biomotion Laboratory
Harvard University

**T. Jock Murray**
Dalhousie Medical School
Halifax, Nova Scotia

**Robert G. Robinson**
Head, Psychiatry Department
University of Iowa

**Richard Rudick**
Director, Mellen Center for Multiple
  Sclerosis Treatment and Research
Cleveland Clinic Foundation

**W. Zev Rymer**
John G. Searle Professor and Director
  of Research
Rehabilitation Institute of Chicago
Northwestern University

**Marca Sipski**
Associate Professor of Clinical
  Rehabilitation Medicine
University of Miami School of
  Medicine

# Appendix C

# Workshop Agendas

**Workshop on New Prospects and Perspectives on MS Research**

November 17-18, 1999
NAS Green Building and Holiday Inn Georgetown
Washington, D.C.

Agenda

**Wednesday, November 17**

| | | |
|---|---|---|
| 6:00 pm | **Henry McFarland**<br>NIH, NINDS | Clinical Picture of MS,<br>including use of imaging<br>in diagnosis and research |
| 7:00 pm | DINNER | |

**Thursday, November 18**

| | | |
|---|---|---|
| 8:30 am | Continental breakfast | |
| 9:00-9:10 am | **Richard Johnston**, Chair<br>National Jewish Medical &<br>Research Center | Introduction |

*Frontiers In Imaging*

| | | |
|---|---|---|
| 9:10-9:25 am | **Chien Ho**<br>Carnegie Mellon University | Tracking Immune Cell<br>Migration Through Imaging |

| 9:40-9:55 am | **Scott Fraser**<br>California Inst. Technology | In Vivo Imaging Of<br>Neuronal Development |
|---|---|---|
| 10:10-10:40 am | General Discussion of<br>Imaging | |
| 10:40-11:00 am | BREAK | |

### Risk Factors and Genetic Tools for Research

| 11:00-11:15 am | **Michael Conneally**<br>Indiana University | Identification Of Risk<br>Factors For MS |
|---|---|---|
| 11:30-11:45 am | **John Roder**<br>Mt. Sinai, Univ. Toronto | Inducible Gene Expression<br>In The Nervous System |
| 12:00-12:15 pm | **Larry Steinman**<br>Stanford University | Analysis Of Gene<br>Expression Using<br>Microarray Technology |
| 12:30-1:15 pm | LUNCH | |
| 1: 15-1:45 pm | General Discussion of<br>Genetic Tools | |

### Experimental Therapeutics and Potential Therapeutic Targets

| 1:45-2:00 pm | **Rhona Mirsky**<br>University College, London | Influence Of Schwann Cells<br>On Neural Development<br>And Repair |
|---|---|---|
| 2: 20-2:40 pm | BREAK | |
| 2:40-2:55 pm | **Marc Peschanski**<br>INSERM, France | Cell And Gene Therapy For<br>Neurodegenerative Diseases |
| 3:10-3:25 pm | **Larry Steinman**<br>Stanford University | Gene Therapy Of<br>Demyelinating Disease |
| 3:40-4:10 pm | General Discussion of<br>Gene Therapy | |
| 4:10-5:30 pm | REFRESHMENTS | |
| 4:30-4:50 pm | **Elliott Kieff**<br>Harvard University | Reflection on the day's<br>discussion through the lens<br>of another field |
| 4:50-5:30 pm | General Discussion | |
| 6:30 pm | DINNER | |

## Workshop on Therapeutic Frontiers:
## Exploring the Options in MS Research

January 14, 2000
Hyatt Regency
Denver, Colorado

Agenda

**Friday January 14**

| | | |
|---|---|---|
| 9:00-9:30 am | Continental breakfast | |
| 9:30-9:35 am | **Richard Johnston**, Chair<br>National Jewish Medical &<br>Research Center | Introduction |
| 9:35-10:15 am | **Ole Isacson**<br>Harvard University | Cellular Transplantation in<br>Neurological Disease |
| 10:15-10:30 am | BREAK | |
| 10:30-11:15 am | **Jeffery Kocsis**<br>Yale University | Neuropharmacological<br>Approaches |
| 11:15-12:00 pm | **Joy Snider** and<br>**Dennis Choi**<br>Washington University,<br>St. Louis | Neuroprotective Strategies |
| 12:00-12:45 pm | LUNCH | |
| 12:45-1:30 pm | **Jay Siegel**<br>U.S. Food and Drug<br>Administration | FDA Perspectives on<br>Clinical Trials in MS |
| 1:30-2:30 pm | General Discussion | |
| 2:30 pm | ADJOURN | |

## Workshop on Quality of Life

February 23-24, 2000
National Academy of Sciences Building
Washington, D.C.

Agenda

**Wednesday, February 23**

| 9:30-10:15 am | **Michael Weinrich** NIH, NICHD, National Center for Rehabilitation Research | Rehabilitation Research Strategies |
|---|---|---|
| 10:15 am | BREAK | |
| 10:30-11:15 am | **Barbara Vickrey** UCLA | Measuring the Quality of Life |
| 11:15 am - 12:00 pm | **Deborah Miller** Cleveland Clinic and Chair, MS Clinical Care Guidelines Committee | The Development and Role of Clinical Care Guidelines |
| 12:00 pm | LUNCH | |

**Thursday, February 24**

| 11:15 am - 12:00 pm | **Mindy Aisen** Rehabilitation Research and Development Service, Department of Veterans Affairs | Research to Maximize Function in MS Patients: Rehabilitation and Beyond |
|---|---|---|

## Individuals That Spoke with the Committee
## About Meeting Patient Needs

January 13, 2000
Hyatt Regency
Denver, Colorado

BRIAN HUTCHINSON          Executive Vice President and Director of Medical
                         Programs at the Jimmie Heuga Center, which pro-
                         vides medical and educational programs for people
                         with MS

PAT KENNEDY              Nurse Practitioner, Rocky Mountain MS Center

CHARLOTTE ROBINSON        Director of Adventures Within, which provides
                         outdoor experience and confidence-building chal-
                         lenges for individuals with MS

ERIC SIMONS              Consultant and Lecturer on living with MS for
                         Berlex Laboratories, Inc, a subsidiary of Schering
                         AG, Germany

PAM SORENSEN             Speech Language Pathologist and President of the
                         Consortium of MS Centers

# Appendix D

# Kurtzke's Expanded Disability Status Scale (EDSS)

| | |
|---|---|
| 0 | Normal neurologic exam |
| 1.0 | No disability, minimal signs in one functional system |
| 1.5 | No disability, minimal signs in more than one functional system |
| 2.0 | Minimal disability in one functional system |
| 2.5 | Minimal disability in two functional systems |
| 3.0 | Moderate disability in one functional system, or mild disability in three or four functional systems though fully ambulatory |
| 3.5 | Fully ambulatory but with moderate disability in three or four functional systems |
| 4.0 | Fully ambulatory without aid, self-sufficient, up and about some 12 hours a day despite relatively severe disability. Able to walk without aid or rest some 500 meters |
| 4.5 | Fully ambulatory without aid, up and about much of the day, able to work a full day, may otherwise have some limitation of full activity or require minimal assistance, characterized by relatively severe disability. Able to walk without aid or rest for some 300 meters |
| 5.0 | Ambulatory without aid or rest for about 200 meters; disability severe enough to preclude full daily activities (e.g. to work full day without special provisions) |

| | |
|---|---|
| 5.5 | Ambulatory without aid or rest for about 100 meters; disability severe enough to preclude full daily activities |
| 6.0 | Intermittent or unilateral constant assistance (cane, crutch, or brace) required to walk about 100 meters with or without resting |
| 6.5 | Constant bilateral assistance (canes, crutches, or braces) required to walk about 20 meters without resting |
| 7.0 | Unable to walk beyond about 5 meters even with aid. Essentially restricted to a wheelchair. Wheels self in standard wheelchair and transfers alone. Active in wheelchair about 12 hours a day |
| 7.5 | Unable to take more than a few steps. Restricted to wheelchair. May need aid to transfer. Wheels self but cannot carry on in standard wheelchair a full day. May require a motorized wheelchair |
| 8.0 | Unable to walk at all, essentially restricted to bed, chair or wheelchair but may be out of bed much of the day. Retains many self-care functions. Generally has effective use of the arms |
| 8.5 | Essentially restricted to bed much of the day. Has some effective use of arm(s). Retains some self-care functions |
| 9.0 | Helpless bed patient. Can communicate and eat |
| 9.5 | Totally helpless bed patient. Unable to communicate effectively or eat/ swallow |
| 10 | Death due to Multiple Sclerosis |

SOURCE: Kurtzke JF. 1983. Rating neurologic impairment in multiple sclerosis: an expanded disability status scale (EDSS). *Neurology.*;33:1444-52.

# Appendix E

# Drugs Used in the Treatment of MS

## APPROVED DISEASE-MODIFYING MEDICATIONS

| Generic Name | Trade Name | Company | Indication | Mechanism of Action | Potential Side Effects |
|---|---|---|---|---|---|
| Beta-Interferon-1a | Avonex, Rebif[a] | Biogen, Serono | RRMS | Beta-interferon-1a is believed to suppress the autoimmune destruction of myelin. Slows accumulation of disability and decreases the frequency of clinical exacerbations. Interferon-β-1a is involved in the regulation of activation, proliferation, migration, and suppressor cell function of T-cells, the modulation of the production of cytokines, including down-regulation of proinflammatory cytokines and up-regulation of inhibitory, antiinflammatory cytokines. | Flu-like symptoms, muscle aches, fever, chills and weakness, pain from intramuscular injection |
| Beta-Interferon-1b | Betaseron | Berlex Labs (Distributor) Chiron (Manufacturer) | RRMS | Possesses both antiviral and immunoregulatory activities, mediated through interactions with specific cell receptors, which results in the expression of interferon-induced gene products. | Redness, pain and swelling and discoloration at injection site, flu-like symptoms, depression, anxiety, depersonalization, suicide attempts |

| | | | | | |
|---|---|---|---|---|---|
| Glatiramer acetate | Copaxone | Teva Marion Partners | RRMS | Blocks myelin-specific autoimmune responses. Non-steroidal, non-interferon. Mechanism uncertain, but it is thought that glatiramer acetate, consisting of the acetate salts of synthetic polypeptides, resembles myelin basic protein (mbp) and serves as a decoy that blocks myelin damaging T cells. | Redness, pain and swelling and discoloration at injection site, flushing, chest pain, weakness, infection, pain, nausea, joint pain, anxiety and muscle stiffness. Immediate postinjection reaction characterized by chest tightness with heart palpitations and difficulty breathing |

Note: Avonex, Betaseron, Copaxone, and Rebif are "orphan drugs." The 1983 Orphan Drug Act (ODA) provides incentives for sponsors to develop products for rare diseases or conditions, by guaranteeing the developer of an orphan product seven years of market exclusivity following the approval of the product by the FDA. The definition of "rare disease or condition" in the Orphan Drug Act:

"...the term rare disease or condition means any disease or condition which (a) affects less than 200,000 persons in the U.S. or (b) affects more than 200,000 persons in the U.S. but for which there is no reasonable expectation that the cost of developing and making available in the U.S. a drug for such disease or condition will be recovered from sales in the U.S. of such a drug."

[a]Rebif has been approved by the European Commission for the treatment of relapsing-remitting multiple sclerosis. The FDA has upheld the Orphan Drug Act and has not granted approval to Rebif. The FDA also had questions about the data filed in the marketing application, which prevented granting tentative approval. If tentative approval is received, Rebif could enter the US market in 2003, when the exclusivity periods for Avonex and Betaseron end.

# AVAILABLE AND EMERGING DISEASE-MODIFYING THERAPIES[a]

### GLOBAL IMMUNOSUPPRESSION

| Medication Options | Status as of 1999 | Putative Mechanisms Of Action |
|---|---|---|
| Cyclophosphamide | Off label use in the U.S. and Europe | Global reduction of T-cell population |
| Azathioprine | Off label use in the U.S. and Europe | As above |
| Glucocorticosteroids | Off label use in the U.S. and Europe | As above |
| Methotrexate | Off label use in the U.S. and Europe | As above |
| Total lymphoid irradiation | Off label use in the U.S. and Europe | As above |
| Paclitaxel | Phase II Clinical Trials | As above |
| 2-Chlorodeoxyadenosine | Phase III Clinical Trials | As above |
| Mitoxantrone | Phase III Clinical Trials | As above |

### IMMUNOMODULATION

| Therapeutic Strategy | Medication Options | Status as of 1999 | Putative Mechanisms Of Action |
|---|---|---|---|
| **1) Inhibit T-cell receptor/peptide/ MHC-II interaction** | Altered peptide ligands | Phase I/II | Block or compete with the binding of encephalitogenic peptides to the MHC-II molecule |
| | Copolymer | Approved for relapsing forms of MS in the U.S. and Europe | Block or compete with the binding of encephalitogenic peptides to the MHC-II molecule |
| | TCR vaccination and TCR peptide vaccination | Phase I | Generation of antibodies against peptides within the TCR |
| | IL-10 , TGF b | Phase I/II | Immunomodulation; reduce MHC-II molecule expression |
| | Interpheron Beta | Approved for relapsing forms of MS in the U.S. and Europe | Immunomodulation; reduce MHC-II molecule expression |
| **2) Induction of T-cell anergy** | Antibodies to B7 or molecules | Preclinical testing | T cells are anergised when TCR/peptide/ MHC-II interaction occurs in the absence of co-signalling |

[a]Adapted from Waubant and Goodkin 1997.

| Therapeutic Strategy | Medication Options | Status as of 1999 | Putative Mechanisms Of Action |
|---|---|---|---|
| | Soluble MHC-II/ peptide complexes | Phase I | T cells are anergised when TCR/peptide/ MHC-II interaction occurs in the absence of co-signalling |
| 3) Deletion of autoreactive T cells | Anti-CD4, anti-CD52 | Phase I/II | Depletion of T cells targeted by the antibodies |
| 4) Reduce T-cell trafficking across blood-brain-barrier (BBB) | Glucocorticosteroids | Unlabelled use in the U.S. and Europe | Decrease the expression of adhesion molecules on T cells and vascular endothelial cells |
| | TGF b | Phase I/II | Decrease the expression of adhesion molecules on T cells and vascular endothelial cells |
| | Interpheron Beta | Approved for relapsing forms of MS in the U.S. and Europe | Decrease the expression of adhesion molecules on T cells and vascular endothelial cells |
| | Antibodies to adhesion molecules (Antegren, anti-CD11/CD18) | Phase II | Decrease the attachment of T cells to vascular endothelial cells |
| | Matrix metalloprotease inhibitors | Phase I | Inhibit proteases that facilitate T-cell trafficking across BBB |
| 5) Alter the balance of pro-inflammatory (Th1) and immunomodulatory (Th2) cytokines | Antibodies to TNFa, IL-1 | Phase I/II | Reduce pro-inflammatory (Th1) cytokine activity |
| | Soluble IL-2 or TNFa receptors | Phase I/II | Reduce pro-inflammatory (Th1) cytokine activity |
| | Antagonists to IL-1 receptor | Preclinical testing | Reduce pro-inflammatory (Th1) cytokine activity |

*continued*

| Therapeutic Strategy | Medication Options | Status as of 1999 | Putative Mechanisms Of Action |
|---|---|---|---|
| | Oral myelin | Testing discontinued; phase III trial revealed no difference between active and placebo groups | Increases immunomodulatory (Th2) cytokine production |
| | Interpheron Alpha | Phase I | Antagonise production of pro-inflammatory cytokines induced by IFNg |
| | Interpheron Beta | Approved for relapsing forms of MS in the U.S. and Europe | Reduce Th1 cytokine secretion and macrophage function |
| | Glucocorticosteroids | Unlabelled use in the U.S. and Europe | Reduce Th1 cytokine secretion and macrophage function |
| | Matrix metalloprotease inhibitors | Phase I | Block cleavage of pro-TNF to TNF |
| | Methotrexate | Unlabelled use in the U.S. and Europe | Reduces level of soluble IL-2 receptor |
| | Intravenous immunoglobulin | Unlabelled use in the U.S. and Europe, Phase III | Reduction of pro-inflammatory cytokines |
| | Anti-CD40 ligand | Preclinical testing | Blocks Th1 differentiation and effector function, inhibits IFNg production |
| | Roquinimex (Linomide) | Testing discontinued; phase III trial revealed an increase in heart attacks associated with this drug | Inhibits TNF production |
| 6) Neuroprotection | Riluzole, Insulin-like growth factor (IGF-1) | Phase I | Prevent neuronal death |
| | Eliprodil | Preclinical testing | Prevent neuronal death |
| 7) Reduces gliosis | Pirfenidone | Phase I | Prevents gliosis, blocks TNF synthesis |

*continued*

| Therapeutic Strategy | Medication Options | Status as of 1999 | Putative Mechanisms Of Action |
|---|---|---|---|
| 8) Promote remyelination | IGF-1 | Phase I | Promotes oligodendrocyte survival and maturation of precursors in vitro |
| | Intravenous immunoglobulin | Unlabelled use in the U.S. and Europe, Phase III | Promote remyelination |
| | Oligodendrocyte grafts | Preclinical testing | Promote remyelination |
| | Eliprodil | Preclinical testing | Promote remyelination |

## ONGOING CLINICAL TRIALS FOR MEDICATIONS IN DEVELOPMENT AS OF AUGUST 2000

| Trade Name | Generic Name | Phase[a] | About the trial | Source |
|---|---|---|---|---|
| Anergix | HLA-DR2 MHC II | I | Anergix consists of complexes of MHC Class II molecules, called Soluble DR2-MBP84-102 Complexes. The complexes contain auto-antigenic peptides that shut down the MBP reactive T cells that damage myelin components, without compromising other T cells required for immune protection of the individual taking the drug. The phase I trial in chronic progressive MS was completed by Anergen in 1998. Anergix was shown to be safe and well tolerated with no signs of generalized immune suppression. Corixa is looking for a partner to initiate Phase II. | PhRMA (Pharmaceutical Research and Manufacturers of America) Database[b] |
| Antegren | Natalizumab | II | Antegren is a humanized antibody that blocks a receptor on leukocytes and thus blocks their migration into the brain. This can reverse paralysis and reduce myelin destruction in the EAE animal model of MS. Ongoing phase II testing has shown that patients treated with Antegren showed a significant reduction in new brain lesions over 12 weeks. | PhRMA Database, UCSF MS Center[c] |
| Fampridine[d] Neurelan | 4-Amino pyridine | II | Fampridine's major action is to block specialized potassium channels on axons. In a demyelinated axon, large numbers of potassium channels are exposed, and nerve transmission is impaired. Fampridine has been shown to increase nerve conduction in impaired and demyelinated axons, and to result in improved neurological function in animal and in vitro studies. A phase II trial was successfully completed in 1998, and additional phase II trials are underway. | FDA—Office of Orphan Products Development |

| Name | Compound | Company | Phase | Description | Source |
|---|---|---|---|---|---|
| Leukarrest | HU23F2G recombinant humanized MAb | ICOS | II | Leukarrest is a humanized antibody that impedes white blood cell movement from the blood stream to the surrounding tissue by binding to CD 11 and CD 18 on the white blood cell surface. Two phase II trials were recently completed in patients with acute symptomatic episodes of MS. | PhRMA Database |
| Leustatin | 2-CDA / Cladribine | Ortho Biotech | III | Cladribine is a potent immunosuppressive drug that has been shown to decrease total lymphocyte count and CD4, CD8 and CD19 subsets. Cladribine may benefit people with Chronic Progressive MS, according to the results of a pilot study, but toxicity is a concern. | PhRMA Database, FDA |
| Myotrophin | Insulin-like growth factor I (IGF-I) | Cephalon | I | IGF-1 promotes the proliferation, differentiation and survival of oligodendrocytes, and reduces inflammation and TNF-alpha induced oligodendrocyte and myelin damage. IGF-I treatment has been shown to reduce lesion severity and promote myelin regeneration in the experimental autoimmune encephalomyelitis (EAE) model. Cephalon is developing Myotropin for use in amyotrophic lateral sclerosis (ALS), and is exploring the drug's potential for use in MS. | ClinicalTrials.gov Database,[e] UCSF MS Center |
| Novantrone | Mitoxantrone | Immunex | III | Novantrone suppresses T cells and B cells, which are key components of the immune system and multiple sclerosis. Immunex has filed a new drug application (NDA) with the FDA for approval to label Novantrone for use in treatment of secondary progressive MS. The FDA has assigned priority review status to the application, indicating that the FDA will act on the application within 6 months of the June 7, 1999 filing date. On January 28, 2000, the FDA Peripheral and Central Nervous System Drugs Advisory Panel unanimously recommended that Novantrone be approved. | PhRMA Database |
| Deskar | Pirfenidone | Marnac | I | Pirfenidone is an anti-fibrotic agent which is also in clinical trials for pulmonary fibrosis. It acts to inhibit the production of tumor necrosis factor (TNF), and reduces gliosis and astrocytosis, which is a proliferation of astrocytes in the area of a degenerative lesion. | UCSF MS Center |

continued

## Ongoing Clinical Trials for Medications in Development as of August 2000 (Continued)

| Trade Name | Generic Name | Company | Phase[a] | About the trial | Source |
|---|---|---|---|---|---|
| Rebif | Recombinant interferon-beta-1a | Serono Laboratories | III | Rebif has been approved by the European Commission for the treatment of Relapsing Remitting Multiple Sclerosis. The FDA has upheld the Orphan Drug Act and has not granted approval to Rebif. The FDA also had questions about the data filed in the marketing application, which prevented granting tentative approval. If tentative approval is received, Rebif could enter the US market in 2003, when the exclusivity periods for Avonex and Betaseron end. | PhRMA Database |
| Rilutek | Riluzole | Rhone Pulenc Rorer | I | Rilutek is neuroprotective in various in vivo experimental models of neuronal injury involving excitotoxic mechanisms. In in vitro tests, Riluzole protected cultured rat motor neurons from the excitotoxic effects of glutamic acid and prevented the death of cortical neurons induced by anoxia. | UCSF MS Center |
| Taxol | Paclitaxel | Angiotech | II | Paclitaxel is an immunosuppressant. According to preliminary results from the treatment extension phase of the phase I/II clinical study of paclitaxel for the treatment of secondary progressive multiple sclerosis, patients showed a significant improvement in all tests undertaken. Study measures included functional testing, quality of life measures and changes in the amount of brain tissue scarring demonstrated by magnetic resonance imaging (MRI). A 189 patient, phase II clinical study is underway. | UCSF MS Center |

| | | | | | |
|---|---|---|---|---|---|
| TM27 | ATM027 humanized Mab | Astra Zeneca/ Avant Immuno-Therapeutics | I/II | T Cell Receptor Monoclonal Antibody (MAb) under development. Astra Zeneca has discontinued the development of this T cell antigen receptor monoclonal antibody because results of a phase II trial suggested that the reduction of disease activity in the trial was not sufficient to warrant further study. The company is considering whether to development the T cell antigen receptor peptide as a MS vaccine. | PhRMA Database |
| Thalidomide | Thalomid | Andrulis Pharmaceuticals | II | Thalidomide suppresses the production of cytokines that are found in the cerebrospinal fluid of patients with MS, and especially Chronic Progressive MS. | PhRMA Database |
| Zenapax | Daclizumab Interleukin-2 Receptor Alpha humanized Mab | Hoffman-La Roche, Inc. | I/II | Zenapax binds to protein receptors on lymphocytes, keeping them from interacting with interleukin-2, a substance necessary for their growth. As a result, the T lymphocytes are unable to attack the myelin sheath. Zenapax was developed as an immune modulating drug for use after transplantation. In two Phase III clinical trials, Zenapax was effective in reducing the incidence of acute rejection episodes within six months of kidney transplantation, the primary endpoint, when administered with standard immunosupressive drug regimens. | ClinicalTrials.gov Database |
| | BB-3364 | British Biotech/ Schering Plough | I | BB-3364 is a matrix metalloproteinase (MMP) inhibitor that also inhibits leukocyte migration to the CNS. Its development is based on the theory that MMPs may contribute to the pathology of MS. BB-3644 also inhibits tumor necrosis factor production. | UCSF MS Center |
| | IR 208 therapeutic vaccine | Immune Response Corporation | I | The vaccine consists of an immunostimulant, Incomplete Freund's Adjuvant, combined with synthetic peptides. The vaccine is designed to halt the T-cell attack on myelin by shutting down specific T cells and inhibit further damage. | PhRMA Database |

continued

# ONGOING CLINICAL TRIALS FOR MEDICATIONS IN DEVELOPMENT AS OF AUGUST 2000 (CONTINUED)

| Trade Name | Generic Name | Company | Phase[a] | About the trial | Source |
|---|---|---|---|---|---|
| | MSP-771 | Neurocrine Biosciences/ Novartis | II | MSP-771 is an altered peptide ligand based on the immunodominant epitope of human MBP. Immune responses directed against this epitope may be involved in the pathogenesis of MS. In vitro, MSP-771 fails to induce T-cell proliferation and selectively reduces the production of inflammatory cytokines by pathogenic T cells. In the EAE model, MSP-771 markedly reduces the severity of disease and induces a specific T-cell response that down-regulates the inflammatory process. The molecule was well tolerated in a phase I study, with the most common side effect being local, transient injection site reactions. The primary endpoint in current clinical trials is the progression or regression of lesions in the brains of these patients as measured by MRI. As a secondary endpoint, clinical investigators will look for the generation of a protective immune response as shown in the Phase I trials. | PhRMA Database |
| | Interleukin-10 (IL-10) | Schering-Plough | I/II | IL-10 has a number of inhibitory functions such as inhibiting interferon g production, antigen presentation, and the production by macrophages of the cytokines IL-1, IL-6 and TNFa. | UCSF MS Center |

## DEFINITIONS

*Preclinical testing.* A pharmaceutical company conducts laboratory and animal studies to show biological activity of the compound against the targeted disease, and the compound is evaluated for safety.

*Phase I.* Tests that involve about 20 to 80 normal, healthy volunteers. The tests study a drug's safety profile, including the safe dosage range. The studies also determine how a drug is absorbed, distributed, metabolized, and excreted as well as the duration of its action.

*Phase II.* Controlled trials of approximately 100 to 300 volunteer patients (people with the disease) assess a drug's effectiveness.

*Phase III.* Tests involving 1,000 to 3,000 patients in clinics and hospitals. Physicians monitor patients closely to confirm efficacy and identify adverse events.

[a]Clinical trial phases are defined at the end of this table.
[b]The PhRMA (Pharmaceutical Research and Manufacturers of America) Database lists only clinical trials being conducted in private firms in the U.S. Clinical trials at academic health centers and universities are not included.
[c]http://mscenter.ucsf.edu
[d]Listed as an orphan drug by FDA, http://www.fda.gov/orphan.
[e]The ClinicalTrials.gov Database contains clinical studies sponsored primarily by the National Institutes of Health. In the future, additional studies from other Federal agencies and the pharmaceutical industry will be included.

## Drugs Used to Treat Various Symptoms: Overview

**Bladder Control**
Capsaicin
Desmopressin
Detrol
Dicyclomine hydrochloride
Hyoscyamine
Imipramine
Oxybutynin chloride
Propantheline bromide

**Depression**
Amitriptyline
Bupropion hydrochloride
Imipramine
Nortriptyline
Paroxetine
Fluoxetine hydrochloride
Sertraline

**Dysesthesia-Paresthesia,
trigeminal neuralgia, pruritis**
Amitriptylene
Carbamazepine
Gabapentin
Hydroxyzine
Phenytoin

**Erectile Dysfunction-Impotence**
Sildenafil citrate
Alprostadil
Papaverine

**Fatigue**
Amantadine
Fluoxetine hydrochloride
Modafinil
Pemoline

**Inflammation**
Azathioprine
Dexamethasone
Methylprednisolone
Prednisone

**Optic Neuritis**
Methylprednisolone
Prednisone
Decadron

**Seizures**
Carbamazepine
Klonopin
Gabapentin
Phenytoin

**Spasticity and Tremor**
Baclofen
Botulinum Toxin A
Klonopin
Dantrolene
Gabapentin

**Urinary Tract Infections**
Methenamine

**Vertigo**
Meclizine hydrochloride

# Appendix F

# U.S. Social Security Administration's Criteria for Qualifying as Disabled from MS

Impairments listed by the SSA for disability evaluation are considered severe enough to prevent a person from doing any gainful activity, and are permanent and expected to result in death. Otherwise, evidence must show that the impairment has lasted or is expected to last for a continuous period of at least 12 months. Only the paragraphs that apply to MS are reproduced here.

## 11.00 Neurological

*C. Persistent disorganization of motor function* in the form of paresis or paralysis, tremor or other involuntary movements, ataxia and sensory disturbances (any or all of which may be due to cerebral, cerebellar, brainstem, spinal cord, or peripheral nerve dysfunction) which occur singly or in various combinations, frequently provides the sole or partial basis for decision in cases of neurological impairment. The assessment of impairment depends on the degree of interference with locomotion and/or interference with the use of fingers, hands and arms.

*E. Multiple Sclerosis.* The major criteria for evaluating impairment caused by multiple sclerosis are discussed in Listing 11.09. Paragraph A provides criteria for evaluating disorganization of motor function and gives reference to 11.04B (11.04B then refers to 11.00C). Paragraph B provides references to other listings for evaluating visual or mental impairments caused by multiple sclerosis. Paragraph C provides criteria for evaluating the impairment of individuals who do not have muscle weakness or other significant disorganization of motor function at rest, but who do develop muscle weakness on activity as a result of fatigue.

Use of the criteria in 11.09C is dependent upon (1) documenting a diagnosis of multiple sclerosis, (2) obtaining a description of fatigue considered to be characteristic of multiple sclerosis, and (3) obtaining evidence that the system has actually become fatigued. The evaluation of the magnitude of the impairment must consider the degree of exercise and the severity of the resulting muscle weakness.

The criteria in 11.09C deal with motor abnormalities which occur on activity. If the disorganization of motor function is present at rest, paragraph A must be used, taking into account any further increase in muscle weakness resulting from activity.

Sensory abnormalities may occur, particularly involving central visual acuity. The decrease in visual acuity may occur after brief attempts at activity involving near vision, such as reading. This decrease in visual acuity may not persist when the specific activity is terminated, as with rest, but is predictably reproduced with resumption of the activity. The impairment of central visual acuity in these cases should be evaluated under the criteria in Listing 2.02, taking into account the fact that the decrease in visual acuity will wax and wane.

Clarification of the evidence regarding central nervous system dysfunction responsible for the symptoms may require supporting technical evidence of function impairment such as evoked response tests during exercise.

**11.01 Category of Impairment, Neurological**

**11.04 Central nervous system vascular accident.** With one of the following more than 3 months post-vascular accident:
B. Significant and persistent disorganization of motor function in two extremities, resulting in sustained disturbance of gross and dexterous movements, or gait and station (see 11.00C).

**11.09 Multiple Sclerosis.** With:
A. Disorganization of motor function as described in 11.04B; or
B. Visual or mental impairment as described under the criteria in 2.02, 2.03, 2.04, or 12.02; or
C. Significant, reproducible fatigue of motor function with substantial muscle weakness on repetitive activity, demonstrated on physical examination, resulting from neurological dysfunction in areas or the central nervous system known to be pathologically involved by the multiple sclerosis process.

**1.01 Category of Impairments, Special Senses and Speech**

**1.02 Impairment of Central Visual Acuity.** Remaining vision in the better eye after best correction is 20/200 or less.

**2.03 Contraction of Peripheral Visual Fields in the Better Eye.**
A. To 10 degree or less from the point of fixation; or
B. So the widest diameter subtends an angle no greater than 20 degrees; or
C. To 20 percent or less visual field efficiency.

**2.04 Loss of Visual Efficiency.** Visual efficiency of better eye after best correction 20 percent or less. (The percent of remaining visual efficiency equals the product of the percent of remaining central visual efficiency and the percent of remaining visual field efficiency.)

**12.02 Organic Mental Disorders:** Psychological and behavioral abnormalities associated with a dysfunction of the brain. History and physical examination or laboratory tests demonstrate the presence of a specific organic factor judged to be etiologically related to the abnormal mental state and loss of previously acquired functional abilities.

The required level of severity for these disorders is met when the requirements in both A and B are satisfied.

A. Demonstration of a loss of specific cognitive abilities or affective changes and the medically documented persistence of at least one of the following:

1. Disorientation to time and place; or
2. Memory impairment, either short-term (inability to learn new information), intermediate, or long term (inability to remember information that was known sometime in the past); or
3. Perceptual or thinking disturbances (e.g., hallucinations, delusions); or
4. Change in personality; or
5. Disturbance in mood; or
6. Emotional liability (e.g., explosive tempter outbursts, sudden crying, etc.) and impairment in impulse control; or
7. Loss of measured intellectual ability of at least 15 I.Q. points from premorbid levels or overall impairment index clearly within the severely impaired range on neuropsychological testing, e.g., the Luria-Nebraska, Halstead-Reitan, etc; AND

B. Resulting in at least two of the following:

1. Marked restriction of activities of daily living; or
2. Marked difficulties in maintaining social functioning; or
3. Deficiencies of concentration, persistence or pace resulting in frequent failure to complete tasks in a timely manner (in work settings or elsewhere); or

4.  Repeated episodes of deterioration or decompensation in work or work-like settings which cause the individual to withdraw from that situation or to experience exacerbation of signs and symptoms (which may include deterioration of adaptive behaviors).

# Appendix G

# Treatments That Have Been Claimed to Be of Benefit in MS[1]

Diet

**Allergen-Free Diet.** Regular use of a diet from which foods are eliminated that are known to produce hives, other skin eruptions, asthmatic attacks, and so on. There is no relationship of MS to external allergens demonstrated. The diet has not been shown to be effective and has dropped out of favor.

**Kousmine Diet.** A low-fat, low-concentrated sugar, high-fiber diet, supplemented by vitamins A, D, E, C, and B complex. There is no scientific evidence that this particular dietary method is effective in treating MS.

**Gluten-Free Diet.** A balanced diet excluding wheat and rye. This diet must be considered ineffective in MS.

**Raw Food, Evers Diet.** A diet containing only natural (unprocessed) foods, including a daily intake of germinated wheat. It appears that this diet should be considered ineffective in MS.

**MacDougal Diet.** This diet combines a low-fat diet with a gluten-free diet and adds supplements of vitamins and minerals. There is no scientific evidence that this diet is effective in MS.

---

[1]This list is based on evaluations made by the Therapeutic Claims Committee of the International Federation of MS Societies. SOURCE: Murray TJ. In Press. Alternative therapies used by MS patients. Polman CH, Thompson AJ, Murray TJ, McDonald WI, eds. *Multiple Sclerosis: The Guide to Treatment and Management.* New York: Demos Publications.

**Pectin-and Fructose-Restricted Diet.** A diet from which unripe fruits, fruit juices, and pectin-containing fruits and vegetables are eliminated, supplemented with menadione (vitamin K3). The methanol hypothesis and the dietary regimen based on it remain unproven.

**Cambridge and Other Liquid Diets.** A balanced, very low-calorie liquid, used in the treatment of obesity. Calorie intake is 330/day with a suboptimal level of protein at 22 g/day. Extra potassium is supplied. This diet is not recommended for the treatment of MS.

**Sucrose-and Tobacco-Free Diet.** Elimination of all food products containing sucrose in the form of cane, brown, or maple sugars, molasses, sorghum, or dates; also products containing propylene glycol or glycol stearate. Tobacco is not to be used in any form. This therapy remains unproven.

**Vitamins.** Individual vitamins or combinations of vitamins are taken in capsule or liquid form as a supplement to a normal diet. Adequate intake of vitamins is advised in all patients with MS, but there appears to be no scientific proof that supplementary doses of vitamins, alone or in combination, favorably affect the course of this disease.

**Megavitamin Therapy.** Massive doses of vitamins. There appears to be no reliable evidence that megavitamin therapy influences the course of MS.

**Megascorbic Therapy.** Massive doses of vitamin C (ascorbic acid), referred to as an orthomolecular treatment. The value of megascorbic therapy in MS is unproven and this treatment is not recommended.

**Minerals.** Addition of various mineral salts to diet. There appears to be no clear evidence that any of these regimens should be considered effective in MS.

**Cerebrosides.** Dietary supplementation with fatty acids of cerebrosides from beef spinal cord. On the basis of published evidence, this treatment is considered ineffective in MS.

**Aloe Vera.** Juice of the aloe vera plant, available over-the-counter, taken by mouth on a regular basis. Aloe vera is not recommended for use in MS.

**Enzymes.** A diet similar to the Evers diet, supplemented with plant and bacterial enzymes, normal digestive enzymes, vitamins, and minerals, lipolytic enzymes, and others. Enzyme supplementation is not recommended.

## Oral Administration

**St. John's Wort.** This plant has been used for hundreds of years and has recently been popularized as a treatment for many conditions. The active ingredient is hypericum. St. John's Wort can be helpful in mild depression. If depression is severe or protracted, standard antidepressants should be used. In the opinion of the committee, St. John's Wort is not a treatment for MS, but might be beneficial in patients who have mild depression or mood change.

**Oral Calcium + Magnesium + Vitamin D.** Inexpensive chemicals available commercially, taken by mouth. The efficacy of this treatment is yet to be determined.

**Hyperimmune Colostrum (Immune Milk).** Pregnant cows are inoculated with measles vaccine or other viruses considered to be related to MS. Colostrum (early milk) is frozen for preservation and taken by mouth. This treatment remains unproven and is not recommended. A clinical trial of adequate size would be required to determine whether it has any value.

**Metabolic Therapy.** A complex program of regimens and medications said to affect mineral balance, diet, and bowel function, e.g., alkalinity of the small intestine; also immune colostrum and high doses of vitamin C, SOD, vitamin A, "thymotropic" tablets to stimulate the immune system, octacosanol, B complex vitamins. This is an unproven, expensive, and possibly dangerous procedure with no known scientific basis.

**Promazine Hydrochloride (Sparine).** A phenothiazine drug. The value of phenothiazine and related drugs in aborting MS exacerbations is unsubstantiated.

**Le Gac Therapy.** Treatment with broad-spectrum antibiotics combined with hot baths. This treatment is not recommended.

**Nystatin.** An antifungal agent usually employed with a yeast-free, low carbohydrate diet. Use of nystatin is not recommended.

## Injected Materials and Oral Administration

**Calcium Orotate, Calcium Aminoethyl Phosphate.** Calcium orotate and calcium animoethyl phosphate (AEP) are calcium salts of synthetic organic compounds, given intravenously and by mouth. In the absence of a properly designed clinical study, the claim of favorable effect remains undocumented.

**Sodium Bicarbonate, Phosphates.** Simple chemicals, given intravenously (sodium bicarbonate) or by mouth (phosphates). These substances are not recommended as treatments. The Committee believes there appears to be no generally accepted scientific basis for use of this therapy; it has never been tested in a properly controlled trial. Risks are undetermined.

## Injected Materials

**Intravenous yeasts (proper-myl).** A preparation of cells from three species of yeast. Administered intravenously, proper-myl appears to be ineffective in the treatment of MS.

**Pancreatic Extract (Deporpanex).** A preparation derived from beef pancreas, given intramuscularly. The exact composition is not known, but it does not contain protein. Due to limited data, this treatment cannot be considered effective in MS. The Committee believes this therapy has been adequately tested and shown to be without value. Risks are undetermined.

**Heart and Pancreas Extract (Pancorphen).** A weak protein solution prepared by digesting beef heart with hog pancreas. It was used as a culture medium for growing bacteria. Pancorphen appears unacceptable as a treatment for MS as there is no evidence of benefit and evidence of side effects and an adverse effect on MS symptoms. The Committee believes that this therapy should not be used.

**Snake Venom (PROven, Venogen, Horvi MS9).** Proven is a processed mixture of cobra, krait, and water moccasin venoms for subcutaneous injection. It has had spectrographic analysis. Although its exact composition is not established, it appears to contain many proteins and some of the numerous enzymatic activities of the original venoms used in the mixture. This therapy is not recommended because of lack of evidence of benefit and because of the side effects and danger of allergic reaction.

**Honey Bee Venom.** Extracts of the bee venom. There are no objective controlled studies. Based on the evidence, this treatment is not recommended. The Committee feels that there is no generally accepted scientific basis for use of this therapy because it never has been tested in a properly controlled trial, and its use carries significant risk.

**Octacosanol.** A simple long-chain alcohol. The Committee believes that there is no generally accepted scientific basis for use of this therapy and that the risks are undetermined.

**Superoxide Dismutase (Orgotein, Orgosein, Palosein).** Superoxide dismutase (SOD) is a metalloprotein enzyme that combines with and "neutralizes" free radicals of oxygen (superoxides) appearing as a normal toxic byproduct of cellular metabolism. It is available in health food stores as an extract of liver in tablet form and is used in veterinary practice as an anti-inflammatory agent (by injection). The Committee believes there appears to be no generally accepted scientific basis for the use of this therapy.

**Procaine Hydrochloride.** Procaine is a simple chemical with anesthetic properties. KH3 is the proprietary name for a procaine compound in capsule form available by prescription in limited areas of the U.S. and in Europe. It is said to improve physical and mental efficiency and to improve the depression of old age. The Committee believes that there is no generally accepted scientific basis for use of this therapy since it has never been tested in a properly controlled trial and its use carries significant risk.

**Dimethyl Sulfoxide.** Dimethyl sulfoxide (DMSO) is a potent solvent for chemicals and has been widely used in industry as a degreaser. The Committee believes that there appears to be no generally accepted scientific basis for use of this therapy. It has never been tested in a properly controlled trial and there are risks of serious side effects.

**Alphasal (formerly Cholorazone or Vitamin X).** A product of electrolysis of a saline solution. If used immediately, contains ozone. Taken orally or by injection. According to the Committee, no scientifically acceptable evidence exists for the usefulness of alphasal in MS.

**Cellular Therapy.** Injection of ground-up brain or other tissues freshly prepared from unborn calves, lambs, or pigs. The little published information suggests that this treatment should be considered ineffective in MS and potentially dangerous.

**Allergens.** Repeated injections of food or other allergens, used in desensitization for asthma and hay fever. The Committee feels that this treatment should be considered ineffective in MS.

**Rodilemid.** A mixture of chelating (metal-binding) agents, developed in Rumania. It includes L-cysteine, the calcium sodium salt of ethylenediamine tetraacetic acid (EDTA), and calcium gluconate. It is taken as a series of six daily intramuscular injections at intervals of one to four months. Rodilemid is unproven as a therapy for MS.

**Autogenous Vaccine.** Vaccine prepared from bacteria growing in or on the patient's own body. Bacterial products may be IFN inducers, including IFN-gamma. Because of this and lack of controlled studies, this treatment should not be used.

**Proneut.** A combination of measles vaccine, influenza vaccine, and histamine phosphate, the dose being individually determined for each patient. There appears to be no convincing evidence at present that this treatment is effective in MS.

**Alpha-Fetoprotein (a-Fetoprotein).** Alpha-fetoprotein (AFP) is a protein produced by the liver of the fetus in the womb to protect it against the mother's immune system. It has been purified and used experimentally. No recommended use at present

**Immunoglobulins (Gamma Globulin, Immunoglobulin G, IgG).** Immunoglobulins are the antibody-containing fraction of human plasma. They are usually injected intramuscularly, but certain special preparations can be given intravenously. The evidence is conflicting as to whether intravenous IgG reduces the frequency of exacerbations in MS. Studies confirming that intravenous IgG might promote remyelination in humans have not been completed.

**Immunobiological Revitalization.** Purified rabbit antibodies against human bone marrow, spleen, and thymus, supplemented by an unidentified "human placental product." This treatment is not recommended.

**Proteolytic Enzymes.** A mixture of digestive enzymes (pancreatin, chymotrypsin, and several others), given intravenously in repeated dosage. Inadequate published information exists to permit informed judgement about this therapy.

**Chelation Therapy with Ethylenediamine Tetraacetic Acid (EDTA).** A simple chemical that chelates metals very efficiently and is used in cases of lead poisoning to remove lead from the body. Must be injected intravenously over several hours. Chelation therapy for MS is not based on acceptable published evidence and is dangerous.

## Physical and Surgical Manipulations

**Acupuncture, Acupressure, Qigong.** These procedures are part of traditional Chinese medicine (TCM). Acupuncture, a 4,000 year old Chinese procedure, is performed by inserting fine needles into specific skin sites with the expectation of influencing the function of underlying organs. The belief is that body energy flows in channels that connect to organs, and an imbalance can be restored by the acupuncture needles inserted into 365 points. Qigong is an approach to restore balance by deep breathing, concentration and relaxation exercises. This treatment is considered to have no effect on the disease process in MS and has not been shown to have any value in the symptomatic management of patients with disease.

**Dorsal Column Stimulation.** The dorsal columns of the spinal cord are large bundles of nerve fibers that carry the sense of touch and the sense of position from the legs, trunk, and arms up to the brain. The spinal cord is protected by a connective tissue wrapping known as dura. Electrical stimulation of the dorsal columns requires implantation of two electrodes on the overlying dura, which is done by passing the electrodes through a special needle. The electrodes are connected with an implanted stimulator or radio receiver. This procedure is ineffective and dangerous. The costs and risks are high. It is not recommended for use in patients with MS.

**Hyperbaric Oxygen.** Breathing oxygen under increased pressure in a specially constructed chamber. Large-scale, double-blind controlled studies have proven that HBO is ineffective as a treatment for MS.

**Transcutaneous Nerve Stimulation.** Transcutaneous nerve stimulation (TNS) is a procedure in which electrodes are placed on the surface of the skin over certain nerves and electrical stimulation is carried out. The dose, varied by changing frequency, pulse width, and intensity, determines which nerve fibers are activated. TNS is a moderately effective treatment for pain, but there is no evidence that it alters the underlying disease in MS.

**Thalamotomy, Thalamic Stimulation.** Destruction of part of the thalamus by surgical means. More recently, electrical stimulation of the thalamus by surgically implanted electrodes has been reported to have a similar effect. Thalamotomy and thalamic stimulation are not recommended for MS except in a small number of carefully selected MS patients.

**Sympathectomy and Ganglionectomy.** Sympathetic nerves and ganglions supplying blood vessels to the head are surgically removed in an effort to increase blood supply to the CNS. There is no convincing evidence that this surgical procedure is effective in treating MS.

**Surgical Spinal Cord Relaxation.** Surgical procedure to fix the cervical spine to restrict forward bending. This therapy is without value in MS.

**Vertebral Artery Surgery.** An operation devised to eliminate kinking or narrowing of the vertebral arteries in the neck. The existing evidence does not support the conclusion that these procedures may be effective in the treatment of MS.

**Ultrasound.** Repeated application of ultrasound, i.e., high-frequency sound, to the area of the back next to the spinal column (backbone). The evidence suggests that this treatment if unlikely to be effective in MS. The high price clearly reflects commercial exploitation.

**Magnetotherapy.** Repeated application of a low-frequency pulsing magnetic field. This treatment is not yet proven. Further controlled studies are underway.

**Dental Occlusal Therapy.** Correction of dental malocclusion with occlusal splints and other procedures, attention to other dental needs, and physical therapy to muscles and structures of the temporomandibular joints. There is neither a scientific basis nor acceptable medical evidence that dental occulusion therapy could favorably influence the MS disease process.

**Replacement of Mercury Amalgam Fillings.** Removal and replacement of all fillings made of silver and mercury amalgam. There is no evidence to suggest that this procedure is of value to MS.

**Implantation of Brain Substances.** Surgical implantation of pig brain in the abdominal wall. The evidence examined demonstrates that this treatment should be regarded as ineffective and dangerous.

**Hysterectomy.** Surgical removal of the uterus. This procedure is not recommended for MS.

# Index

AMPA/kainate receptors, 243, 244, 287, 290
Amputation, 247, 250
Amytrophic lateral sclerosis (ALS), 13, 14,
        115, 330, 339, 365
    treatment, 283, 285, 286, 287, 289, 300,
        305, 366, 367
Anergix, 394
Animal models, *ix*, 84, 90-104, 396
    bone marrow transplants, 296
    brain, 96, 103
        encephalomyelitis, 7, 43, 72-73, 84-
            86, 99; *see also* Experimental
            autoimmune encephalomyelitis
            (EAE)
        demylenation, 7, 91-99 (passim), 102-103,
            357
        immune system, general, 7, 21, 48, 91,
            97, 103
        magnetic resonance imaging, 262
        major histocompatibility complex (MHC),
            91, 103
        neurons, 6, 7, 95
        remyelination, 243-244
        research recommendations, 4, 6-7, 356-358
        spasticity, 131
        T cells, autoreactive, 251-252, 355
        tolerance strategies, 21
        transgenic, 91, 93, 97, 100-104, 280, 355,
            356-357
        transplantation, 292
        viruses, 21, 91, 357-358
            mouse hepatitis virus (MHV), 95, 98-
                100
            Theiler's murine encephalomyelitis
                virus (TMEV), 48, 91, 92, 95-98,
                99, 269, 357
Antegren, 294
Antibiotics, 407
Antibodies, 42, 68, 255, 349, 350, 394, 410
    *see also* Antigens; Immunoglobulins;
        Vaccines
    autoantibodies, 66, 73, 74, 92, 93, 251,
        255, 266, 355
    neutralizing, beta-interferon, 51, 52, 97
    T cells, antigen-specific, 60, 70, 93, 252-
        253, 254, 257-258, 260, 263-265,
        279, 280, 354, 355, 397
Antigens, 60, 68, 263
    *see also* Major histocompatibility
        complex
    astrocytes, 244-245, 350

autoantigens, 5-6, 7, 42, 44, 45, 50, 60,
        66, 67, 71-74 (passim), 82, 88, 91,
        93, 100, 244, 251-255, 257, 279,
        280, 354, 355, 357, 398
    superantigens, 67, 92, 93, 95, 254
    cerebrospinal fluid (CSF), 42, 45
    neutralizing antibodies, 51, 52, 97
Anxiety, 122, 123, 152, 200, 211, 217, 224
    *see also* Depression
    side effects of treatment, 50, 125, 126,
        127, 135, 388
    treatment, 227, 229
Apoptosis, 7, 98, 243, 254, 255, 259, 269,
        281, 284-285, 286, 287, 295, 351,
        358-359, 392
Arthritis, 14, 44, 69, 122, 145, 152, 153, 297,
        299, 328, 329, 337, 366
Asians, 48, 77, 79, 83, 85, 87
Assistive technology, *ix*, 199, 205-210, 385-
        386
    catheterization, 143, 206
    cognitive impairment, 119, 209
    cost and cost-effectiveness, 205, 206, 207,
        210
    defined, 205
    employment, 193, 207-208
    environmental control technology, 206, 207
    health screening, 222-223
    insurance coverage, 206, 209, 222
    wheelchairs, 128, 188, 199, 206-207, 209,
        220, 222, 386
Astrocytes, 3, 4
    antigens, 244-245, 350
    biological features of MS, 45, 62, 64, 71,
        87
    blood-brain barrier, 257
    cytokines, 257, 258, 259, 350
    disease mechanism research, 241, 245,
        253, 257, 258, 259, 267
    glial scars, 3, 241, 350
    inflammation, 258
    research recommendations, 241, 244-245,
        253, 257, 258, 259, 267, 349, 350
    treatment, 282, 284, 286, 294
Asymptomatic MS, 6, 30, 35-36, 88, 115, 177
Ataxia and tremor, 128, 138-140, 163
    assistive technologies, 209
    employment and, 191
    experimental autoimmune
        encephalomyelitis (EAE) *vs* MS,
        92

# M